W0227535

# Management of Adult Glioma
# in Nursing Practice

Ingela Oberg
Editor

# Management of Adult Glioma in Nursing Practice

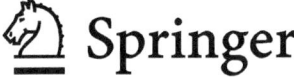 Springer

*Editor*
Ingela Oberg
Department of Neurosurgery
Cambridge University Hospitals NHS Foundation
Cambridge
Cambridgeshire
UK

ISBN 978-3-319-76746-8    ISBN 978-3-319-76747-5    (eBook)
https://doi.org/10.1007/978-3-319-76747-5

Library of Congress Control Number: 2018964421

© Springer Nature Switzerland AG 2019
This work is subject to copyright. All rights are reserved by the Publisher, whether the whole or part of the material is concerned, specifically the rights of translation, reprinting, reuse of illustrations, recitation, broadcasting, reproduction on microfilms or in any other physical way, and transmission or information storage and retrieval, electronic adaptation, computer software, or by similar or dissimilar methodology now known or hereafter developed.
The use of general descriptive names, registered names, trademarks, service marks, etc. in this publication does not imply, even in the absence of a specific statement, that such names are exempt from the relevant protective laws and regulations and therefore free for general use.
The publisher, the authors, and the editors are safe to assume that the advice and information in this book are believed to be true and accurate at the date of publication. Neither the publisher nor the authors or the editors give a warranty, express or implied, with respect to the material contained herein or for any errors or omissions that may have been made. The publisher remains neutral with regard to jurisdictional claims in published maps and institutional affiliations.

This Springer imprint is published by the registered company Springer Nature Switzerland AG
The registered company address is: Gewerbestrasse 11, 6330 Cham, Switzerland

# Foreword

Anyone whose life has been touched by a brain tumour diagnosis understands the impact of this indiscriminate disease.

Alongside debilitating ill health, it often brings crippling fear and feelings of isolation for those diagnosed and for their families.

At The Brain Tumour Charity we hear every day from people seeking answers and support, searching for options and asking what to expect as the months and years roll by.

Every one of them deserves the best possible treatment and care at each stage of their brain tumour journey.

Every one of them needs access to experts in the field of neuro-oncology who are committed, as we are, to improving the lives of all those affected by a brain tumour.

This book, compiled and written by just such experts to share knowledge and best practice for adult glioma patients from diagnosis to end-of-life care, is a major step towards that goal.

Sarah Lindsell
The Brain Tumour Charity
Farnborough, Hampshire, UK

# Preface

There are over 150 different kinds of documented brain tumours, yet despite the disparity between their grading and tumour type, the malignant brain tumours behave in a very similar way in the adult population, often associated with poor survival rates. The most frequent of the adult malignant brain tumours remains the glioma, which is what this book focuses on.

The role of ward-based nurses is ever evolving and over the last few decades has become less patient focused and more 'managerial' with onus on flowcharts, assessments, documentation, audits, drug (medicine) rounds and aiding patient flow—as well as supporting junior and senior colleagues alike, be they nursing or medical. In the United Kingdom, the introduction of clinical nurse specialists has helped greatly in bridging the gap between ward-based nurses and consultant-led patient care. Specialist nurses are highly skilled members of a multidisciplinary team (MDT) who work to ensure decisions are made with the patient's best interest at heart.

Caring for a glioma patient is complex and multifaceted, and for the novice (and/or specialist) nurse, it can seem a daunting and sometimes overwhelming task filled with arduous decisions, poor outcomes and high patient turnover. However, it can also be a truly rewarding experience as you help the patient and their loved ones navigate through the myriad of questions, concerns and treatment options, enabling them to make informed decisions which are right for them at any given time point, whether this consists of surgery, active treatment, palliation or best supportive care.

The overarching aim of neuro-oncology nurses, be they ward based or specialist, is to support patients and their families and loved ones, through the disease trajectory, and provide them with appropriate and timely information, enabling them to self-manage as much as possible. Patients and carers also need to know when, where and how to seek additional help and support, as well as to recognise transition from one care phase to another, including transition to the end-of-life phase. To help patients achieve this, the neuro-oncology nurse requires a deeper understanding of their diagnosis, prognosis and treatment options, along with their side effects, whilst also maintaining realistic expectations and facilitating hope. To enable this to happen, neuro-oncology nurses must possess robust communication skills to facilitate open and honest conversations to occur in a sensitive and empathic manner.

This book helps the reader navigate through these variable segments and helps them gain insight and knowledge around adult gliomas. The aim of this book is to equip the novice neuro-oncology nurse and other healthcare professionals (including nursing and medical students) with the tools required to adequately care for an adult glioma patient from the start of his or her disease trajectory right through to end-of-life scenarios, providing clinical overviews and setting learning outcomes within each chapter.

The first few chapters of this book look at the role of the multidisciplinary team (MDT) and its core (as well as extended) membership, providing a typical presentation pathway of a patient with a suspected glioma. Other chapters cover anatomy and physiology; the role of neuroimaging and histopathology, along with neurological presentations and medical management of gliomas; and the importance of knowing how to best capture patient's needs and concerns at varying stages in their treatment pathway and how to act on these results—a process known as holistic needs assessment (HNA) frameworks.

Vital communication skills and key elements required on how to facilitate a skilled conversation are explored in depth in this book. It will help equip the novice nurse with important skills required to communicate well, keeping the patient at the centre of the discussions. Surgical management of gliomas, along with commonly encountered pre- and post-operative complications, is also explored in greater detail. Treatment options with radiotherapy and chemotherapy (and their side effects) are detailed, including a portrayal of a patient scenario to enable visualisation of a patient's journey. Exploring the vital role allied health professionals (AHPs) provide, alongside the concept of specialised and specific, targeted neuro-rehabilitation, is also looked at in this section. Furthermore, we gain first-hand insight from a patient on what daily life is like living with a glioma and how her experience of being diagnosed abruptly shaped her perception of the healthcare system. It provides a very rare (and vital) alternative perspective—from that of a patient.

The final chapters of this book take us through the legalities that surround a patient's mental capacity—why and how this can be affected and what we as nurses need to consider in order to protect their rights and act as patient advocates. The transition from paediatrics to adult care—something referred to as TYA (Teenage and Young Adult) services within the United Kingdom—is also explored, alongside their behaviour and developmental stages, leading to a greater understanding of this vastly under-represented patient cohort. Other chapters explore the difference between palliative and end-of-life care, including clinical manifestations of when the patient is entering this final stage in their disease trajectory. Another vital chapter is the views of a carer and spouse—in this instance, a wife, helping to look after her husband who is living with a transforming glioma. This is also whilst she is a parent, as well as the main income earner for the family. This is a very moving and insightful chapter on the vastly extended role carers take on. It provides us with new insights into their deeply personal journeys, hopefully equipping the reader with a new sense of compassion and empathy, stretching beyond the hospital setting.

It is hoped this book will equip the newly qualified healthcare professional with qualities to help manage a complex glioma patient well, placing their well-being at the forefront of clinical practice. Whilst it is recommended this book is read as a whole, chapters can be accessed individually, as a form of reference, to help gain deeper insight into specific aspects of the care pathway. Enjoy!

Cambridge, UK                                                                          Ingela Oberg

# Acknowledgements

This book would never have come to fruition if it wasn't for the determination, dedication and hard work of every individual, contributing author. My sincerest, heartfelt thanks to them all for agreeing to not only write their chapter(s) but also for making my role in editing so straightforward as a result, due to their personal engagement and boundless professionalism. My greatest thanks, however, go to *Zara Lorenz* who wrote about caring for a loved one with a malignant brain tumour and *Isabella Robbins* as a patient's perspective. Their reflective accounts are heartfelt and give us real insight into daily life and struggles with a glioma. As a direct result, both these chapters have changed how I not only engage and communicate with patients but also how I engage with carers.

Thanks also go to those behind the scenes, to those colleagues who have helped me edit and proof-read chapters. In particular, thanks go to my colleagues at Cambridge University Hospital NHS Foundation Trust (Addenbrooke's), Dr. Sarah Jefferies (consultant clinical oncologist) and Mr. Tom Santarius (consultant neurosurgeon), for helping me edit the oncological, surgical and anatomical chapters, and to Helen Bulbeck (Brainstrust) for helping with the editing process for the holistic needs assessment chapter.

I would like to extend my personal thanks to Sarah Lindsell (CEO, The Brain Tumour Charity) who did not flinch when asked to write the foreword for this book but indeed jumped at the chance with great enthusiasm! I am also enormously grateful and very humbled that Springer Publishing (and all those within) from the very start of this process believed a novice editor like myself could produce a relevant book on gliomas. I hope I have managed to do them all proud.

Finally, my thanks go to my partner Adam who was left to manage our busy household looking after our young twin boys, enabling me to work from home (and at home), at any given opportunity, for months on end. You are my rock.

# Contents

# Neuroanatomy and Physiology

## Christina Amidei and Sarah Trese

**Abstract**

Knowledge of the anatomy and physiology of the nervous system and its related components is critical to the safe and effective care of the patient with a glioma. Topics covered in this chapter include cranial anatomy, cell types and related physiology to assist in understanding of functional deficits, cerebrovascular anatomy and unique aspects of cerebral circulation, the meninges, the ventricles and cerebrospinal fluid production, and functional anatomy of the cerebrum, diencephalon, and brain stem. Finally, physiologic concepts of cerebral haemodynamics and intracranial pressure are reviewed.

**Keywords**

Neuroanatomy · Gliomas · Neurophysiology · Functions of brain lobes · Intracranial pressure · Astrocytes · Oligodendrocytes

**Learning Outcomes**
- Be able to differentiate the different brain lobes and name some of their more important functions.
- Be aware of some of the more intricate and complex brain structures and their functions, such as the temporal lobe, central motor and sensory cortex.

C. Amidei (✉)
NMH/Arkes Family Pavilion, Chicago, IL, USA
e-mail: christina.amidei@nm.org

S. Trese
Northwestern Memorial Hospital, Chicago, IL, USA
e-mail: Sarah.Trese@nm.org

© Springer Nature Switzerland AG 2019
I. Oberg (ed.), *Management of Adult Glioma in Nursing Practice*,
https://doi.org/10.1007/978-3-319-76747-5_1

- Understand how a glioma can affect these parts of the brain and how subsequently patients may present to clinicians with symptoms.
- Gain deeper understanding of how gliomas arise from oligodendrocytic or astrocytic cells and the role and impact of oedema as a natural defence barrier.

## 1.1 Introduction

Providing appropriate care for a person diagnosed with a glioma depends on an understanding of the anatomy affected as well as consequences of the tumour on physiologic mechanisms within the brain. The brain is a complex organ that is responsible for most aspects of life. When the brain is affected by a glioma, changes may occur in movement, emotion, problem-solving, judgement, memory, language, thinking, consciousness, and even autonomic function. This chapter will review cranial anatomy, cells of the nervous system, the structure and role of the meninges and ventricular system, as well as blood vessel anatomy within the brain in addition to autonomic anatomy and function. Functional anatomic components of the brain are reviewed, and physiologic concepts of cerebral haemodynamics and intracranial pressure are presented to provide a basis for understanding care provided to patients with this challenging problem.

## 1.2 Cranial Anatomy

The brain and its supporting structures are housed within the skull, also known as the cranium. The cranial bones have an inner and outer table of compact bone with a spongy layer in between. This anatomic configuration affords protection to the intracranial contents without adding weight to the cranium.

Although the cranium is thought of as a single structure, it is actually comprised of several bones that originate as bony islands during prenatal development that eventually fuse together to form the skull. The areas where the bony islands fuse together are known as sutures. The sutures are partially fused at birth and eventually close completely by about 3 years of age [1].

Eight bones comprise the cranium as follows: the *frontal* bone forms the top third, front (forehead), and inferior cranium, including the bony ridge above the eyes and roof of the orbits. There are air-filled spaces within this bone above the orbit known as frontal sinuses. There are paired *parietal* bones that form the middle and posterior top and sides of the head. The *occipital* bone forms the posterior and inferior portion of the cranium. Paired *temporal* bones form the medial and inferior portions of the cranium.

The skull base is comprised of the inferior portions of frontal, temporal, and occipital bones. Two additional bones contribute to structure of the cranial base: the ethmoid and sphenoid bones. The ethmoid bone sits between and above the orbits, and its horizontal portion, the cribriform plate, forms the roof of the nasal cavity and the thin medial potion of the floor of the anterior cranial fossa. The sphenoid bone forms the central skull base and the floor of the middle cranial fossa. A midline indentation in the sphenoid bone, the sella turcica, holds the pituitary gland [1, 2].

The exterior portion of the cranium is relatively smooth. However, the interior surface of the cranium has furrows that accommodate blood vessels on the surface of the dura. The most pronounced of these is the furrow in the temporal bone that accommodates the middle meningeal artery. Damage to bone or dura in this area can cause arterial bleeding that accumulates on the surface of dura, known as an epidural (also known as extradural) haematoma.

There are also numerous ridges in the interior cranial base. These ridges provide cuplike compartments known as anterior, middle, and posterior fossae. The anterior fossa is made of the inferior frontal bone, the cribriform plate of the ethmoid bone, and the sphenoid ridge and holds the frontal lobes of the brain. The greater wing of the sphenoid bone and petrous bone as far posteriorly as the petrous ridge forms the floor of the middle fossa which holds the temporal lobe. The inferior occipital bone and petrous bone posterior to its ridge form the posterior fossa which holds the cerebellum and the brain stem. Finally, the cranial base has openings through which blood vessels and nerves enter and exit the cranium, called foramina.

Surgical opening into the cranium is known as a craniotomy. Surgical access to resect a glioma requires a craniotomy to be performed. A craniotomy is performed by drilling one to four small holes, called burr holes, into the cranium. The holes are connected, allowing a small tailored piece of bone to be removed for access. Once tumour resection is complete, the bone is replaced and held in place with sutures, wires, or plates and screws until it heals. The burr holes often close over time but will always be visible on imaging. The term craniectomy is used to denote situations where the bone is removed and not replaced at the time of surgery. Craniectomy may be performed for posterior fossa cranial access or may occur when the brain is too oedematous to allow bone to be safely replaced at the time of surgery. Delayed cranial repair, known as cranioplasty, may be required in this circumstance.

## 1.3    Meninges

The meninges are a series of three membranes surrounding the brain and spine: dura mater, arachnoid, and pia mater (Image 1.1). The outermost membrane, the dura mater, is a two-layer tough fibrous material that folds around and in between areas of the brain. The outer layer adheres to the inner table of the cranium. Embedded between the two dural layers are large cerebral veins known as sinuses. The inner dural layer suspends and stabilises the brain inside the skull, producing compartments within the cranium. The dural fold between the cerebral hemispheres is known as the falx cerebri, while the dural fold separating the cerebellar hemispheres is known as the falx cerebelli. The diaphragma sellae is a dural fold that covers the pituitary gland within the sella turcica. It has a small opening for the pituitary stalk that connects the pituitary gland to the hypothalamus. Another dural infolding separates the occipital lobes from the cerebellar hemispheres and is known as the tentorium. The cerebral hemispheres are located above the tentorium in the supratentorial

**Image 1.1** Overview of the meninges, and their relationship to the skull and brain (Reproduced with permission TeachMeAnatomy)

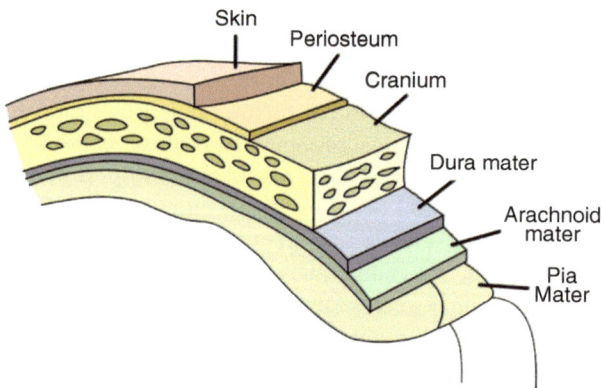

compartment, while the cerebellum is located in the infratentorial compartment, below the tentorium. There is an opening in the tentorium called the tentorial incisura, or the tentorial notch, through which midbrain passes from the supra- to the infratentorial compartments. Increased volume in one of these compartments can cause herniation of brain tissue around the tentorium, leading to potentially irreversible tissue damage.

The middle membrane, the arachnoid, has a weblike appearance with trabecular fibers that connect to the pia mater on the brain surface. Cerebrospinal fluid is contained in the subarachnoid space between the arachnoid and pia mater. The innermost membrane, the pia mater, tightly surrounds the brain surface. The arachnoid and pia mater together are often referred to as the leptomeninges. Occasionally, glial and other tumours metastasise along the surface of the arachnoid membrane, a complication of cancer known as leptomeningeal metastasis.

## 1.4 Functional Anatomy of the Brain

### 1.4.1 Divisions of the Nervous System

The nervous system is divided into the central nervous system and peripheral nervous system. The central nervous system is comprised of the brain and spinal cord. The peripheral nervous system is comprised of 31 paired peripheral nerves and 12 paired cranial nerves [2]. These systems, although anatomically separate, are integrated to generate and process sensory (afferent) information, generate motor and autonomic activity, and store information.

### 1.4.2 Cells of the Nervous System

Two types of cells are found in the nervous system: *neurons* and *neuroglial* cells. Neurons are functional units of the nervous system, while neuroglial cells serve as the support system for neurons [3, 4].

Neurons have several important components. At the proximal end of the neuron is the *cell body*, also known as soma. The cell body is comprised of a cell membrane which encases the cytoplasm and nucleus. The endoplasmic reticulum, mitochondria, and Nissl bodies are contained within the cytoplasm; these areas regulate metabolic function in the cell. The nucleus contains RNA and DNA which convey the genetic information of the cell. *Dendrites* protrude from the cell body and serve to receive impulses from the adjacent cells. The *axon* extends distally from the cell body and ultimately extends to the nerve terminal. Some axons are covered with a myelin sheath that serves to insulate the AXON while accelerating impulse transmission. The *nerve terminal*, also known as the presynaptic terminal, stores neurotransmitters substances so they may be released through the presynaptic membrane into a space between cells known as the synapse.

Neurons produce neurologic function as they receive chemical impulses from other cells, electrically conduct those impulses, and then release chemicals that communicate with other cells. Neurons transit impulses in the following manner. Chemicals in the synaptic space bind to dendrites, initiating a change in cell membrane permeability, allowing sodium to move into the cell while potassium moves out. This chemical change generates an action potential and causes electrical depolarisation of the cell. In turn, the impulse is conducted from the neuron to the adjacent cell. Following impulse conduction, cell membrane permeability is stabilised, sodium is pumped out, and potassium moves into the neuron, causing repolarisation [4, 5]. Tumours can cause metabolic alterations in the extracellular space around neurons and predispose to disrupted depolarisation which may be manifest as a seizure.

Neurotransmitters are chemical substances released from the nerve terminal into the synapse during the process of depolarisation. Neurotransmitters diffuse across the synapse and bind with an adjacent cell, propagating an impulse. Once in the synapse, neurotransmitters are repackaged and actively transported back into the presynaptic terminal for future use. The specific neurotransmitter released is determined by the neuron that releases it and type of cell it communicates with. Neurons communicate with other neurons, muscle cells, and endocrine cells [5]. Known neurotransmitters are listed in Table 1.1.

Neuroglial cells support, nourish, protect, and repair neurons. There are more than 3.5 times more glia than neurons within the nervous system. Types of neuroglial cells and their functions are: [4, 5]

- Astrocytes are star-shaped cells that form a support structure between capillaries and neurons. They play a role in blood-brain barrier function and nourish the neurons.
- Ependymal cells form the lining of the ventricles and facilitate production of cerebrospinal fluid.
- Oligodendrocytes are cells within the brain that build and maintain the myelin sheath.
- Microglia are located sporadically around the brain that phagocytise materials and remove waste products.
- Schwann cells are located along axons of the peripheral nerves. They produce myelin.
- Satellite cells provide support for neurons in the peripheral nervous system.

**Table 1.1** Neurotransmitters and their functions

| Neurotransmitter | Function |
| --- | --- |
| Acetylcholine | Primary parasympathetic transmitter; mostly excitatory effect in motor cortex; inhibitory effect on some of parasympathetic nervous system |
| Norepinephrine | Primary sympathetic transmitter; mostly excitatory |
| Dopamine | Controls behaviour and fine motor function; inhibitory |
| Serotonin | Controls mood, hunger, sleep, behaviour, temperature; inhibits pain |
| Glutamate | Sensory actions; excitatory |
| Gamma-aminobutyric acid (GABA) | Excitatory; excess may cause seizures |
| Substance P | Controls pain sensation; excitatory |
| Endorphin | Excitation to pain inhibition systems |
| Enkephalin | Excitation to pain inhibition systems |
| Glycine | Inhibits at spinal cord synapses |

Tumours can arise from any cell of the nervous system. Tumours arising from neurons are termed neuromas. Astrocytes give rise to astroctyomas, oligodendrocytes to oligodendrogliomas, ependymal cells to ependymomas, Schwann cells to schwannomas, and so forth. Further information on cellular origin and classification of glial tumours is found in Chap. 7.

### 1.4.3   Brain Anatomy

The brain is a dynamic organ that changes over the lifespan. Overall brain weight changes (quadrupling from birth to the age of 3 years), reaching its maximum in early adulthood, when brain development is largely completed [3]. Brain weight starts to decrease at about age 45–50 years, with maximum loss of weight at about age 89.

The brain is responsible for generating or controlling the most basic of bodily functions to the highest level of executive function. It is divided into three major areas: the cerebrum, the cerebellum, and the brain stem. The surface of the brain has a wrinkled appearance, due to the many sulci and gyri of on the brain's surface. The gyri are folded ridges of brain tissue, and the sulci are the valleys in between the gyri. This structure provides a greater surface area for the brain, allowing a greater number of neurons to be packed into these areas to facilitate information processing. Very deep sulci are called fissures and these separate major areas of the brain [1, 5].

### 1.4.4   The Cerebrum

The cerebrum is comprised of paired cerebral hemispheres and a central core with thalami, basal ganglia, and the hypothalamus. The cerebral hemispheres are incompletely separated by the great longitudinal fissure, in clinical practice most commonly referred to as the interhemispheric fissure. Each hemisphere has an overlying layer of cerebral cortex. The cerebral cortex consists of grey matter (unmyelinated neurons). Neurons are densely packed into the cortex which is about 3–5 mm in depth. White matter lies underneath the cortex and is made of axons covered in myelin, which gives it the white appearance. White matter is comprised of many pathways, known as tracts, which connect with other areas within the brain structures, facilitating integration throughout the nervous system. Association tracts connect areas within the hemisphere of origin. Projection tracts serve to connect the cortex to the lower brain and spinal cord, and transverse tracts connect the hemispheres. The largest transverse tract is a structure that serves to connect right and left cerebral hemispheres and is located at the base of the great longitudinal fissure. It is called corpus callosum. The right and left hemispheres are further organised into the frontal, parietal, temporal, and occipital lobes. Together, they are generally responsible for our movement, speech, reasoning, and memory, among many other things [1–5].

The largest and most anterior of these is the *frontal lobe* (Image 1.2). The frontal lobe is bordered posteriorly by the central sulcus, which separates it from the parietal lobe. This region can be furthered divided into the prefrontal and frontal eye fields, precentral gyrus, and motor speech areas. The prefrontal region contributes to our individual personalities, judgement, and abstract thinking. Patients with impairment to this area may present with mood lability as well as impulsive ideas, actions, or behaviours. Since so many aspects of higher cognition and reasoning depend on this area, patients exhibiting symptoms of frontal lobe damage may experience difficulty with tasks that require decision-making, planning, or focus. The precentral gyrus, or motor strip, is necessary for the processing, initiation, and control of fine motor movements. Just anterior to the precentral gyrus is the supplemental motor cortex, which serves to refine movement. Patients with a tumour in the precentral gyrus or supplementary motor cortex and associated tracts may present with impaired motor skills. Whether those impairments are temporary or not will depend on extent of involvement. Broca's area is located in the inferior aspect of the precentral gyrus and is necessary for the motor aspect of speech production. Injury

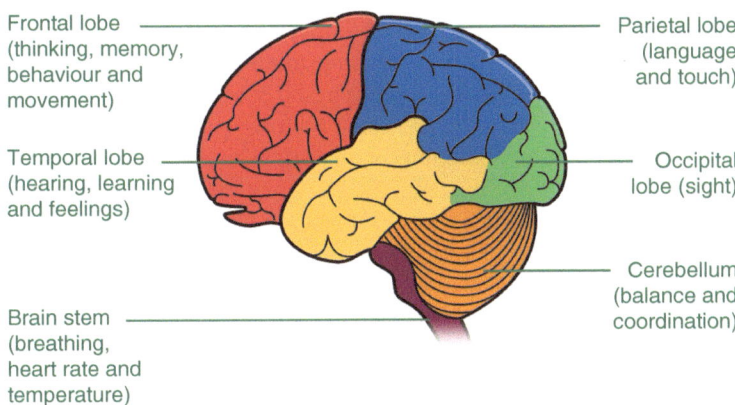

Frontal lobe (thinking, memory, behaviour and movement)

Parietal lobe (language and touch)

Temporal lobe (hearing, learning and feelings)

Occipital lobe (sight)

Cerebellum (balance and coordination)

Brain stem (breathing, heart rate and temperature)

**Image 1.2** Macmillan depicting the brain lobes. Reprinted with permission (Macmillan image)

to Broca's area may produce expressive aphasia. In this disorder, motor output of speech is impaired.

Immediately posterior to the frontal lobe is the *parietal lobe* (Image 1.2), also known as the somatosensory cortex. Adjacent to the precentral gyrus (motor strip) of the frontal lobe, the post central gyrus in the dorsal aspect of the parietal lobe is commonly referred to as the sensory strip. This area parallels motor function in the adjacent frontal lobe precentral gyrus. It allows for interpretation of not only temperature discrimination and pain but also for proprioception and allows us to discern how finely innervated our skin is through our ability to differentiate that two sharp points of contact are in fact two separate objects and not one. Consequently this area contributes to spatial awareness, and therefore dysfunction may present as a lack of coordination or spatial perception. Overall, a person with damage to the parietal lobes may struggle to name objects, write words, perform simple mathematics, distinguish left from right, or follow directions.

Motor and sensory functions are not evenly represented across the precentral and postcentral gyri, as delineated in the homunculus diagram (Image 1.3). The finest motor and sensory functions are carried across the greatest area. Foot and leg functions are located medially, hand and arm functions are carried superiorly, while facial functions are located more lateral.

The *temporal lobes* (Image 1.2) are inferior to and separated from the frontal and parietal lobes by the lateral or Sylvian fissures. The temporal lobes contain both the primary and secondary auditory areas and are imperative for communication and memory. The location of the primary auditory cortex in the superior margin of the temporal lobe is responsible for reception of sound which is then processed in the auditory association area, where we interpret the sounds heard, based on memory or previous recognition. This includes Wernicke's area, and if damaged, the patient may exhibit receptive aphasia. The temporal lobe also contains the hippocampus, crucial for memory functioning, as well as the olfactory cortex and gustatory cortex in the insula, the medial portion of the temporal lobe. The frontal, but especially the temporal and insular, lobes are especially vulnerable to seizure production. As a result, a tumour in this area and scar tissue from surgery may cause a patient to present with symptoms that range from barely noticeable to severe. A seizure beginning in this area may be manifest as experiencing strange smells, euphoria, or déjà vu. Other patients may experience receptive aphasia, confusion, or inability to remember simple phrases or recent events. Some patients present with complex partial seizures and exhibit repetitive motions or alterations in their level of consciousness. Often, patients and their families may admit to noticing these symptoms more in retrospect upon receiving a diagnosis.

The *occipital lobes* (Image 1.2) are posterior to the parietal and temporal lobes. The parieto-occipital sulcus serves as the anterior border for the occipital lobes; the occipital lobes are the most posterior portion of the cerebrum. In the most posterior region of the occipital lobe is the largest of all cortical sensory areas: the primary visual cortex. The visual association area, similar to the auditory association area, allows the visual input we receive to be translated and then associated with images we have previously seen or may remember. An example would be object or facial

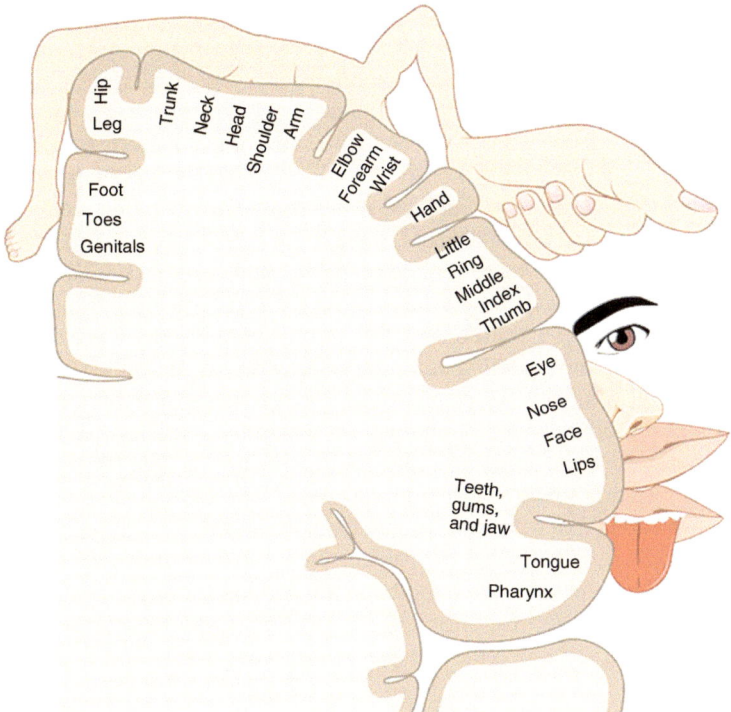

**Image  1.3** Motor/sensory    homunculus    (https://commons.wikimedia.org/wiki/File:1421_
Sensory_Homunculus.jpg)

recognition. Damage to the occipital lobe, particularly the visual association area, could potentially manifest through the inability to recognise a familiar face, hallucinations, poor depth perception and lack of spatial awareness, difficulty with balance, cortical blindness, or agnosia.

While both hemispheres may appear anatomically alike, one hemisphere may have different abilities than the other. Just as most people demonstrate dominance with one hand, lateralisation allows for cerebral dominance of various tasks or abilities. For the majority of patients, their left cerebral hemisphere is dominant for language and calculation, whereas their right has greater influence on emotion, insight, and artistry. Therefore, two patients with a tumour in the same anatomical location may present with very different clinical presentations based on their respective cerebral dominance. It is also worth noting that a tumour can afflict both hemispheres and various structures simultaneously.

Below the cerebral hemispheres is the central core, which consists of several subcortical structures that connect the cerebral hemispheres to the brain stem. The *basal ganglia* are located deep within the cerebral hemispheres and are actually a series of nuclei that are responsible for refining fine movements and speech. In the ventromedial aspect of the brain lie the thalami, hypothalami, and pineal gland, which are collectively known as the diencephalon. The *thalamus* is by far the largest structure within the diencephalon. These structures work together to relay and integrate sensory function to the higher cortical structures, including the perception of pain. They also play a significant role in attention, arousal, alertness, social behaviour, food seeking, and emotions. A tumour in the thalamic area may cause pronounced sensory disturbance, central pain syndrome, altered social behaviour, inattentiveness, and emotional lability. Also located in this area is the *internal capsule*. The internal capsule is comprised of white matter tracts that connect afferent fibers to the cortex and efferent fibers to the brain stem and spinal cord.

Inferior to the thalami and more centrally located is the *hypothalamus*. Despite its small size, the hypothalamus has important regulatory functions. It controls water balance, body temperature, appetite, thirst, and the sleep-wake cycle. In addition, it plays a role in regulating autonomic function, including vasomotor dilation of the blood vessels, slowing of heart rate, peristalsis, and pupillary constriction. Hypothalamic glioma can cause autonomic instability, excessive appetite or thirst, body temperature alterations, and altered sleep patterns. The hypothalamus connects to the pituitary gland via the pituitary stalk. The hypothalamus manufactures releasing hormones that trickle down into the anterior pituitary gland where they are stored until release is triggered by a feedback system regulated by the hypothalamus. Also manufactured in the hypothalamus and stored in the posterior pituitary are antidiuretic hormone (responsible for controlling water reabsorption in the renal tubules) and oxytocin, which plays a role in lactation, libido, and overall mood.

## 1.4.5 Cerebellum

The cerebellum lies inferior to the occipital lobes, from which it is separated by a sheet of dura called tentorium, and posterior to the brain stem (Image 1.2). Cerebellar peduncles connect the cerebellum to the midbrain, pons, and medulla. The cerebellum is divided into right and left cerebellar hemispheres that are connected by the midline cerebellar vermis. The cerebellum has a grey matter cortex with a white matter interior, similar to the cortex. Proprioceptive input from the vestibular system allows the cerebellum to assess body position in space and provide corrective actions that increase preciseness of movements or dampening movements as needed. Thus, the cerebellum is responsible for posture, coordination, and muscle tone [3]. Gliomas that affect the cerebellum can cause incoordination, increased or exaggerated muscle tone, and speech problems, especially dysarthria.

## 1.4.6 Brain Stem

The brain stem exterior is comprised primarily of white matter with grey matter nuclei located in the central portion of the brain stem. Most major motor and sensory tracts pass through the brain stem and cross to the opposite side, rendering the brain stem a major relay center. All but two of the cranial nerves (olfactory and optic nerves) have attachments to the brain stem, corresponding with relay and integration of related functions at those levels.

Brain stem is arbitrarily divided into the midbrain, pons, and medulla (Image 1.2). The midbrain is the uppermost part of the brain stem and plays a role in the sleep-wake cycle. It also serves as a center for auditory and visual reflexes and contains nuclei for cranial nerves III and IV. The pons lies in the middle of the brain stem and plays an important role in respiratory regulation with the medulla. It also contains nuclei for cranial nerves V–VIII. The medulla lies in the most inferior part of the brain stem, containing nuclei for cranial nerves IX–XII. Centers that control basic heart rate and rhythm, vasomotor activity, and swallowing, sneezing, coughing, and vomiting are located in the medulla. Initiation of inspiration and expiration is controlled by the medulla, while the pons regulates the rhythm of the inspiratory-expiratory process [2, 4].

Gliomas affecting the brain stem produce symptoms based on specific location. Because the brain stem has major relay and integration functions, even a small tumour can produce substantial symptoms. Bilateral cranial nerve deficits, along with abnormalities of the sleep-wake cycle and major sensory dysfunctions, are common. Respiratory disturbances are often seen at the terminal stage of illness.

## 1.5    The Ventricles and Cerebrospinal Fluid

Four fluid-filled cavities, known as ventricles, are found within the brain (Image 1.4). The lateral ventricles are located on the medial aspect of each of the cerebral hemispheres. The third ventricle is medial to the thalami and its floor is formed by the hypothalamus and midbrain. The fourth ventricle is located posterior to the pons and medulla and anterior to the cerebellum. Narrow pathways connect the ventricles. The interventricular foramina (also known as foramina of Monro) connect the two lateral ventricles to the third ventricle, and the cerebral aqueduct of Sylvius connects the third with the fourth ventricles. Additional foramina, two foramina of Luschka and the foramen of Magendie, open from the fourth ventricle into the subarachnoid space [1, 3].

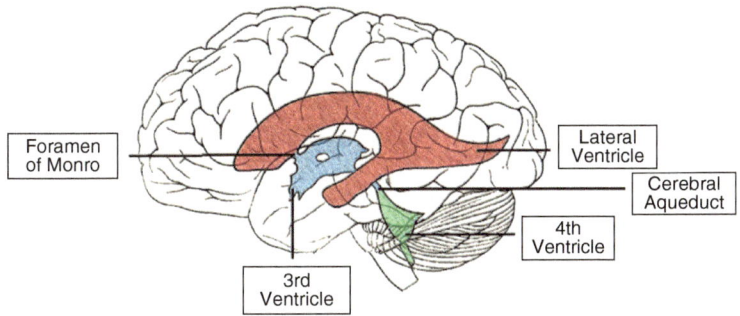

**Image 1.4** Anatomical positioning of the ventricles of the brain (Reproduced with permission from TeachMeAnatomy)

The ventricles are lined with ependymal cells. Ependymal cells cluster in the ventricles with capillaries to form a structure known as the choroid plexus. The choroid plexus produces cerebrospinal fluid (CSF) as a filtrate from blood plasma. Once produced, CSF flows through the ventricular system and out from the fourth ventricle into the subarachnoid space. Subarachnoid CSF is then absorbed into the venous system through tubules in the arachnoid membrane known as arachnoid villi. The villi penetrate the dura and lie adjacent to the venous sinuses. Absorption occurs via a pressure gradient; as CSF pressure rises, it is absorbed into the venous system. The villi act as one-way valves, allowing only CSF outflow while not allowing blood to pass into the villi. The process of CSF production, flow, and absorption is relatively continuous, with CSF production rate at about 20 ml/h. About 150 ml of CSF is contained within the ventricular system and subarachnoid space [4, 5].

The function of CSF is not well understood. Beyond acting as a shock absorber for brain tissue, it is likely that CSF plays a role in metabolic homeostasis within the cranium. It is thought to play a role in pH balance, active transport of substances into brain tissue, neuroendocrine regulation, and maintenance of the blood-brain barrier. CSF has chemical similarities to plasma and may actually serve as an additional source of glucose for the brain if needed.

Gliomas can affect the ventricular system. Because of the abundance of ependymal cells within the ventricles, ependymomas typically occur in proximity to the ventricles. Tumours can obstruct flow within the ventricular system, either by compressing or obstructing the ventricular system. This can lead to obstructive hydrocephalus. Blood or infection in the subarachnoid space can prevent absorption of CSF; this can lead to communicating hydrocephalus.

## 1.6    Circulation in the Brain

There are several unique aspects of cerebral circulation. One is that blood vessels in the brain have two layers as compared to blood vessels elsewhere in the body. This may be due to the role blood vessels play in the blood-brain barrier. However, this anatomic variant can predispose damage to blood vessels, making them more prone to bleeding. Cerebral veins also do not have a muscle layer or valves. Another unique aspect is that arterial and venous vessels in the brain do not run in parallel as they are found in other structures in the body. This is due to venous circulation having an additional role of draining cerebrospinal fluid in addition to draining deoxygenated blood. The third unique aspect is a vascular structure known as the circle of Willis. The circle of Willis is a circle of blood vessels at the base of the brain that serves to connect anterior and posterior circulation, as well as circulation between the otherwise anatomically separate right and left sides of the brain. Within this circle of arteries, blood can be redirected on demand [1]. For example, should the left carotid artery be narrowed or occluded, blood flow from the right side can be shared with the left side of the brain through the anterior communicating artery, thus preserving blood flow throughout the brain. This "adjustable" circulation cannot always to be relied on as the connecting arteries may be small or absent or not otherwise able to provide adequate blood flow as needed.

Arterial blood supply to the brain originates from the two carotid arteries, supplying anterior circulation to the brain, and two vertebral arteries, supplying posterior circulation to the brain. The right common carotid originates from the brachiocephalic artery, while the left common carotid artery originates from the aortic arch. Both common carotid arteries bifurcate in the neck just below the jaw to form the internal and external carotid arteries. The external carotid arteries supply blood to the face and scalp. The internal carotid arteries enter the cranium through the anterior skull base and feed into the circle of Willis, bifurcating to form the anterior and middle cerebral arteries. The anterior cerebral arteries supply blood to the medial motor cortex and anterior frontal lobe, while the middle cerebral arteries supply blood to the temporal, parietal, and remainder of the frontal lobes. The right and left anterior cerebral arteries are connected via the anterior communicating artery [5].

Posterior circulation begins in the two vertebral arteries, originating from the subclavian arteries and coursing through the upper cervical vertebrae. The vertebral arteries enter the cranium through the foramen magnum and join to form a singular basilar artery. The basilar artery has small branches that supply blood to the brain stem and cerebellum, and eventually it bifurcates into two cerebral arteries which supply blood to the temporal and occipital lobes. Posterior communicating arteries connect the posterior cerebral arteries to the internal carotid arteries, thus completing the circle of Willis [5].

Venous circulation is embedded between the two layers of the dura and found adjacent to the ventricular system, highlighting the role that venous circulation plays in drainage of cerebrospinal fluid. Veins draining cerebral hemispheres drain blood into the large superior sagittal and inferior sagittal. Blood from the deep brain structures, such as basal ganglia and thalamus, are drained via the vein of Galen. Vein of Galen join with inferior sagittal sinus to form the straight sinus. The straight sinus joins with the superior sagittal sinus at the confluence of the sinuses which is drained by the left and right transverse sinuses. These then continue as the sigmoid sinuses, which when reaching the skull base become internal jugular veins. The cavernous sinuses are located on either side of the pituitary gland and serve as a junction of a number of venous channels draining mostly inferior brain surface and orbits veins. Although nearly all venous blood is normally drained via the sigmoid sinus/internal jugular vein route, numerous alternative drainage channels exist and can become important in certain pathological states. Neurosurgeons must be cautious during surgical resection of gliomas so as not to compromise venous circulation. Compromise may create venous congestion, haemorrhage, and increased intracranial pressure.

Gliomas can affect blood vessels within the brain in several ways. A major blood vessel can course through a tumour, making it challenging to remove the tumour without damaging cerebral circulation and causing a stroke. Manipulation of major blood vessels in the vicinity of a tumour during a tumour resection surgery can cause spasm of the vessel leading to stroke. Alternatively, damage to the blood vessel may lead to intra- or postoperative haemorrhage. Gliomas can also be very vascular lesions, with tumours developing their own blood supply off of major vessels. This may be manifest as a "tumour blush" on angiographic studies, including computed tomography and magnetic resonance imaging.

Blood vessels play an important role in the blood-brain barrier [1, 4]. At the capillary level, blood vessels of the brain maintain very tight junctions with adjacent cells. These junctions have highly selective permeability, which allows small molecules to readily cross but prevents larger molecules, toxins, and disease-causing elements from crossing into the brain. Blood-brain barrier permeability can be influenced by physiologic alterations and certain disease states but remains an important protective mechanism for the brain. This barrier may be altered when tumours are present in the vicinity.

## 1.7 Brain Systems

Two integrated systems that are less anatomically distinct deserve special mention: the limbic system and the reticular activating system. The limbic system represents a series of connections between the cingulate gyri, hippocampi, and amygdalae in the medial temporal lobes, the thalamus, and the hypothalamus. The limbic system collectively is responsible for attention, cognition, long-term memory, and learned behaviours, as well as the emotions of pleasure, fear, and self-preservation. Damage to this area from a tumour or surgery can produce socially inappropriate behaviours, failure to recall old information or form new memories, or even violent behavioural outbursts. The reticular activating system is a complex system with components located within the pons, midbrain, hypothalamus, thalamus, and frontal lobes. This system collectively is responsible for arousal and sleep-wake cycles. Involvement of the superior components produces sleep-wake disorders, while inferior involvement leads to disorders of arousal and impaired consciousness.

## 1.8 Cranial Nerves

Although the cranial nerves originate in the brain, they are actually part of the peripheral nervous system (Image 1.5). Key points about cranial nerves include: [1, 5]

- There are 12 pairs of cranial nerves that innervate the head and neck structures. Cranial nerve deficits can be unilateral or bilateral.
- The nerves have sensory, motor, or combined sensory motor function. Cranial nerves III, IV, VI, XI, and XII are motor nerves; cranial nerves I, II, and VIII are sensory nerves; and cranial nerves V, VII, IX, and X are mixed nerves with both mixed motor and sensory functions.

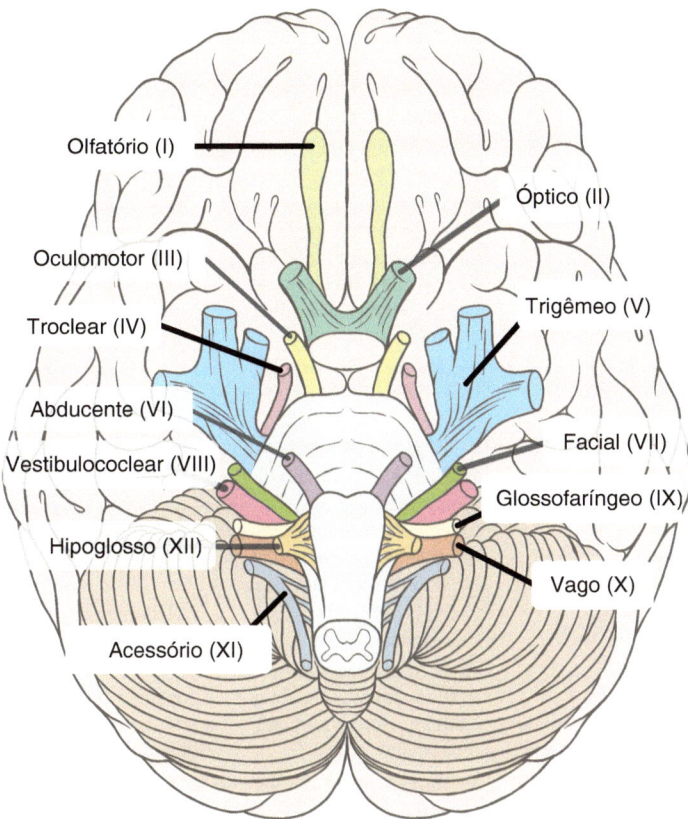

**Image 1.5**  Location of the cranial nerves on the cerebellum and brainstem. Courtesy of Patrick Lynch (https://commons.wikimedia.org/wiki/File:Brain_human_normal_inferior_view_with_labels_pt.svg)

- Nerves are numbered in descending order based on their point of connection within the brain. Cranial nerves I and II are inserted in the cerebral hemispheres. Cranial nerves III and IV are inserted in the midbrain, cranial nerves V–VIII are located in the pons, and cranial nerves IX–XII are inserted in the medulla.
- With the exception of cranial nerve IV, the cranial nerves do not decussate (cross). It is also the only cranial nerve originating from the dorsal side of the brain stem. Function of cranial nerves can be used to localise anatomic area of involvement in the brain, particularly when other neurologic functions cannot be assessed.
- Cranial nerves enter or exit through the cranial base to reach the structures they innervate. Damage to the skull base or increased pressure within the cranial compartment can damage cranial nerves.

Functions for each of the cranial nerves are found in Table 1.2.

**Table 1.2** Cranial nerves and related functions and dysfunctions

| Number | Name | Function | Dysfunction |
|--------|------|----------|-------------|
| I | Olfactory | Sense of smell (also related to taste) | Loss of sense of smell and taste |
| II | Optic | Visual acuity and visual field | Decreased visual acuity; hemianopia |
| III | Oculomotor | Control of iris sphincter (pupil constriction, accommodation, reflex activity); eyelid elevation; medial, superior and inferior eye movement | Pupil dilation and loss of pupillary reactivity to light; inability to open the eyelid; lateral deviation of the eye at rest; inability to move eye medially |
| IV | Trochlear | Medial and inferior eye movement | Lateral and superior eye deviation at rest; inability to move eye medially and inferiorly |
| V | Trigeminal | Sensation of pain, touch, and temperature for the skin and mucous membranes of the head and teeth; palpebral and corneal reflexes; mastication | Loss of palpebral and corneal reflexes; pain in the skin of the face or facial numbness; inability to chew |
| VI | Abducens | Lateral (outward) eye movement | Medial eye deviation at rest; inability to move eye laterally |
| VII | Facial | Taste in anterior two-thirds of the tongue; salivation; eyelid closure and facial movement | Loss of sense of taste; decreased salivation; incomplete eyelid closure; facial weakness |
| VIII | Acoustic | Hearing; proprioception and balance | Loss of hearing and balance |
| IX | Glossopharyngeal | Taste in posterior third of the tongue; motor and sensory function in the throat; gag and swallow reflexes (sensory) | Loss of gag and swallow reflexes; dysphagia |
| X | Vagus | Parasympathetic function in the thoracic and abdominal organs; gag and swallow reflexes (motor) | Parasympathetic dysfunction; loss of gag and swallow reflexes |
| XI | Spinal Accessory | Head rotation and shoulder shrug | Weakness of shoulder shrug and head turn |
| XII | Hypoglossal | Tongue movement (speech and swallowing) | Tongue weakness; if unilateral, deviation away from weak side; dysphagia |

## 1.9    Autonomic Nervous System

The autonomic nervous system (ANS) is part of the peripheral nervous system, although major components are located within the cranium. Centers within the hypothalamus, brain stem, and spinal cord are the primary areas that activate the ANS. Most organs of the body are innervated by the motor neurons comprising the ANS, highlighting the primary role of the ANS in maintaining a stable internal milieu. The neurons in the ANS work as a two-neuron system, with preganglionic neurons originating in the hypothalamus or brain stem and postganglionic neurons with which they connect located either in the organ innervated or ganglia.

There are two divisions of the ANS that work in synergy: the sympathetic and parasympathetic divisions [2]. The sympathetic nervous system may also be termed the thoracolumbar system because preganglionic neurons emerge ventrally though the spinal cord and synapse with ganglia adjacent to the spinal cord in thoracic and lumbar regions. Thoracic ganglia 1–5 innervate the head and neck, while the remaining ganglia down to L2 innervate the abdominal organs. The sympathetic system is activated in situations of physiologic or emotional stress and is commonly thought of as the "fight or flight" system. Preganglionic neurons in the sympathetic division release acetylcholine, while postganglionic neurons release noradrenalin and are termed adrenergic neurons. Adrenergic activity increases blood pressure and heart rate, dilates the pupils, and vasoconstricts the peripheral blood vessels to increase cardiac output.

The parasympathetic division is also known as the craniosacral system because neurons emerge along with cranial nerves III, VII, IX, and X and from cell bodies at the second through fourth sacral levels of the spinal cord. The cranial component innervates the face, pupils, parotid glands, and abdominal organs, including the bowel down to the splenic flexure. The sacral component innervates the lower colon, rectum, bladder, and genitalia. The parasympathetic division responds to very specific stimuli and has a short duration. Both preganglionic and postganglionic neurons in the parasympathetic division release acetylcholine and are termed cholinergic neurons. Cholinergic activity constricts the pupils, releases fluids from glands in the head and neck, slows heart rate, and contributes to bowel and bladder emptying.

## 1.10   Cerebral Physiology

Two important physiologic concepts relevant to care of patients with gliomas are cerebral haemodynamics and intracranial pressure. Both may be altered by gliomas.

### 1.10.1  Cerebral Haemodynamics

The brain requires a nearly constant supply of oxygen and glucose as it is unable to produce energy by anaerobic metabolism. A continuous cerebral blood flow (CBF) supplies the necessary oxygen and glucose, and at rest, about 20% of blood supply may be found circulating through the brain. Blood flow in grey matter is usually greater than blood flow in white matter. CBF is usually maintained at a rate that matches metabolic demand. As metabolic demand increases, so does blood flow and, subsequently, blood volume. Conversely, blood flow and volume decrease when metabolic demands are low. Increased CBF beyond what is required to maintain metabolism causes hyperaemia. Should CBF not be able to keep pace with metabolic demands, then ischaemia occurs. Both hyperaemia and ischaemia can injure the brain [1].

Several physiologic factors may affect CBF. Carbon dioxide is a potent vasodilator that can dramatically increase CBF, with increase in arterial partial pressure of carbon dioxide having a concomitant effect on increasing cerebral blood flow. An increase in hydrogen ion concentration also impacts CBF in the same manner. Decreased partial pressure of oxygen also can trigger an increase in CBF, but less dramatically than carbon dioxide. Seizures may markedly increase brain metabolism and subsequently CBF; pain can also increase CBF. These physiologic factors are important in patient care. Preventing seizures, hypercarbia (hypercapnia), hypoxia, and pain is a crucial measure in promoting adequate cerebral blood flow [1].

Cerebral autoregulation is a mechanism related to CBF. Autoregulation is the maintenance of CBF across a wide range of blood pressure. When systemic blood pressure increases, CBF will remain stable. Autoregulation preserves CBF for a short period during times of decreased systemic blood pressure. When autoregulation is lost, CBF becomes passive and depends on systemic blood pressure. Blood pressure extremes, cerebral oedema, increased intracranial pressure, ischaemia, hypercarbia, and hypoxia may all impair autoregulation [2, 4, 5].

## 1.10.2 Increased Intracranial Pressure

*Intracranial pressure* (ICP) is the pressure exerted by the intracranial components within the closed intracranial compartment [1, 5]. The cranium is a non-distensible box that is filled to capacity with blood, brain tissue, and CSF. Volumes of each of these components remain in a dynamic equilibrium. Brain tissue comprises about 88% of the intracranial volume, while CSF and blood comprise about 8% and 4% of volume, respectively. The modified *Monro-Kellie hypothesis* presents that an increase in volume of one or more of the intracranial components without a subsequent decrease in one or more of the components can lead to an increase in ICP [5]. Sneezing, coughing, choking, and the Valsalva maneuver can temporarily increase ICP as well.

Compensatory mechanisms exist that allow adaptation to volume and subsequent pressure changes. CSF production may be decreased, absorption may increase, or CSF may be displaced into the spinal canal. Cerebral vasoconstriction and increased venous return are additional compensatory mechanisms. There are finite limits to the compensation that these mechanisms provide before ICP will increase. Compliance is the term used to denote the functioning of these compensatory mechanisms. When compliance is intact, increases in volume have little effect on ICP. However, when compensatory mechanisms have been used to capacity, compliance is poor and a small increase in volume can create a substantial increase in ICP. Small volume changes over time are better tolerated that acute large volume changes. This is one reason that slowly growing tumours may grow to large size before becoming symptomatic, and rapidly growing tumours have progressive symptoms.

Any one of the intracranial components can increase in volume, contributing to an increase in ICP [1, 5]. The most common cause of increased brain tissue volume is cerebral oedema. *Cerebral oedema* is characterised by an increase in fluid volume of the extracellular or intracellular spaces or both. Two types of cerebral oedema exist. *Vasogenic oedema* occurs predominately in white matter and is thought to occur due to increased permeability of the cerebral blood vessels. Plasma and proteins leak into the extracellular space. *Cytotoxic oedema* occurs predominately in grey matter and is thought to occur due to increased permeability of the cell wall membranes. Intracellular fluid volume and intracellular sodium increase. Vasogenic oedema is commonly associated with brain tumours or other masses within the brain, although certain drugs can alter blood vessel permeability. In contrast, cytotoxic oedema is associated with ischaemia and hypoxia, although hyponatraemia of any cause can also cause this type of oedema. Both types of oedema may occur simultaneously or sequentially. The mass effect produced by cerebral oedema can initially cause vasogenic oedema, but can decrease blood flow, contributing to ischaemia and subsequent cytotoxic oedema.

Treatment of cerebral oedema focuses on understanding of the contributing factors. Corticosteroids are helpful in treating vasogenic oedema as the function to restore normal permeability in blood vessels. Corticosteroids are ineffective in treating cytotoxic oedema. Acute cytotoxic oedema responds best to osmotic diuretics which serve to pull fluid from the intracellular to extracellular space. Fluid is then actively transported into the intravascular space where it is excreted upon circulation through the kidneys.

Other problems can increase brain tissue volume and subsequently increase ICP; these are generally known as "mass" lesions (because they add to mass and exert mass effect) or "space-occupying" lesions (because they occupy space within the closed intracranial compartment). Brain tumours are by far the most common space-occupying lesions, although brain abscess and haemorrhage are other examples. Procedures that decompress or remove these mass lesions can immediately improve ICP.

Excessive volume of CSF, known as hydrocephalus, can increase ICP. CSF overproduction is very rare. Much more common is reduced CSF return to the vascular system, essentially by two mechanisms: CSF flow out of the ventricular system may be decreased or obstructed while production continues (obstructive hydrocephalus) or CSF may fail to be reabsorbed into the venous sinuses (communicating hydrocephalus) [3]. Since CSF mechanisms are used to compensate for increases in ICP, compliance may be quickly altered in the face of hydrocephalus, regardless of the cause. Hydrocephalus may be associated with interstitial oedema whereby CSF diffuses out of the ventricles into the periventricular extracellular space. CSF diversion, either through an external ventricular drainage system or an internally placed shunt, may be used to decrease intracranial CSF volume. Any factor that increases blood flow can also increase blood volume. Those factors are mentioned in Sect. 1.10.1 [1, 2].

Herniation may be localised or affect the entire brain. A tumour mass may increase pressure unilaterally, causing herniation of the cingulate gyrus underneath the falx cerebri, creating a "shift" of brain tissue that will be visible on a computed tomography or magnetic resonance imaging scan. This is known as subfalcine or cingulate herniation and may be asymptomatic or associated with mild neurologic symptoms [5]. Herniation of the uncus of the temporal lobe around the tentorial notch is known as uncal herniation. Cranial nerve III sits adjacent to the tentorial notch so early herniation of tissue around this notch can produce a unilateral cranial nerve III deficit of a dilated, nonreactive pupil. Symptoms can progress rapidly with uncal herniation, to include decreased level of consciousness, hemiplegia, increased muscle tone, posturing, and vital sign instability. The cerebellum may herniate upward around the tentorium or down into the spinal canal when there is mass effect in the infratentorial compartment. This is usually associated with rapidly progressive neurologic deficit. If a craniectomy is performed in the presence of increased intracranial pressure, the brain may also herniate through the cranial opening. In this circumstance, bone is usually not replaced until the pressure decreases and the brain is more relaxed. Finally, bilateral cerebral oedema may be associated with central herniation, which is a shift of the cerebral structures down through the tentorium, placing pressure on the brain stem. Central herniation is manifest by progressive neurologic deficit including decreased level of responsiveness, posturing, and unstable vital signs.

Attempts should be made to prevent increased ICP where possible, and when present, intervene early. Treatment of increased ICP will depend on specific pathophysiologic processes in play.

## References

1. Stewart-Amidei C. Nervous system alterations. In: Introduction to critical care nursing. 7th ed. Philadelphia, PA: Saunders; 2017. Chapter 14.
2. Bader MK, Littlejohns LR, Olson D, American Association of Neuroscience Nurses. Anatomy of the nervous system. In: AANN core curriculum for neuroscience nursing. 6th ed. St. Louis, MO: Saunders; 2016. Chapters 1–3.
3. Marieb E, Nicpon Hoehn K. The central nervous system. In: Human anatomy & physiology. Boston, MA: Pearson; 2010. Chapter 12.
4. Grossman S, Porth CM. Organization and control of neural function. In: Pathophysiology: concepts of altered health states. 9th ed. Philadelphia, PA: Wolters Kluwer; 2014. Chapter 17.
5. Hickey J. Overview of neuroanatomy and physiology. In: The clinical practice of neurological and neurosurgical nursing. 7th ed. Philadelphia, PA: Lippincott, Williams and Wilkins; 2013. Chapter 5.

Elliott Rees and Tilak Das

**Abstract**

Neuroimaging is paramount in the medical management of glial tumours. Through various imaging modalities, radiologists provide essential information about tumours and guide treatments. Alongside tumour location and complications, imaging is also able to give a strong indication of tumour grade, a key factor in determining treatment pathways. Once a diagnosis has been established, neuroimaging is then often relied on for monitoring low-grade tumours for transformation as well as post-treatment follow-up of higher-grade tumours.

**Keywords**

Neuroimaging · Neuroradiology · Glioma · Glial tumour · CNS tumour

**Learning Outcomes**
- Be able to differentiate between CT and MRI scans and understand the clinic setting and relevance where each modality may be used.
- Understand the importance of contrast-enhanced imaging in diagnosing gliomas.
- Be able to visually differentiate oedema from cerebral spinal fluid (CSF) using T1- and T2-weighted MRI imaging.
- Gain a deeper understanding and insight into the varying MRI techniques used for surveillance imaging, in order to detect early recurrence or transformation of a low-grade glioma into a high-grade glioma.

E. Rees · T. Das (✉)
Department of Radiology, Addenbrooke's Hospital, Cambridge University Hospitals
NHS Foundation Trust, Cambridge, UK
e-mail: tilak.das@addenbrookes.nhs.uk

© Springer Nature Switzerland AG 2019                                                    21
I. Oberg (ed.), *Management of Adult Glioma in Nursing Practice*,
https://doi.org/10.1007/978-3-319-76747-5_2

## 2.1    Introduction

Imaging plays a critical role in the diagnosis, management and follow-up of glial tumours. Consequently, the radiologist, a doctor specialising in the interpretation of medical imaging, is a fundamental member of the multidisciplinary team and patient care pathway. Radiology is a rapidly evolving medical specialty that is based on using a range of imaging techniques to diagnose and sometimes treat conditions. Radiographers (radiology allied health professionals) are the technicians that produce imaging of a diagnostic quality and work in parallel with radiologists.

## 2.2    Imaging Modalities

The aim of medical imaging is to generate a visual representation of the internal structure of the body to allow for the non-invasive investigation of tissues, the planning of interventions as well as evaluating organ functions. Whilst the range of modalities is vast, this review will concentrate on those relevant to brain tumours. The physics that underpins imaging techniques is complex; a brief overview will be made in this chapter.

Neuroimaging, or neuroradiology, is a subspecialty within radiology concentrating on the imaging of conditions affecting the brain, spinal cord and peripheral nerves. Relevant imaging modalities within clinical neuroradiology are primarily those that focus on structure—computed tomography (CT), magnetic resonance imaging (MRI) and to a lesser extent ultrasound (US) and plain radiography. Modalities focussing on function are more recent developments and include positron emission tomography (PET) and functional MRI. Physiological processes are the target of functional imaging, and although there is a role in glioma characterisation, their predominant use in the central nervous system relates to research within cognitive neuroscience and psychology.

### 2.2.1    Computed Tomography (CT)

CT images are obtained using a rotating X-ray machine that takes measurements from multiple angles around the patient. Through computer processing, this information is used to create a 2D (two-dimensional) cross-sectional series of images resulting in a 3D representation. As X-rays are variably prevented from penetrating the body depending on tissue densities, the images produced by CT will be a representation of this. CT is very useful for assessing cortical bone and calcification but somewhat limited when evaluating the posterior fossa and cerebellum, due to artefact from the thick skull surrounding this area.

CT is the most commonly performed imaging technique for the investigation of neurological conditions and is often the first radiological test in a suspected brain tumour. It is relatively cheap, rapid (usually taking no more than 15 min) and widely available. The main drawback of CT is that it involves exposure of the patient to radiation, which can damage cells leading to an increased risk of developing cancer. The current effective dose for a CT of the head is equivalent to 1 year of natural background radiation (2.7 mSv) which equates to an additional risk of fatal cancer of 1 in 10,000 [1]. Another risk of CT relates to whether intravenous contrast agents are used (iodine-based compounds that increase the visibility of body tissues). Typical CT head examinations do not use contrast as the most common indications would be to exclude haemorrhage or infarction. If there is suspicion of metastases or other mass lesions, a CT 'pre-' and 'post-'contrast is obtained. The main risk of giving contrast is an allergic reaction, most worryingly, anaphylaxis. However, this is a lesser risk with the current low-osmolar contrast agents (1 in 10,000) compared to the previously used ionic agents (1 in 100) [2]. Other reactions that occur more frequently but are of lesser concern include skin rashes. Historically, contrast-induced kidney damage has also been a concern, although the literature continues to debate whether this is a legitimate worry [3].

## 2.2.2 Magnetic Resonance Imaging (MRI)

MRI is an imaging technique that uses powerful magnetic fields and radio waves to produce images of the body. The physics of MRI is based around the fact that the body contains a large amount of water molecules, each containing two hydrogen nuclei (protons). When placed in a strong magnetic field, the protons align with the direction of the field. A radio wave pulse 'knocks' the protons out of alignment, and the process of realigning with the magnetic field produces radio signals, which are recorded and processed into images. By altering the parameters of the application of radio waves, different 'sequences' can be created. Each sequence provides different information in the form of differences in the contrast between tissue types (Fig. 2.1).

A significant advantage of MRI over CT is that no radiation is used in MRI. MRI of the brain gives better tissue contrast than CT and has greater specificity and sensitivity for abnormalities. MRI is the test of choice for characterising brain tumours

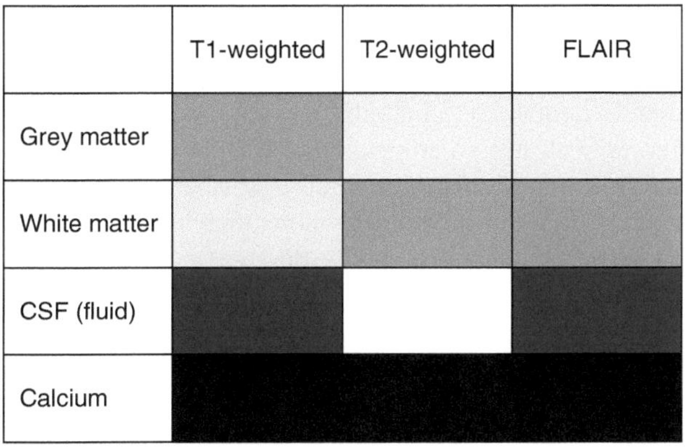

|  | T1-weighted | T2-weighted | FLAIR |
|---|---|---|---|
| Grey matter |  |  |  |
| White matter |  |  |  |
| CSF (fluid) |  |  |  |
| Calcium |  |  |  |

**Fig. 2.1** Table demonstrating different tissue characteristics (intensities) on standard MRI sequences

and has greater sensitivity for identifying tumours. Some disadvantages are that the examination itself is usually much longer, taking between 15 and 90 min to perform, with greater susceptibility to movement artefact. The cylinder containing the scanner components is larger than that used in CT, and so the bore that the patient passes through is often smaller. This can be an issue with larger patients and those with claustrophobia. There is also a contraindication in those with certain implantable devices, such as cardiac pacemakers or nerve stimulators, due to the strong magnetic field used.

## 2.3    Analysis of a Brain Tumour: A Systematic Approach

There is a wide range of radiological appearances of tumours of glial origin such that the primary role of imaging is to identify the presence of a tumour, give an indication of grade, and assess complications. Certain tumours will show characteristic features from time to time, and inferences can be made about which type of glial tumour is present, but as with most of radiology, the cell type is ultimately determined by tissue diagnosis. The multiple types of glial tumour and their classification will be covered in a later chapter.

The most basic manifestation of a glial tumour will be an intra-axial mass lesion (arising from the brain tissue as opposed to the lining of the brain), sometimes with mass effect on the adjacent brain. Tumours will originally start small, and those with similar appearances to the surrounding tissue will not be appreciated until they reach a certain size or cause a reaction such as inflammation of the surrounding brain. Certain tumours infiltrate normal tissues and will appear as diffuse lesions. These ideally need to have a different signal characteristic to the surrounding normal tissue or they would not be perceived. Once a lesion can be seen, the differential for the potential causes can be narrowed by assessing several characteristics as listed below.

### 2.3.1    Patient Factors

Although this book is focussed on adult gliomas, it is worthwhile appreciating that different types of brain tumours occur at different ages and that the incidence of tumours generally increases with age. Astrocytoma, the most common glial neoplasm, can occur at any age, whereas glioblastoma is more prevalent in older adults. There is also a gender difference with gliomas occurring more often in men. The clinical history will also impress on the differential, for example, duration and speed of onset of symptoms, evidence of sepsis, immune status and known malignancy in another part of the body.

### 2.3.2    Location

Location is important to establish, not only for aiding with the differential but also as it is paramount in planning a biopsy, radiotherapy or surgery. The initial assessment is usually to determine whether the lesion is intra- or extra-axial, that is, whether it is originating from the brain parenchyma itself or not. If not, the lesion is not a true brain tumour but arising from the tissues surrounding the brain, most commonly a meningioma that originates from dura or schwannoma from cranial or peripheral nerves. Establishing the origin of the lesion is usually straightforward but can at times be challenging, and much has been written about the different signs that can be helpful. More detailed localisation can then be considered in terms of which lobe the lesion is in, whether it is cortically or medullary based and if there are nearby or involved eloquent areas or vessels. Gliomas are most often found in the frontal and temporal lobes and usually centred on the subcortical white matter which contains the greatest number of glial cells. Examples of cortically based glial tumours are oligodendrogliomas and gangliogliomas.

### 2.3.3   Pattern of Spread

The way brain lesions behave can often aid in determining the likely type. Whilst some tumours will have mass effect and compress surrounding structures, others grow in an infiltrative manner along white matter tracts. Of the glial tumours, the low-grade infiltrative astrocytoma is one of the more common examples that show the infiltrative pattern. Another feature that can add specificity when it comes to pattern of spread is whether the lesion crosses the midline via the corpus callosum. Glioblastoma is an example of this, also known as a butterfly glioma for the shape it forms although primary central nervous system (CNS) lymphoma can look similar. Multifocal disease patterns are most commonly caused by metastases although glial tumours (multifocal glioblastoma) would also be in the differential.

### 2.3.4   CT Characteristics

The main feature that can be determined on CT is tissue density as it affects the degree of X-rays penetrating tissue. As most glial tumours tend to be of similar density to normal brain, CT assessment is not as helpful in defining tumour extent. They may be 'hyperdense' relative to brain, which can aid their identification. Certain glial tumours contain calcification which is extremely dense and typically represented by the colour white on CT (oligodendrogliomas commonly and astrocytomas occasionally). More usefully, oedema in the tissue surrounding the tumour, represented by low density (dark grey), or the effect of pressure from the tumour ('mass effect'), is readily identified and may prompt further investigation with MRI. CT is also useful to identify complications such as haemorrhage or obstruction of the ventricular system.

### 2.3.5   MR Characteristics

Multiple sequences are obtained in a typical brain tumour protocol, which may vary slightly between institutions but will generally include T1- and T2-weighted, fluid-attenuated inversion recovery (FLAIR), diffusion-weighted imaging (DWI) and post-contrast T1-weighted imaging. The signal intensity of the different parts of an MR image is determined by multiple factors. The various shades of white, grey and black are therefore referred to as intensities (hypo-, iso- or hyperintense). Parts that are lighter grey or white are described as hyperintense, whereas the other end of the scale, dark grey or black, is described as hypointense (Fig. 2.1). This terminology is also used when comparing a lesion to the background 'normal' tissue.

**T1-weighted** This sequence is useful for anatomical assessment and as a good general overview. As a rule, substances that are bright or 'hyperintense' on T1 weighting include fat and proteinaceous material. Fluids, commonly cerebrospinal fluid (CSF) or cystic lesions, are dark or 'hypointense'. Most glial tumours will be iso- or slightly hypointense compared to a normal brain.

**Contrast-enhanced** Contrast-enhanced imaging is typically T1-weighted as contrast agents (gadolinium-based) are paramagnetic (affecting the magnetism of nearby tissues) and, when taken up by tissue or tumour, appears hyperintense on this sequence. Pre- and post-contrast sequences are compared to look for 'enhancement'. Contrast medium given in both CT and MR imaging will act in the same way. As contrast medium passes through the circulatory system, it will be limited from entering the brain tissues by the blood-brain barrier, which acts to maintain a constant environment and protect the brain from pathogens. When this barrier is disrupted, by tumour, for example, contrast medium leaks into the tissues and is seen as enhancement, i.e. signal intensity that is different, usually brighter, than before contrast medium is administered (Fig. 2.2).

**T2-weighted** T2 is good at demonstrating pathology. Most brain tumours will be hyperintense to brain on T2-weighted imaging (Fig. 2.3). Other substances that are hyperintense on this sequence include fluid (CSF) and oedema (increased fluid content). Fat is typically intermediate to slightly hyperintense. Substances that produce hypointense signal include calcification and highly cellular tumours (e.g. high-grade glioma and lymphoma).

**FLAIR** This is a T2-weighted sequence but with suppressed CSF signal, meaning the CSF appears dark. By doing this, brain pathology that is adjacent to the ventricles or subarachnoid spaces (CSF containing) can be more easily appreciated as it is no longer adjacent to similarly hyperintense signal.

**SWI** Susceptibility-weighted imaging (SWI) and gradient recalled echo (GRE) are differently acquired sequences with similar results. Within neuroimaging, their main function is to demonstrate small amounts of blood products or calcification, which image as very low signal with 'blooming' artefact (appearing larger than the true size).

**DWI** There are many uses within neuroradiology for diffusion-weighted imaging (DWI), traditionally used in assessing stroke as it is very sensitive at picking up early and small areas of infarction. It has also been shown to be useful in grading glial tumours.

DWI relies on slightly different physics than the usual MRI sequences. It is based around the ability of water molecules to diffuse locally. When there are no boundaries to diffusion, such as in CSF, diffusion is very 'facilitated' and the signal is represented as very low. Within cellular tissue, diffusion will be comparatively

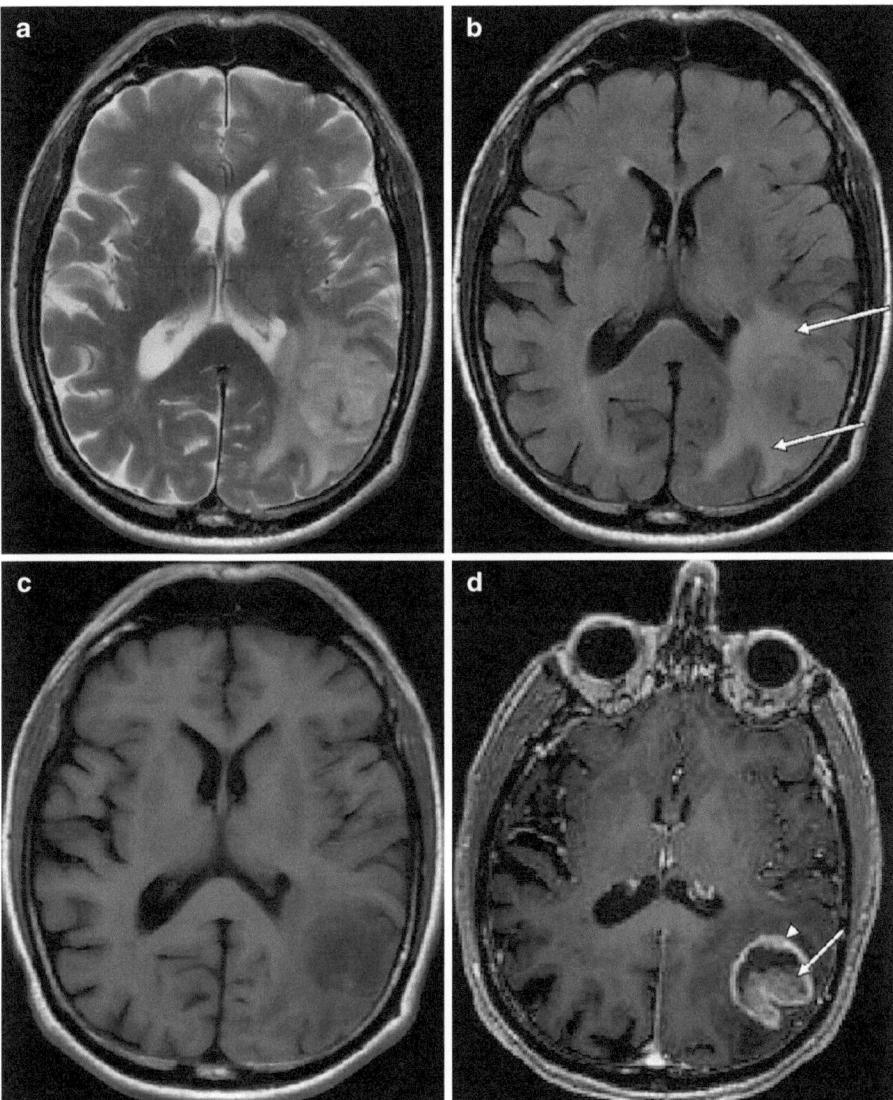

**Fig. 2.2** High grade glioma. (**a, b**) T2-weighted and FLAIR sequences show a mixed signal lesion in the left parieto-occipital convexity involving the white matter and overlying cortex. There is surrounding vasogenic oedema (arrows). (**c, d**) Pre- and post-contrast T1-weighted sequences demonstrate irregular ring enhancement (arrowhead) as well as patchy central enhancement (arrow)

'restricted' due to cell membranes limiting diffusion and is therefore of more intermediate signal. In hypercellular tissues or when cells are swollen (such as in certain tumours or after stroke), diffusion is even more restricted and represented as very high signal comparatively.

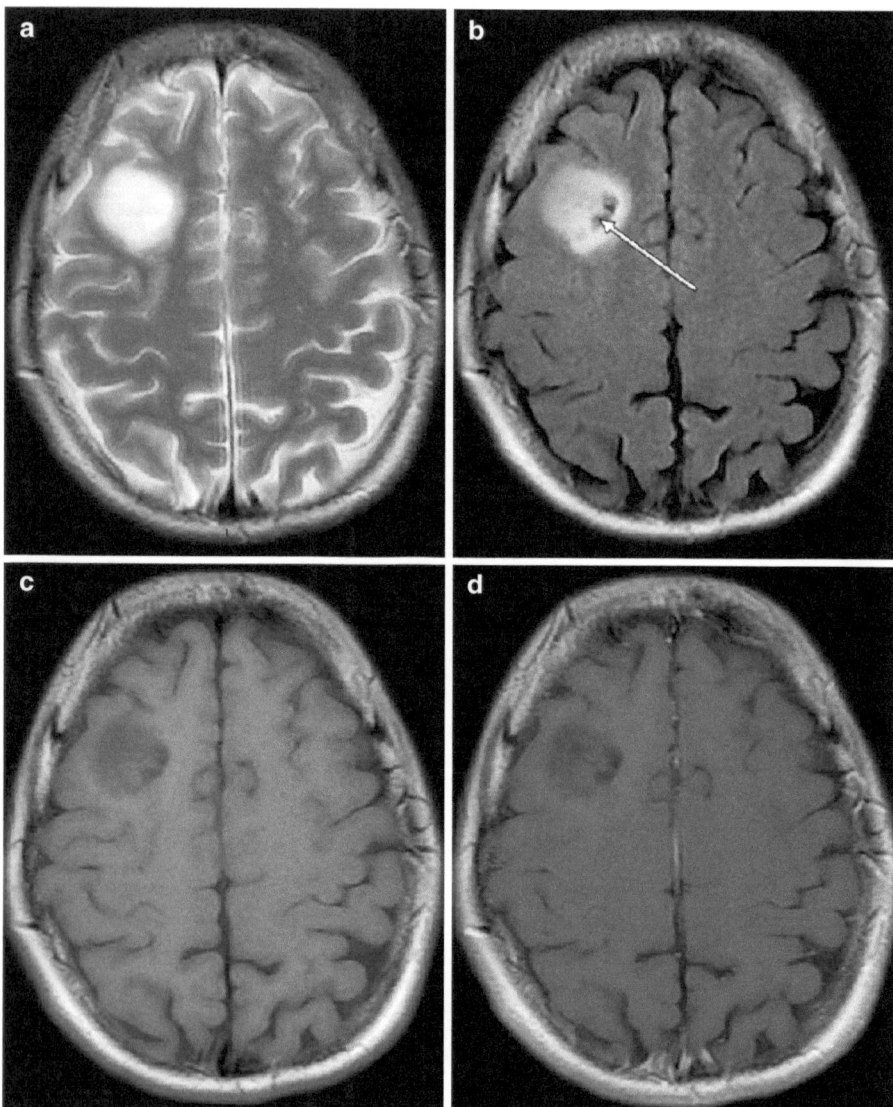

**Fig. 2.3** Low grade glioma. (**a**) T2-weighted sequence demonstrates a well defined hyperintense lesion in the superior aspect of the right frontal lobe in the subcortical white matter. There is no surrounding oedema. (**b**) FLAIR sequence shows areas of nulled signal (arrow) in keeping with cystic material. (**c, d**) Pre- and post-contrast T1-weighted sequences demonstrate a low signal lesion with no contrast enhancement

Higher-grade tumours generally show more restricted diffusion. DWI is also useful in distinguishing abscesses from necrotic tumours, which can appear similar. Abscesses tend to have restricted diffusion centrally, likely due to the viscosity of pus, whilst necrotic tumours have restricted diffusion in the cellular peripheries but not in the fluid centrally.

DWI typically generates several sets of images including images with different *B*-values (an important parameter in generating the images) and a calculated apparent diffusion coefficient (ADC) map, which should be interpreted together.

**Perfusion MRI** Perfusion dynamic susceptibility contrast (DSC)-MRI is a type of functional imaging that can help grading of tumours and potentially assess therapeutic response. Although there are many types of perfusion imaging, one of the most common uses gadolinium-based contrast agents alongside rapid sequence acquisition to evaluate cerebral microvasculature. Images are acquired rapidly and repeatedly whilst injecting contrast, and from the data, the blood concentration can be plotted for different regions of the brain. Relative cerebral blood volume (rCBV)—the volume of blood that passes through a given region in a given time—is of particular interest with tumour imaging as high grade; aggressive tumours generally have increased rCBV (Fig. 2.4). This is postulated to occur secondary to disruption of the blood-brain barrier as well as angiogenesis. As well as grading tumours, perfusion imaging is useful to guide biopsies, targeting the higher-grade areas most likely to yield positive results. Treatment response to the more recent anti-angiogenic drug therapies can be assessed. There is also a role for perfusion MRI in monitoring low-grade gliomas for transformation into high-grade tumour.

## 2.4    Features of High-Grade Tumours

### 2.4.1    Oedema

This refers to excessive amounts of water due to inflammatory processes within the brain parenchyma. The type of oedema that is relevant to brain tumours in radiology is known as vasogenic oedema (Fig. 2.2), which results from disruption of the blood-brain barrier and subsequent leakage of fluid from capillaries into the extracellular space. It predominantly affects the white matter and has been said to resemble spreading fingers as the cortical grey matter tends to be unaffected. Compared to normal white matter, oedema appears as hypodense on CT and hyperintense on T2-weighted or FLAIR MRI. There is also often swelling of the brain as might be expected from fluid leakage, and the CSF spaces become effaced. Higher-grade glial tumours, such as glioblastoma, tend to elicit peritumoural oedema, one theory being that the malignant cells induce this response to provide a suitable environment for growth [4].

### 2.4.2    Enhancement

Glial tumours that do not disturb the blood-brain barrier will show similar amounts of enhancement to background normal brain (low-grade diffuse gliomas). New enhancement of a previously non-enhancing tumour implies high-grade transformation. When abnormal enhancement is present, it can help to classify this into patterns. Typical radiological descriptors include 'ringlike', 'solid' and 'patchy'

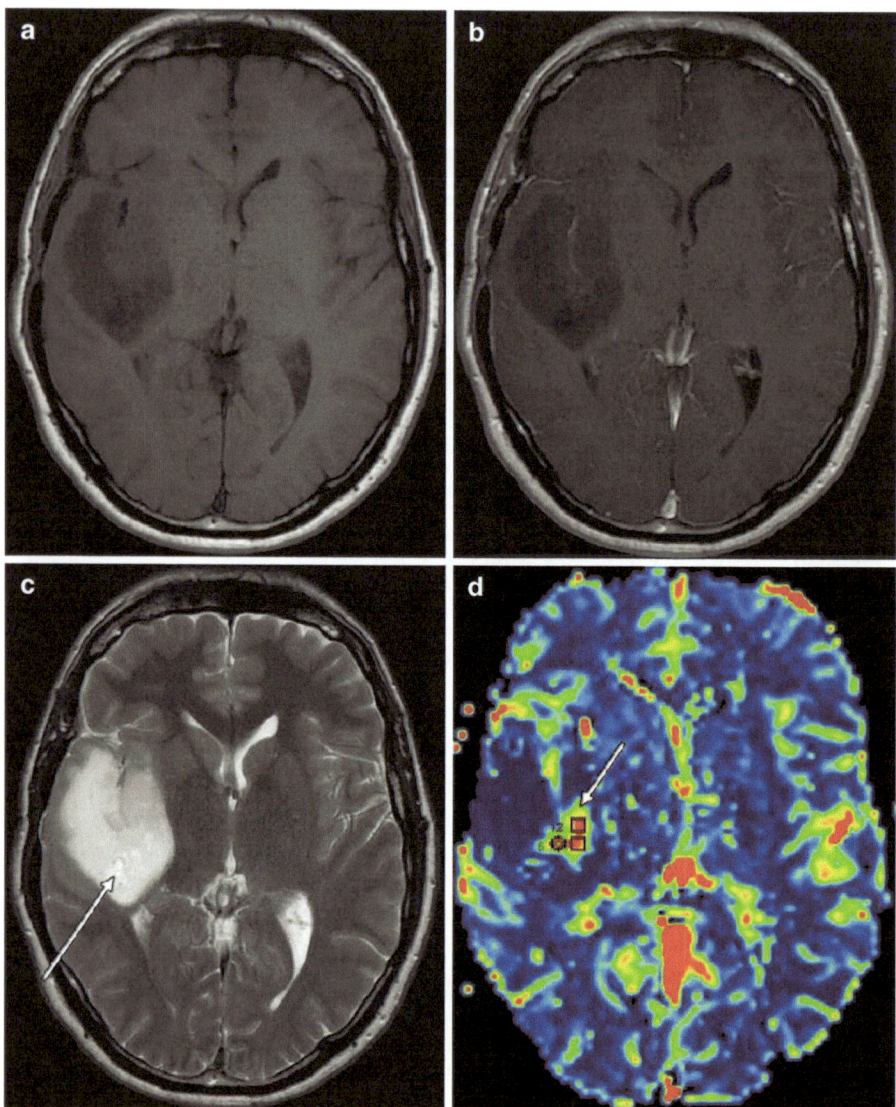

**Fig. 2.4** Low grade glioma, grade II astrocytoma with high grade transformation. (**a**, **b**) Pre- and post-contrast T1-weighted sequences demonstrate a non-enhancing, diffusely infiltrative lesion in the right anterior temporal lobe and insula. (**c**) T2-weighted sequence shows the well defined hyperintense lesion with a small cystic focus posteriorly (arrow). (**d**) Cerebral blood volume image from a DSC perfusion study demonstrates several 'hotspots' at the posterior aspect of the insula. Region of interest measurements from these areas were compared with normal contralateral white matter to give a maximum relative cerebral blood volume of 14.8. This indicates high grade transformation

enhancement. Although the differential for ring-enhancing lesions is long, glioblastoma is the classic glial tumour that can have this pattern. Solid-enhancing glial tumours tend to be high-grade astrocytomas with surrounding non-enhancing areas that can lead to the true size being underestimated. Patchy enhancement can be present in diffuse gliomas including oligodendrogliomas. Although enhancement in a glial tumour often correlates with grade, not all enhancing tumours are high grade, and conversely, some non-enhancing tumours are high grade. Rarer WHO grade 1 ('benign') tumours, such as juvenile pilocytic astrocytomas or ganglgliomas, can have enhancing components.

### 2.4.3  Leptomeningeal Metastases

Leptomeningeal metastases appear as increased sulcal signal on FLAIR and small enhancing nodules along the meninges or meningeal thickening on post-contrast T1-weighted imaging. Typically, there is a clinical suspicion before imaging, and CSF sampling for malignant cells via lumbar puncture can also aid in diagnosis. Meningeal metastases are a rare complication that can arise from many different tumour types. Glioblastoma and anaplastic astrocytoma are the more common glial tumours that metastasise to the meninges, and it can be a sign of transformation to a higher grade. There are several different mechanisms by which metastases can develop including direct extension from the original tumour and haematogenous spread. Once malignant cells are in the meninges, dissemination can occur via the CSF. As the CSF circulates around the brain and spinal cord, it is important to include spinal imaging whenever there is suspicion of leptomeningeal metastases.

## 2.5  Surgery-Related Imaging

### 2.5.1  Image-Merged Neuro-navigation

When planning neurosurgical biopsy or resection, it is critical to pinpoint the lesion accurately and minimise damage to surrounding brain. MRI as well as CT protocols can be tailored to demonstrate the lesion of interest, with reference to a 3D coordinate system that can be paired with the stereotactic surgical frame to give precise localisation. These can in turn be registered with functional imaging techniques that allow identification and avoidance of eloquent brain areas.

### 2.5.2  Post-operative Imaging

Routine post-operative imaging is important to assess the presence of residual tumour and establish a baseline (Fig. 2.5). The protocol will typically be the same as standard brain tumour sequences with post-contrast T1- and T2-weighted and DWI being of greatest interest. The timing of imaging is debated and will vary

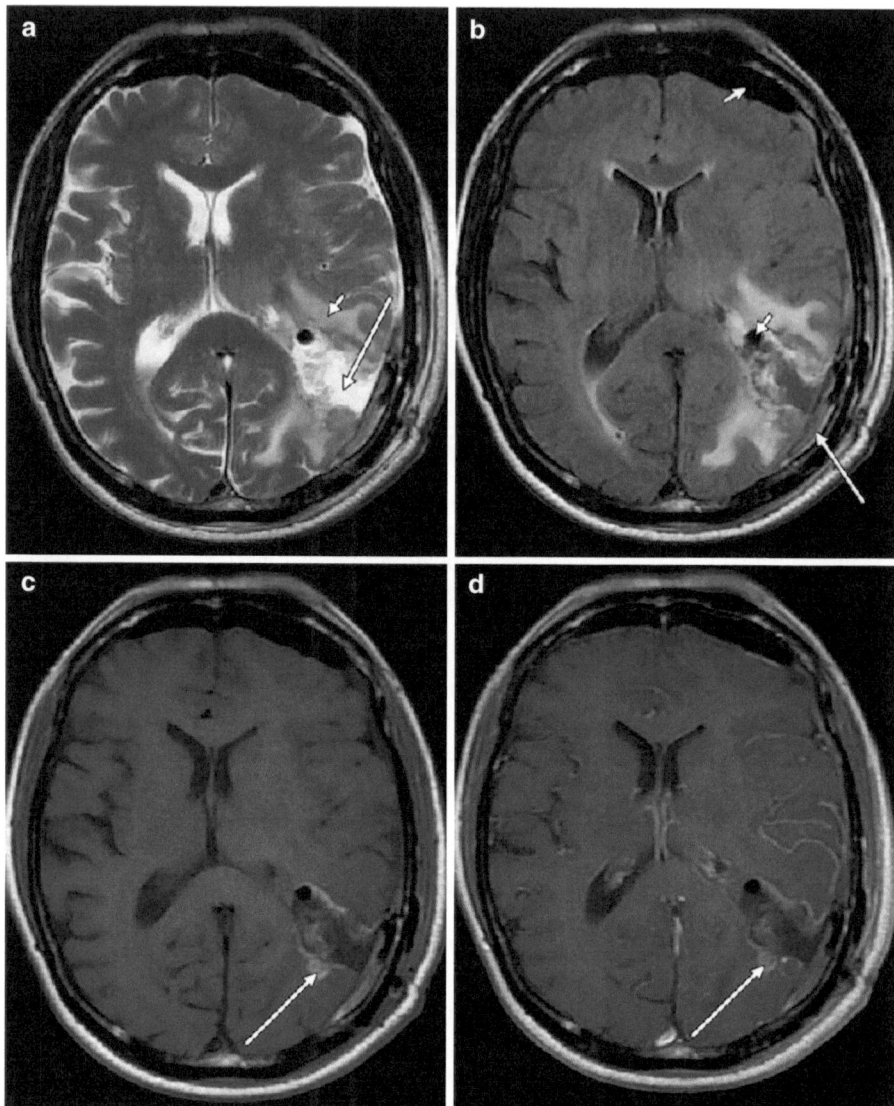

**Fig. 2.5** Post-operative study after tumour resection. (**a**) T2-weighted sequence demonstrates a resection cavity containing CSF (arrow) and other mixed signal material representing blood degradation products. There is residual white matter oedema (short arrow). (**b**) FLAIR sequence shows expected post-operative changes including low signal intracranial gas (short arrow) and shallow extra-axial haematoma (arrow). (**c**, **d**) Pre- and post-contrast T1-weighted sequences shows no evidence of residual tumour. High signal areas at the resection margin are present on the pre-contrast images in keeping with a small amount of haemorrhage (arrows)

between institutions. As surgery disrupts the blood-brain barrier, there is usually a certain amount of 'normal' parenchymal enhancement that can last for months after the operation. For high-grade enhancing tumours, early post-operative imaging (within 72 h) is important to estimate residual disease before additional enhancement related to the surgery confounds the radiological appearance. The pattern of enhancement is important in assessing residual tumour, with thick linear or nodular patterns more likely to represent disease rather than thin linear enhancement. Correlating with DWI also aids in differentiating perioperative brain insult from tumour. Follow-up imaging in the longer term is decided by the multidisciplinary team and will depend on the tumour type, patient symptoms and treatment.

## 2.6 Differential Diagnoses

Once a lesion is identified in the brain, it is important to consider the multiple possible causes. Using the imaging characteristics can help to narrow down the differential, but the clinical findings are paramount, and so information provided by the referring team is critical. Limiting the differential as much as possible helps when forming a management plan and estimating prognosis. The following neurological conditions are some of the more commonly encountered. They can exhibit many features that primary brain tumours demonstrate and therefore can create diagnostic dilemmas with significant implications on treatment decisions.

### 2.6.1 Demyelination

When discussing demyelination, multiple sclerosis is the archetypal disease that comes to mind, although the term demyelinating simply refers to the loss of normal myelin in a region of the brain. An aggressive demyelinating disease known as tumefactive demyelination is difficult to differentiate from tumours due to its ring-enhancing appearances and often subject to biopsy for this reason. Tumefactive demyelinating lesions (TDL) are usually large and solitary and can be confused with high-grade glioma. Useful distinguishing features from glial tumours are that TDLs often have an incomplete enhancing ring, less surrounding oedema and mass effect and a lower rCBV on perfusion imaging.

### 2.6.2 Ischaemic Stroke

Depending on when an ischaemic stroke or infarct is imaged, the appearances will vary in a predictable manner. The subacute phase (10–15 days) is one period that can be confused with a tumour due to mass effect and irregular areas of enhancement. If there is haemorrhage into an infarct, this can also prove a challenge. In these cases, the history is very helpful as strokes usually have characteristic history and examination findings. It can help to perform follow-up imaging as findings of infarction will evolve. CT is often sufficient for this as evolving or established infarction becomes more evident on CT with time and CT can also be used to assess for complications of infarction such as haemorrhage. Infarcts will not have elevated rCBV unlike a high-grade tumour on perfusion imaging.

### 2.6.3 Metastases

Brain metastases are a common cause of intracranial mass lesion and have a variety of manifestations. If there is a known primary elsewhere, that will obviously have a strong bearing on the differential. Multiplicity is a feature that would typically point towards metastases rather than a primary brain tumour. However, multifocal glioblastoma appears as multiple enhancing tumours. Metastases are normally located at the grey-white matter interface and glioblastoma in the subcortical white matter extending along white matter tracts. Perfusion imaging can sometimes aid with differentiating metastases from high-grade glioma.

### 2.6.4 Lymphoma

Primary lymphoma of the brain is a relatively rare tumour and like most tumours can have a variety of appearances. The classic mimic of a glial tumour is when lymphoma crosses the corpus callosum and has similar appearances to the 'butterfly' glioma. Features that can help to distinguish are that gliomas more frequently have central necrosis and haemorrhage, whereas lymphoma tends to enhance more homogeneously. Lymphoma is often, but not always, located around and adjacent to the ventricles. Because the management of lymphomas is radically different from that of gliomas, it is often helpful to be able to suggest the diagnosis before a biopsy is available.

### 2.6.5 Abscess

An abscess can form when a pathogen grows in the brain. This will usually start as an area of inflammation (cerebritis), which becomes encapsulated as the body attempts to prevent the infection spreading. As an abscess often appears as a ring-enhancing lesion, the differential will include tumours. One of the more useful signs of an abscess is high DWI signal centrally (restricted diffusion).

### 2.7 Conclusion

Neuroimaging has become critical in the diagnosis and management of glial tumours. Non-invasive techniques are now able to integrate structural, functional, metabolic and haemodynamic information into tumour evaluation. By working together in multidisciplinary teams, the radiologist can help in deciding the best techniques to establish tumour grade and plan treatment. Newer imaging techniques and improved understanding of the biology of brain tumours mean that the patient will ultimately benefit through earlier, more specific diagnosis and tailored treatments.

## References

1. Watson SJ, Jones AL, Oatway WB, Hughes JS. Ionising radiation exposure of the UK population: 2005 review. Didcot: Health Protection Agency; 2005.
2. Drain KL, Volcheck GW. Preventing and managing drug-induced anaphylaxis. Drug Saf. 2001;24(11):843–53.
3. Katzberg RW, Newhouse JH. Intravenous contrast medium–induced nephrotoxicity: is the medical risk really as great as we have come to believe? Radiology. 2010;256:21–8.
4. Lin ZX. Glioma-related edema: new insight into molecular mechanisms and their clinical implications. Chin J Cancer. 2013;32(1):49.

# Neurological Assessment of Patients with Gliomas

# 3

Timothy Ham and Timothy Rittman

**Abstract**

In this chapter we look at how to approach the neurological assessment of a person with a brain tumour. We discuss the symptoms they may present with, in particular cognitive impairment, headache and seizures. We introduce the neurological examination of motor function, eyes and cognition, concentrating on the most useful aspects of these assessments for patients with a brain tumour.

**Keywords**
Examination · History · Headache · Seizure · Cognition

**Learning Objectives**
- Gaining a deeper knowledge and insight into some of the most common presenting signs and symptoms of a glioma patient and how to manage them.
- Understanding the importance of undertaking a full neurological examination and what the findings may imply in terms of a glioma diagnosis versus differential diagnosis.
- Understanding the importance of using various neurological assessment tools in relation to glioma patients.

## 3.1 Presenting Symptoms of Gliomas

People with gliomas can present with a wide range of symptoms depending upon the part of the brain affected. The three commonest symptoms that lead people to seek medical attention are cognitive impairments/problems, headaches and seizures [1–3].

T. Ham · T. Rittman (✉)
Department of Neurology, Addenbrookes Hospital, Cambridge, UK
e-mail: timothy.ham@addenbrookes.nhs.uk; timothy.rittman@addenbrookes.nhs.uk

© Springer Nature Switzerland AG 2019                                          37
I. Oberg (ed.), *Management of Adult Glioma in Nursing Practice*,
https://doi.org/10.1007/978-3-319-76747-5_3

## 3.2    Cognitive Impairment

Up to 90% of people with a brain tumour have impaired cognition at the beginning of their illness, although they themselves may be unaware of this [4]. Added to this, cognitive impairment may not be immediately apparent during normal conversation. Relatives may describe someone being "not quite right" or having a "bad memory" which can describe a wide range of cognitive symptoms, not just memory problems. For these reasons formal cognitive testing is a helpful addition to the assessment of patients with a glioma.

In the same way that arm or leg weakness can help localise a brain lesion to a specific part of the brain, cognitive problems can be viewed in a similar way. Table 3.1 shows the cognitive symptoms and signs that are associated with the different lobes of the brain. The principal domains of cognition include: memory, executive function, language and visuospatial function.

Memory impairment is usually volunteered by relatives and caregivers. Features in the history may include repetitive questioning and forgetting how to perform well-practiced tasks such as using the TV or using a phone. Language dysfunction is frequently misinterpreted as memory loss or "confusion". People may use the wrong words, make up new words or repeat well-rehearsed catchphrases. People who struggle to comprehend language may complain about their hearing.

Among the cognitive domains, executive function is the most commonly impaired cognitive function in gliomas [4]. This refers to the ability to organise,

**Table 3.1** Localisation of cognitive function to cortical lobes

| Brain lobe | Cognitive functions | Clinical manifestations |
|---|---|---|
| Frontal | Executive function<br>Rule learning<br>Inhibition | Disorganised, chaotic life<br>Behavioural change/inappropriate behaviour<br>Difficulty understanding simple instructions<br>Impulsiveness |
| Temporal | Language<br>Object recognition<br>Memory | Poor memory<br>Difficulty naming objects (anomia)<br>Poor grammar<br>Difficulty reading and writing |
| Parietal | Dominant lobe:<br>– Language<br>Nondominant lobe<br>– Constructional praxis<br>Both hemispheres<br>– Visuospatial function<br>– Motor praxis | Dominant hemisphere:<br>– Gerstmann's syndrome: alexia (unable to read), agraphia (unable to write), dyscalculia (unable to perform simple arithmetic), finger agnosia (unable to name fingers), left/right disorientation<br>Nondominant hemisphere:<br>– Dressing apraxia (struggles to put on clothes)<br>– Neglect/sensory extinction<br>Either hemisphere:<br>– Sensory disturbance<br>– Apraxia<br>– Visuospatial disturbance |
| Occipital | Visual | Hemianopia<br>Visuospatial disturbance |

inhibit and prioritise tasks. Executive dysfunction typically arises from lesions in the frontal lobe of the brain but also occurs in any disease process that affects substantial areas of white matter. The manifestation of executive dysfunction can be varied but usually leads to a change in behaviour and a more chaotic, disorganised life. The consequence is increased anxiety levels for the patient and those around them. In this regard, obtaining a history from a relative or carer is essential. One can ask whether the patient has difficulties organising themselves, behaves out of character or struggles to understand simple instructions.

Visuospatial function results from lesions of the parietal or occipital lobes. Patients often have difficulty describing visuospatial symptoms and frequently visit the optician only to be told there is nothing wrong with their eyes, particularly if there is no accompanying visual field impairment. However, they may trip, misjudge stairs or struggle to drive (particularly reversing). On assessment in the clinic, patients may struggle to sit down because they cannot judge the distance to the chair behind them.

Assessing cognition can help in the diagnosis of a brain tumour but can also be used to assess the response to treatment or monitor for disease recurrence. This is particularly true of people who first present with cognitive symptoms or who have tumours away from the motor areas of the brain. Knowing the location of a brain tumour can help tailor specific cognitive testing, for example, assessing visuospatial function in a patient with a parieto-occipital lesion or memory function in a patient with a lesion near the hippocampus.

Radiation-related cognitive impairment may occur many years after treatment resulting in a slow decline in memory and general ability. This is becoming less common since radiotherapy has become more targeted allowing lower doses to be used. Patients most at risk of cognitive decline related to radiotherapy are those who received whole brain radiotherapy, high-dose radiotherapy (particularly above 2 Gy) [5] and with a pre-existing brain condition (e.g. cerebrovascular disease or multiple sclerosis).

## 3.3    Headaches

Headaches are a common feature of brain tumours, but they are not usually the principle symptom when people present to a healthcare professional. Although in retrospect nearly half of people with gliomas report headaches as their first symptoms [2] by the time they are seen in hospital, the headache is nearly always associated with other symptoms and signs. It is estimated that only 2–4% of patients with brain tumours present to hospital with headache alone, although the number is higher in general practice and this percentage would likely increase if the diagnosis was made earlier [1, 2].

The headaches associated with brain tumours are due to raised intracranial pressure. "Red-flag" features suggesting that a headache is caused by raised intracranial pressure are:

- Worse on lying flat, leaning forward or straining
- Worse in morning (i.e. after sleeping flat overnight)
- Waking a patient from sleep
- Associated with effortless vomiting

The best bedside test to check for raised intracranial pressure is fundoscopy (see below). It is unusual for a tumour to be large enough to cause raised intracranial pressure without other associated neurological findings on examination unless it is in a clinically silent area of the brain (e.g. the frontal lobe where a large tumour may cause subtle personality change and executive cognitive problems but little else). Small pituitary tumours may also cause headaches disproportionate to their size. Importantly, raised intracranial pressure headaches followed by loss of consciousness in patients with a brain tumour can indicate imminent obstruction of cerebrospinal fluid drainage from the ventricles, brainstem herniation and death. For this reason, any episode of loss of consciousness in a patient with a brain tumour should be taken seriously.

## 3.4    Seizures

Epileptic seizures are a common presenting symptom in brain tumours and are more often seen in low-grade rather than high-grade tumours. Seizures are caused by the uncontrolled spread of electrical activity in the brain; if the activity spreads widely enough, then it will cause symptoms related to the affected brain region (Table 3.2), and if it spreads to the whole cortex, it will cause loss of consciousness and a

**Table 3.2**  Localisation of seizures semiology to cortical lobes

| Brain lobe | Clinical manifestations of seizures |
|---|---|
| Frontal | Head turning away from the affected hemisphere (head version) Shaking of the opposite arm or leg Strange posturing of the arms and legs (e.g. cycling legs or "fencing posture" in the arms) Dominant hemisphere seizures can cause aphasias and speech arrest |
| Temporal | Déjà vu (a feeling of familiarity) and jamais vu (a feeling that you are in a familiar environment for the first time) Epigastric rising sensation (often described as "butterflies in the stomach") Unusual smell or taste that patients may find difficult to describe Psychic sensations (i.e. a feeling or panic or euphoria) Complex patterns of movements called automatisms (e.g. picking at clothes, pacing, spitting, chewing or lip-smacking) Auditory hallucinations (hearing music or noises) |
| Parietal | Sensory disturbance (tingling, electric shocks or pain in the opposite side of the body) Feeling that the opposite half of the body is larger or smaller than it really is |
| Occipital | Visual disturbance (normally coloured shapes) Partial blindness Palinopsia (seeing multiple copies of a single objects) |

generalized convulsion. Seizures can present in a multitude of ways depending upon where in the brain a tumour sits. The table below lists some of the commonest manifestations of seizures from the different parts of the brain:

Seizures are unpredictable, and while they are more likely to occur after provoking factors (e.g. alcohol, recreational drug use and sleep deprivation), they frequently occur without an obvious trigger. Seizures are normally short lived and last for a few seconds or at most a few minutes. Although seizures have a wide variety of presentations, they tend to be stereotypical in that a patient will describe the same or very similar symptoms during each attack. They may describe symptoms that sound bizarre or unusual, but if they are short lived and stereotypical, then seizures should always be considered.

Patients often lose awareness during a seizure and may have no memory of an attack so obtaining a witness history can be invaluable. With smartphones being so common, it is often possible for witnesses to film a seizure providing an extra source of information. Even if a patient loses consciousness during an attack, they may still be aware that a seizure has occurred because they have lost time, been incontinent of urine or simply feel unwell and fatigued.

## 3.5    Neurological Examination and Assessment

### 3.5.1    Levels of Consciousness

#### 3.5.1.1 Glasgow Coma Scale (GCS)

The GCS is a score out of 15 that gives a quick measure of a patient's alertness [6]. Its main advantage is that the score is quick to calculate, and most medical staff are familiar with it and understand the clinical implications of the score. The GCS score has three components: a 6-point motor score, a 5-point verbal score, and a 4-point eye score (see below). The motor sub-score is the most sensitive to changes in conscious level. The score is calculated as the best score that can be achieved.

The motor component is normally assessed by asking a patient to perform simple one-step motor tasks (e.g. "touch your nose", "stick out your tongue" or "squeeze my fingers"). Gripping an object placed in the palm can be a reflex action seen after frontal lobe injury. Therefore, if a patient is only able to squeeze your fingers, then you should also check that the patient will also let go to command before concluding that they are performing a voluntary movement. If a patient does not respond to verbal commands, then apply a painful stimulus in the form of a "trapezius squeeze" and gauge their response (see Table 3.3). The trapezius squeeze is unpleasant but has a lower potential to cause injury than some of the older forms of painful stimuli (e.g. nail bed pressure or supraorbital pressure). When assessing the motor component of the GCS, it is important to ensure that the person is capable of moving and feeling on the assessed side. If they have no response on one side of their body, then the other side should be assessed in case the patient is hemiplegic or has hemiparaesthesia.

**Table 3.3** Glasgow coma scale

| Motor score | |
|---|---|
| 6 | Obeys commands (e.g. stick out tongue, squeeze fingers) |
| 5 | Localises to pain (i.e. purposeful movement towards painful stimulus) |
| 4 | Withdraws from a painful stimulus |
| 3 | Flexion in response to pain—also called decorticate posturing |
| 2 | Extension in response to pain—also called decerebrate posturing |
| 1 | No response to pain |
| Verbal score | |
| 5 | Normal speech (i.e. orientated to self and environment) |
| 4 | Confused but able to answer questions |
| 3 | Inappropriate words only |
| 2 | Incomprehensible speech or sounds |
| 1 | No verbal response |
| Eye score | |
| 4 | Eyelids open spontaneously |
| 3 | Eyelids open to speech or command |
| 2 | Eyelids open to painful stimulus |
| 1 | No response to pain |

The GCS was originally designed for assessment of level of consciousness after traumatic brain injury and should be used with caution with other conditions as its scores can be misleading (6). A patient may score poorly on the GCS if they do not understand the command due to communication problems (e.g. hearing loss, dementia, non-native language speaker or aphasia), and the GCS should always be interpreted in the context of the individual patient. For example, an aphasic patient who is unable to speak or understand commands may have a GCS of 10/15 ($V = 1$, $E = 4$, $M = 5$) despite being fully alert.

### 3.5.1.2 The FOUR (Full Outline of UnResponsiveness) Score

The FOUR score has gained increasing popularity in recent years, replacing the GCS in some hospitals (see Table 3.4). Although it is less well known than the GCS outside the intensive care community, the FOUR score has advantages in being able to assess non-verbal aspects of consciousness and patients who are intubated.

## 3.5.2   General Observations

If large enough, a tumour and its surrounding oedema can cause herniation of the brainstem into the foramen magnum at the skull base. The process of brainstem herniation is referred to a "coning" and is a life-threatening neurological emergency causing a reduced level of consciousness (see above for GCS and FOUR score assessment), dilated pupil(s), raised blood pressure and slowed heart rate. The blood pressure and heart rate can change dramatically with changes in posture as lying down can cause further elevation in the intracranial pressure and worsening brainstem herniation.

**Table 3.4** FOUR score

| Eye response score | |
|---|---|
| 4 | Eyelids open or opened, tracking or blinking to command |
| 3 | Eyelids open but not tracking |
| 2 | Eyelids closed but opens to loud voice |
| 1 | Eyelids closed but opens to pain |
| 0 | Eyelids remain closed with pain |
| Motor response score | |
| 4 | Thumbs up, fist or peace sign to command |
| 3 | Localising to pain |
| 2 | Flexion to pain |
| 1 | Extensor posturing |
| 0 | No response to pain or generalized myoclonus status epilepticus |
| Brainstem response score | |
| 4 | Pupil and corneal reflexes present |
| 3 | One pupil wide and fixed |
| 2 | Pupil *or* corneal reflexes absent |
| 1 | Pupil *and* corneal reflexes absent |
| 0 | Absent pupil, corneal, and cough reflex |
| Respiration score | |
| 4 | Not intubated, regular breathing pattern |
| 3 | Not intubated, Cheyne-Stokes breathing pattern |
| 2 | Not intubated, irregular breathing pattern |
| 1 | Breathes above ventilator rate |
| 0 | Breathes at ventilator rate |

### 3.5.3 Fundoscopic Examination

The immediate life-threatening complications of a glioma are mainly due to the effects of raised intracranial pressure, which can be assessed indirectly through fundoscopy. A fundoscope or ophthalmoscope is a simple piece of equipment that allows you to look into a person's eye and directly visualises the retina, optic nerve head and retinal blood vessels. To the trained eye, examining these features can show early signs of raised intracranial pressure in the form of papilloedema and loss of the normal venous pulsations (Fig. 3.1). Fundoscopy should be performed routinely on every patient with a suspected brain tumour. Examining the retina with an ophthalmoscope is arguably the most important part of the examination in patients with brain tumours. Unfortunately, fundoscopy is also considered by many to be the most difficult part of the neurological examination because it is technically challenging, and it needs to be performed regularly for a person to become proficient.

People with raised intracranial pressure usually have preserved visual acuity even when extensive changes are seen on fundoscopy. They may only report visual symptoms when either the macula is affected or the intracranial pressure is sufficiently elevated to restrict blood flow to the optic nerve. At this point they may

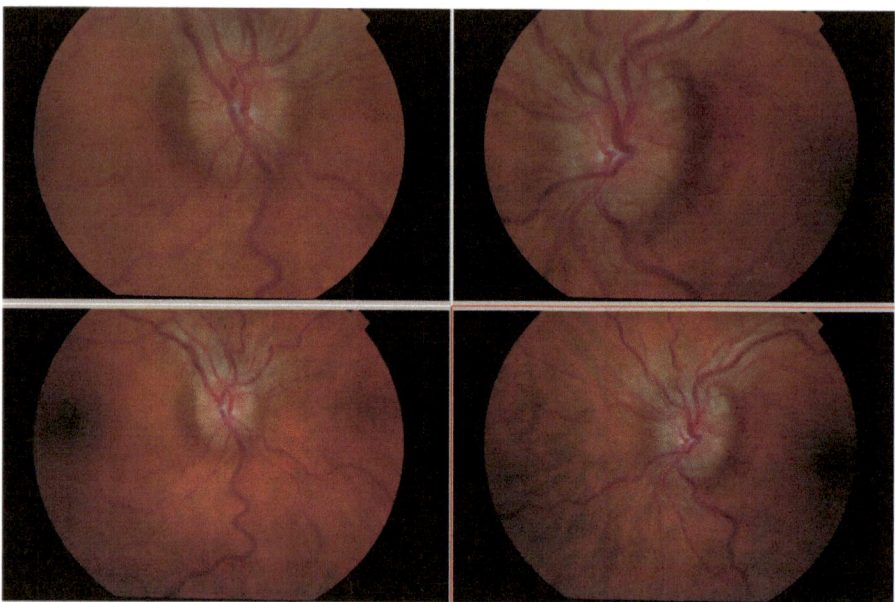

**Fig. 3.1** Papilloedema

report transient blurring of their vision after sudden changes in posture or straining. These events are called "visual obscurations" and are a concerning symptom suggesting that the intracranial pressure is significantly elevated.

### 3.5.4 Motor Examination

The part of the brain that controls movement is called the primary motor cortex or the motor strip. The motor strip is located in the precentral gyrus directly in front of the central sulcus. The central sulcus is the border between the frontal and parietal lobes, and the motor strip makes up the posterior border of the frontal lobe. There is a motor strip in each hemisphere that controls movements on the opposite side of the body through the corticospinal tracts. When the motor strip or corticospinal tracts are damaged, it causes weakness to the face, arm and leg on the opposite side of the body. The strength of each muscle group is measured in a standardised way on the Medical Research Council (MRC) scale from 5 to 0 (Table 3.5):

A complete description of the neurological examination is beyond the scope of this chapter, but the following will hopefully provide useful information and a screening test for assessment. Strength in the face, arms and legs are tested individually.

Facial weakness can be obvious (e.g. some patients have a marked facial droop leaving them unable to close their eyes or control their saliva), and others may have subtler weakness that only becomes apparent when you ask them to mime facial gestures. To test the muscles of facial expression, patients are typically asked to perform the following facial gestures:

**Table 3.5** Medical research council grades of muscle power

| Medical Research Council (MRC) grade | |
| --- | --- |
| 5 | Full power (i.e. what you would expect in a normal person) |
| 4 | Subjective reduction in power (i.e. able to lift a limb but can be overcome by examiner) |
| 3 | Anti-gravity movement only (i.e. able to lift limb but not against resistance) |
| 2 | Can only move in the plane of gravity |
| 1 | Twitch of movement |
| 0 | No movement |

- Raise their eyebrows
- Close their eyes against resistance
- Smile
- Purse their lips or blow out their cheeks

Weakness in the face caused by a unilateral brain injury does not affect the frontalis muscle that elevates the eyebrow because it is bilaterally innervated from both hemispheres. Therefore, patients with a brain tumour affecting the motor strip may have a droopy face, but they are still able to raise their eyebrow on the affected side. This is called forehead sparing.

Testing strength in the arm is done by asking the patient to raise their arms in the air and perform a variety of arm movements against resistance from the examiner. Sometimes weakness is obvious and volunteered by patients but can be more subtle. Subtle arm weakness can be best assessed by looking for pronator drift. Pronator drift is an unconscious movement of the arm caused by the fact the flexor muscles in the arm are stronger than the extensor muscles. It can be most easily demonstrated by asking a patient to hold their hands out in front of them palm up (i.e. "as if you are balancing a tray on your hands") and then asking a patient to close their eyes and keep their arms still. If there is damage to the motor strip or corticospinal tract, then the fingers on the affected hand may curl up and the hand may turn over (i.e. the palm turns downwards) and the arm may drop. This unconscious movement is a useful subtle sign of injury to the motor strip.

Leg strength is best assessed by asking a patient to walk, stand on tiptoes and stand on each leg individually. If a patient is able to do all of these actions, then the power in their legs is most likely normal. If a patient is unable to do these actions easily, then each muscle group should be tested individually.

## 3.5.5 Coordination

Coordination is broadly controlled by the cerebellum. Incoordination is often referred to as ataxia and can be subtle or very marked. Testing for ataxia can be done quickly in the arms by the finger-nose test where a patient is asked to alternate between touching your finger and their nose. In the legs, the corresponding assessment is the heel-shin test where a patient is asked to carefully run their heel up and down their shin. When performing this task, we are checking to see if patients miss the target when making these repetitive movements. It should be noted that tests of coordination are very difficult to interpret if a limb is weak or numb. If a limb is strong and has normal sensation, then incoordination in performing these movements may suggest an ipsilateral (same side) cerebellar injury. Cerebellar injury may be associated with other features summarised in the DANISH acronym (i.e. **D**ysmetria or Dysdiadochokinesia, **A**taxia, **N**ystagmus, **I**ntention tremor, **S**lurred/Staccato speech and **H**eel-shin incoordination).

### 3.5.6  Sensory Examination

The primary sensory cortex or sensory strip is located in the post-central gyrus in the anterior border of the parietal lobe directly behind the motor strip. Each sensory strip processes sensations from the opposite side of the body via the spino-thalamic tracts and dorsal columns. When the sensory strips are damaged, they cause altered sensation on the opposite half of the body. Testing sensation as part of the neurological examination can become a very long and protracted process testing the various sensory modalities of light touch, pin-prick, temperature and joint position sensation. In practice, extensive assessment of sensation in patients with brain tumours is largely unnecessary; these in-depth tests are more useful when assessing lesions of the spine or peripheral nerves, whereas in people with brain tumours, the sensory loss is due to cortical injury. Checking that sensation is intact to light touch in all four limbs and either side of the face is usually sufficient [7].

Sensory neglect is one of a small group of unusual conditions called anosognosia where a person may be unaware of their disability even though it may be obvious to an observer. It is normally due to damage of the nondominant parietal lobe. A person with neglect may be weak or unable to feel the contralateral side of their body but unaware of any disability. Likewise, a person may be unable to see in the contralateral visual hemifield but unaware of their impairment. On testing sensation, a patient with complete neglect will not be able to move their limb to command but may be able to move as a reflex when an unpleasant stimulus is applied. There are subtler forms of neglect where a patient may be able to feel or see objects on the affected side, but they are unable to detect them when a simultaneous stimulus is placed on the unaffected side. This milder form of neglect is called "extinction" and is easily tested by ensuring that a patient can feel your touch, in both sides of the body, and then asking them which side you are touching when you touch both sides of the body simultaneously.

### 3.5.7  Language

Conceptually neurologists break up language into speech and written language. Impairment in speech is referred to as *aphasia*, and impairment in reading or writing are *alexia* and *agraphia*, respectively.

Early work on language from single brain lesions identified two areas of the brain involved in language. These are Broca's area in the frontal lobe and Wernicke's area in the temporal lobe resulting in "expressive" and "receptive" aphasia, respectively. Language comprehension and speech production is now understood to be vastly more complex than the involvement of these two areas alone. It would therefore be tempting to dismiss this oversimplified model in favour of a more realistic modern understanding of language. However, for many people with a glioma, the identification of a primary problem with either comprehension or speech production can be helpful in understanding their impairment. In reality, a pure expressive or receptive aphasia is rare, and most people will have elements of both.

To assess expressive aphasia, one can ask simple questions to which you are confident the patient will know the answer:

- Start with the patient's name and address.
- Move on to topics familiar to people such as where they live and recent holidays.
- Listen for mistakes in pronunciation, using the wrong words and hesitation.

People may describe that they know what they want to say but cannot "get the words out".

In contrast, people with receptive aphasia speak fluently, but do not address the question asked of them.

For a more detailed assessment, language can be broken down into the elements of grammar, semantics and fluency. Semantics refers to knowledge of the meaning of words, e.g. recognising that "salmon" is a type of fish. For the careful listener, much can be picked up from hearing normal conversation on a topic familiar to the patient. For language impairments in these domains listen for:

- Grammar: words in the wrong order, short simple sentences
- Semantics: "empty" sentences with few nouns and little content
- Fluency: hesitation, pauses between words and a loss of the usual "smoothness" of speech

Bedside assessment of language is helpful to identify a problem with language and may help patients and their carers to understand the effect of a brain tumour. For an in-depth assessment of language, a formal neuropsychological assessment is required. Speech and language therapists can also be helpful providing practical advice where communication is difficult, e.g. using picture boards, educating relatives to ask simple questions.

### 3.5.7.1 Cognitive Assessment

There are vast arrays of cognitive tests that can assess the minutiae of executive function, memory, language, visuospatial function and behaviour used by psychologists that are beyond the scope of this chapter. For practical purposes, most people require a brief bedside screening test that takes a few minutes and is repeatable on subsequent visits. For this, we recommend either the Montreal Cognitive Assessment (MoCA, www.mocatest.org) or the Addenbrookes Cognitive Examination-III (ACE-III, https://sydney.edu.au/brain-mind/resources-for-clinicians/dementia-test. html). Both of these tests are freely available to professionals without copyright issues.

The MoCA is a slightly shorter test (5–10 min) scored out of 30 which has strengths in assessing executive function and language. The ACE-III takes slightly longer (10–15 min) scored out of 100 and assesses a wider range of cognitive domains with strengths in working memory, language and visuospatial function.

The Mini-Mental State Examination (MMSE) is a widely used brief test of cognition scored out of 30, though its use is limited in the assessment of people with brain tumours. It has strengths in orientation and working memory which are either obvious on bedside assessment or more relevant to acutely delirious patients rather than those with a glioma.

## 3.6    Conclusion

There is much to learn from a careful history and bedside assessment of people with a brain tumour. We have demonstrated that elements of the history can point to the location of a tumour, and that monitoring cognition and motor signs can be useful in monitoring progression or response to treatment. We have emphasised how the history and fundoscopy can pick up the warning signs of intracranial hypertension. We go on to discuss simple, repeatable tests that can be applied in most clinical situations.

## References

1. Kurtzke JF. Neuroepidemiology. Ann Neurol. 1984;16(3):265–77.
2. Grant R. Overview: brain tumour diagnosis and management/Royal College of Physicians guidelines. J Neurol Neurosurg Psychiatry. 2004;75(2):18–23.
3. Posti JP, Bori M, Kauko T, Sankinen M, Nordberg J, Rahi M, et al. Presenting symptoms of glioma in adults. Acta Neurol Scand. 2015;131(2):88–93.
4. Tucha O, Smely C, Preier M, Lange KW. Cognitive deficits before treatment among patients with brain tumors. Neurosurgery. 2000;47(2):324–34.
5. Klein M, Heimans JJ, Aaronson NK. Erratum: Effect of radiotherapy and other treatment-related factors on mid-term to long-term cognitive sequelae in low-grade gliomas: a comparative study. Lancet. 2002;360:1361–8.
6. Teasdale G, Jennett B. Assessment of coma and impaired consciousness. A practical scale. Lancet. 1974;304(7872):81–4.
7. Smith P. Open eyes to sensory testing. Pract Neurol. 2017;(17):167.

# Multidisciplinary Team Working

**4**

Ingela Oberg

**Abstract**

The ever-changing face of modern healthcare has brought out the requirement to form a team of experts to help plan, coordinate and communicate the best possible care for cancer patients, reducing inequalities and increasing overall effectiveness. In most western countries, this structure and membership of skilled individuals are referred to as a multidisciplinary team (MDT). MDTs increase communication and decision-making, increase patient satisfaction, aid recruitment into clinical trials, enhance continuity of care and, not least, ensure the patient receives the best advice on appropriate treatment options.

This chapter will aim to explore some of the key roles and responsibilities within an MDT to help equip the novice nurse with a deeper understanding of both how the process works and how they can positively contribute to the patient's cancer treatments and care pathway.

**Keywords**

Multidisciplinary team · Cancer waiting times · MDT referral · Cancer guidance

**Learning Outcomes**

The MDT process:

- Gain an understanding of the referral pathways of a radiologically diagnosed glioma patient.
- Understand and differentiate between the varying professionals that make up an MDT team and how they individually contribute to the MDT process.
- Gain basic insight into UK-based national cancer waiting time targets.

I. Oberg (✉)
Department of Neurosurgery, Addenbrooke's Hospital, Cambridge University Hospitals NHS Foundation Trust, Cambridgeshire, UK
e-mail: ingela.oberg@addenbrookes.nhs.uk

© Springer Nature Switzerland AG 2019
I. Oberg (ed.), *Management of Adult Glioma in Nursing Practice*,
https://doi.org/10.1007/978-3-319-76747-5_4

## 4.1    Introduction

Despite the rising incidence of cancer, more people are surviving and living with and beyond this disease; and as a population people are getting increasingly older, putting further pressures onto the National Health Service (NHS). At the same time, the NHS has to cope with increased pressures and demands, more subspecialisations and new innovations in both treatments and technologies. All of these combinations brought out the requirement to form a team of experts within a multidisciplinary team (MDT) to help plan, coordinate and communicate the best possible care for cancer patients, reducing inequalities and increasing overall effectiveness.

MDTs are now the cornerstone of cancer care and management not just in the UK but in most western countries. It increases communication and decision-making, increases patient satisfaction, aids recruitment into clinical trials, enhances continuity of care and, not least, ensures the patient receives the best advice on appropriate treatment options.

This chapter will aim to explore some of the key roles and responsibilities within an MDT to equip the novice nurse with a deeper understanding of both how the process works and how they can positively contribute to the patient's pathway.

## 4.2    Background

The concept of MDT working initially came about in the late 1980s in the UK with the development of the National Health Service (NHS) breast cancer screening programme where radiologists, radiographers and oncologists came together to discuss the findings of the mammograms identifying possible tumours [1]. However, it was not until the national improving outcomes guidance (IOG) series was launched a decade later that there was any impetus in ensuring MDT working was implemented across the bigger cancer sites known as the 'Big 4': breast, lung, colorectal and prostate [1, 2]. In 2006, the IOG for the brain and central nervous system was launched, and for the first time, this document detailed the composition of teams required to run an effective, multidisciplinary team. Furthermore, this document indicated who were so-called core members and who could be considered an 'extended member' and set out minimum standards of attendance and requirements [2].

In today's practice, MDT discussions have become the cornerstone of every cancer service not only in the UK but predominantly also across many other western countries including America and Australia. An effectively run MDT increases communication and shared decision-making across boundaries such as primary, secondary and tertiary care. It increases patient satisfaction by providing early access to imaging and decreasing time to diagnosis, aids recruitment into clinical trials, enhances continuity of care and, not least, ensures the patient receives the best advice on appropriate treatment options [1].

Presenting symptoms of brain tumours can be both very varied and nondescript, meaning it can be very difficult for a general practitioner (GP) to accurately predict a suspicion of a brain tumour. The vast majority of patients registered with a GP suffer headaches at some stage in their lives—this does not mean everyone needs to be screened for a possible brain tumour. Altered behaviour and mood changes can indicate stress or depression, not necessarily the presence of a brain tumour, and progressive neurological deterioration can indicate other neurological diseases such as multiple sclerosis over a tumour. It has been estimated that a GP may only see one primary brain tumour in every 7 years of clinical practice. However, the combination of new neurological symptoms accompanied with new neurological signs is more suggestive of pathology than symptoms alone and should trigger the GP or health professional to seek out urgent clinical advice and request the appropriate imaging [3]. A significant proportion of brain tumour patients still present acutely with seizures, for example, via accident and emergency (A&E) departments, prompting a brain scan and a subsequent brain tumour diagnosis via an emergency route.

To try and minimise emergency presentation routes, and to try and support GPs in clinical decision-making if they suspect the presence of a brain tumour, the NHS devised minimum targets and cancer waiting times for referrals [3, 4]. These targets, along with the published IOG series, have revolutionised how cancer patients are dealt with both by individual trusts and the NHS in general, with the introduction of MDTs.

The following sections will explore the *core memberships* and their individual roles within the brain/CNS MDT in more detail. For the purposes of avoiding confusion, clinical nurse specialists (also abbreviated CNS) have been referred to as 'key workers', something which will be used in this chapter for continuity purposes.

## 4.3  Neurosurgeon

A core member neurosurgeon working in the field of neuro-oncology is someone who spends at least 50% of their clinical programmed activities on neuro-oncology cases. Furthermore, they also need to be 'regularly involved' in speciality clinics helping to care for these patients [2]. Most of the UK neurosurgical centres have fully subspecialised since the introduction of the IOG, meaning most (if not all) of the specified surgeon's time is allocated to caring for the neuro-oncology patient. Having a neurosurgeon present at MDT discussions where surgical techniques, risks, benefits and size/location of the tumour(s) are taken into account is pivotal, and a fully formed MDT will not run without the presence of at least one consultant neurosurgeon.

As part of this subspecialisation, regular surgical clinics have been established to review and consent patients having previously been discussed in the MDT, whether they are new patient referrals or rediscussions. One rationale for having surgical clinics is that it is not a neurologist or GP, for instance, who decides when the timing is right for a patient to have a recommended surgical procedure—that is a joint decision taken by the patient and their neurosurgeon. Another more obvious reason is to have a clinic where the histopathological results are relayed to the patient and their families by the surgeon who performed the operation, prior to commencing any oncology treatments. The surgeon and key worker can thus ensure they have a complete understanding of their diagnosis and prognosis, as well as undertaking a thorough wound review, removal of staples/sutures and sign posting to support services and third sector organisations.

## 4.4 Neuroradiologist

A radiologist is a medical doctor who specialises in interpreting imaging from computed tomography (CT) or magnetic resonance imaging (MRI) scans. Most radiologists subspecialise, so some become specialists at breast imaging (mammograms), and others are specialised in interpreting brain imaging or images of the central nervous system, hence the terminology neuroradiologist.

Much like the neurosurgeon, the neuroradiologist also needs to spend at least 50% of their clinical programmed activities working specifically with neuroradiology imaging. The position also needs to be a substantive one (i.e. not a locum post) [2]. As can be read about in the chapter dedicated to neuroimaging, a neuroradiologist is pivotal to the smooth running of the MDT. It is his/her opinion about what imaging may represent that is documented in the MDT outcomes, and they determine whether this may represent a glioma, metastasis, a benign tumour or even in some cases other malignancies such as lymphoma or even infections such as an abscess. The majority of clinical prioritisation of surgical cases is done on the basis of the opinion given by the neuroradiologist—in other words, a suspected high-grade glioma will be given surgical preference to a benign meningioma or even a suspected small brain metastasis.

## 4.5 Neuropathologist

A pathologist is a medical doctor who has specialist training in being able to identify diseases by studying cells and tissues under a microscope. A neuropathologist specialises in diseases of the central nervous system, like high-grade gliomas. Unlike the previous two members, a neuropathologist has no minimum requirements for their clinical programmed activities. They simply need to be a registered, accredited pathologist or neuropathologist with specialist expertise in neuro-oncology [2].

Obtaining the grade and type of various brain tumours is a very complex process, especially given the updated pathology guidelines that came into circulation in March 2017, giving added importance to molecular markers such as 1p19q, MGMT and IDH statuses to name but a few [5]. These markers help subspecialise gliomas into astrocytomas and oligodendrogliomas and help predict the tumour's behaviour and how well it may respond to oncology treatments. A pathologist would hence need to have specialist knowledge on more than just a basic cellular level, so most neuropathologists attending an MDT are solely subspecialised in the field of brain/CNS tumours and conditions.

Most core members stay for the duration of the entire MDT discussion, but in some centres, the pathology cases are reviewed first to ascertain the patient's histopathological diagnosis and their individual molecular tumour profile, which, as stated, helps predict the patient's prognosis and will also help formulate a patient's treatment plan. Once the cases requiring neuropathology input have been discussed in their entirety, the new referrals that have come in to the MDT are discussed, and at that stage the neuropathologists are free to leave should they so wish, as their direct input is no longer required. Please see Chap. 7 for a more detailed analysis on how the pathology process works and the grading system and classification used for adult gliomas.

## 4.6    Oncologist

According to the IOG, and within the UK, a specialised neuro-oncologist is a clinical oncologist with a specialist interest in tumours of the central nervous system. There are dedicated neuro-oncologists that predominantly work with *primary* brain tumour patients (and other central nervous system tumours) [2]. Patients with *secondary* (metastatic) brain tumours will still be discussed at the MDT, but their overall management remains under the care of the oncologist looking after their primary disease such as breast or lung oncology. This is irrespective of whether or not their tumour(s) require neurosurgical input or not.

In recent years, the introduction of stereotactic radiosurgery (SRS) means the aspect of an overall treating consultant is even further diluted, with some neuro-oncologists now treating small volume brain metastases before passing the patients back to their primary oncologist once again. Please see Chap. 14 for more details on SRS and other radiotherapy techniques.

A neuro-oncologist is deemed pivotal at MDT as surgery would normally only be offered if there was a reasonable chance the glioma patient would do well with post-operative oncology treatments such as chemotherapy, radiotherapy or (increasingly used) immunotherapy. Putting a glioma patient through high-risk neurosurgery with little to no oncological input at the end of the process seems a rather futile undertaking otherwise. Hence, an oncologist's opinion and discussion around treatment options (both pre- and post-operatively, along with expected overall survival) and likely benefits of any recommended treatments are vastly important in the MDT.

It is important to highlight that in the UK, the vast majority of doctors treating brain tumour patients with chemotherapy and radiotherapy are general clinical oncologists. In many other European countries and across the world, it would be specialised neurologists who undertake these treatments. This is on the basis neurologists have specialist training in central nervous system diseases and disorders and are also trained to dispense and administer medicines to do with these conditions, brain tumours included. It would therefore make sense if they also administered the anticancer treatments and monitored them for side effects. In the UK, the administration of anticancer treatments is strictly limited to oncologists.

## 4.7    Clinical Nurse Specialist/Key Worker

Clinical nurse specialists (or key workers) are pivotal to the patient's pathway, and as such it is no surprise they are also regarded as key, core members of the MDT. According to the IOG, they must possess specialist knowledge of CNS tumours and hold relevant skills in communication [2].

Specialist nurses coordinate care across the primary, secondary and tertiary settings and often liaise with family and next of kin. A lot of neurosurgical centres are tertiary referral centres, meaning several hospitals spread across a wide geographical area refer directly in to a regional MDT. In a lot of cases, discussions around patients will be held for the first time at local, specialist MDT where any input from the neuro-oncology clinical nurse specialist may be limited as they have previously not met the patient. However, a significant proportion of discussions are around patients who have relapsed after completion of treatment, in which case the specialist nurse is ideally situated in informing the MDT of their patient's current clinical condition (sometimes referred to as performance status—see Chap. 15 for more details), individual treatment preferences and overall patient wishes. They can inform MDT how they coped during previous treatments and any side effects the patient may have experienced—all important information for the MDT to consider.

Alongside the above, clinical nurse specialists are also well equipped to help the MDT coordinator (see below) in triaging the referrals, making sure all referring information and imaging is available to the MDT panel for discussion. In particular, the specialist nurse can ascertain if the patient has improved neurologically on high-dose dexamethasone, for example, what medications they are on and any past medical history (PMH) of note or of clinical relevance. Having as much updated clinical information made available to the MDT panel for discussion, the less chance there will be of overlooking a vital piece of information or for the requirement of a rediscussion due to missing information at the time of referral into MDT. Ultimately, this will benefit the patient regarding timely decision-making and may minimise delays to post-operative treatments such as radiotherapy or chemotherapy.

## 4.8    Neurologist

A neurologist is described as someone with expertise in neuro-oncology, epilepsy and/or neuro-rehabilitation [2]. They would be able to give invaluable advice, for example, on seizure medication or if the location of the lesion would be responsible for the patient's symptoms. They can offer advice on other neurological tests that may provide additional information prior to surgical intervention (like a lumbar puncture), especially if the diagnosis remains uncertain and could represent inflammatory lesions over viable neoplasia. In many instances, a patient is primarily referred to a neurologist for primary investigations into their presenting neurological signs to see if their symptoms are in keeping with a suspected brain tumour or more in keeping with a neurological condition such as demyelination, inflammation or infection.

## 4.9    Palliative Care

This has been defined by the IOG as being a healthcare professional who has relevant experience and expertise in the provision of palliative care services for patients with CNS tumours [2]. Some centres have combined this requirement with the role of the key worker (specialist nurse) as they are often the patients and families' primary point of contact right through to end of life liaising with primary palliative care services and hospices.

## 4.10    Neuropsychologist

A clinical neuropsychologist with a specialist interest in tumours of the brain is a very valuable resource to have at MDT, especially when discussing low-grade gliomas with a prolonged disease trajectory. A neuropsychologist can undertake a baseline assessment of the patient's memory and verbal recall, as well as seeing if their speech or mobility is affected by either the use of some medication or as a result of the tumour or even the oedema. A neuropsychologist will assess the patient's literacy and overall cognition and put together a treatment plan for both the patient and the clinicians to adhere to. They then follow the patients up a few months after surgery to see if any of the parameters have shifted, by either showing signs of improvement or sometimes even a slight worsening of memory or verbal recall. Should this be the case, an adjusted treatment plan will be adapted and necessary onward referrals instigated as appropriate—to areas such as neuro-rehabilitation or for cognitive behavioural therapy (CBT), counselling or specialist speech and therapy services.

In many cases, a neuropsychologist (having undertaken a baseline assessment of the patient) is very well equipped to help out with speech and language mapping during awake surgery. This is done if a tumour is situated in the speech and language cortex (predominantly found in the left frontal lobe in most right-handed people).

## 4.11    Specialist AHP

Every MDT is meant to have representation from a specialist in the allied health professional (AHP) field, meaning either physiotherapists, occupational therapists, dietetics or speech and language teams. In reality, many MDTs have struggled with this core requirement as this cohort of AHPs is significantly understaffed in the UK, and they simply do not have the capacity to attend weekly MDTs with very little required input—their clinical priority remains the inpatients and helping patient flow by assessing those ready for discharge home. There are, however, ward-based MDTs involving these specialist AHPs that look at all the current neurosurgical (and neuro-oncological) inpatients, including those with tumours, and what can be done to support their recovery, promote self-independence and enable safe, early discharge. Should ongoing support from an AHP be required following discharge home from hospital, they would make the necessary onward referrals to community-based AHPs for continued rehabilitation in the community.

## 4.12   Coordinators

The MDT coordinator is a vital team member and ensures the patients' referring clinical details, presenting information and personal demographics are registered with a 'hospital number' and relevant contact details, as well as GP details are documented. They are administrators as opposed to having a clinical background, so they would not be equipped to make clinical decisions as part of the wider MDT group.

MDT coordinators ensure all the referring information is available at the time of discussion, along with any brain images and subsequent local radiology reports. They collate all the clinical outcomes following the MDT discussion and ensure timely distribution to the referring teams/clinicians and the patient's GPs. They ensure patients are relisted for discussion as required and chase outstanding scan dates and reports. They undertake robust data collection as part of MDT audits and service improvement programmes, and some even undertake cancer tracking within their remit, to ensure brain tumour patients are treated within national cancer waiting time guidelines and targets [2].

## 4.13   Other Extended Members

Some MDTs, for example, have a dedicated neuro-oncology trials nurse present who can indicate if a patient would be a suitable candidate for any particular research trials. They are aware of the trials portfolio and have access to inclusion and exclusion criteria. This has helped the recruitment of patients into clinical trials greatly as this discussion (and trial eligibility) is then documented in the MDT outcomes which are widely circulated. There are sometimes multiple trials open via neuroimaging, neurosurgery and neuro-oncology—all with their own inclusion and exclusion criteria, so having a dedicated trial person who can navigate around the myriad of options has proven to be very useful for many tertiary neurosurgical centres.

## 4.14   The Referral Process

Within the UK, most neurosurgical centres are tertiary centres, meaning they can accept referrals from a wide catchment area, in some areas between 10 and 15 referring hospitals. The UK comprises of very spread out geographical areas, such as Wales, Scotland and East Anglia. Having a very dispersed population in remote areas makes it even more important to have a robust referral process, to not only provide a comprehensive MDT service but also to provide a solid basis for support and information for those hospitals (or GPs) referring directly to a regional MDT. As such, minimum criteria for referral standards have been established within MDTs, which include core standards for imaging requirements. If a patient presents with a suspected brain tumour, a contrast CT followed by a contrast MRI (unless clinically contraindicated as with some pacemakers) would be required to make a radiological diagnosis. For suspected brain metastasis, an updated staging CT chest, abdomen and pelvis to source the primary lesion, along with a cancer treatment plan and anticipated overall survival from the treating primary physician, would be required [2, 3].

Although imaging is vitally important for the basis of a robust MDT discussion, it is equally important to ascertain the current clinical condition of the patient and have to hand all the relevant reports and information around past medical history and comorbidities that may be required for the MDT discussion. This is one area where the key worker (specialist nurse) plays a pivotal role—they are ideally placed with their clinical nous and specialist background to highlight any missing information prior to the MDT to help minimise pathway delays, for example, finding out how long the patient has been on dexamethasone, if any clinical improvements in their neurological condition have been noted, etc. Furthermore, they can advise the local teams looking after the patient about side effects of medication and where to signpost family and carers for advice and information prior to any neurosurgical review. For some, this is a model that has worked well, in that the key worker really does become a key player and is the point of contact for patients, carers, other health professionals and the MDT team throughout that patient's entire pathway.

## 4.15 The MDT Discussion

Once the coordinator has registered and listed all patients due for discussion, a list is often circulated to the core MDT members prior to the meeting. This is a very sensitive document with patient identifiable information and clinical details that must be given due patient confidentiality status and disposed of in the correct manner. The radiologists in particular use these lists to prepare for the MDT meeting by triaging the imaging and correlating presenting symptoms to the location of the tumour, to ensure the two add up and that nothing further needs to be considered, such as a dual pathology.

Within certain geographical areas, the tertiary centre covers neurosurgery for the whole geographical region, but neuro-oncology treatments can be delivered in several satellite centres [6]. Hence, the satellite centres in many UK units log in via remote video access on a weekly basis to partake in MDT discussions. As a result, the structure of the MDT is often such so that the pathology cases are presented first, followed by new referrals and return discussions.

In the pathology section, their tumour grading, molecular status, how the patient is (neurologically and cognitively) following surgery and any onward treatment plans like chemotherapy or radiotherapy are discussed in relation to their nearest treatment centre. Those patients whose pathology is due to be discussed in MDT are normally made clinic appointments to discuss the results ahead of the MDT in order to minimise delays to their treatment pathways.

Following on from the pathology discussions, new referrals are then discussed, allowing for the other centres video linking in, to present some of their cases and partake in discussions. The radiology opinion and MDT discussions are documents in real time often by the specialist nurse or MDT coordinator, and following the MDT, the outcomes and action points are circulated to the attendees, and an outcome is also sent to the patient's general practitioner and referring physician for information. Which ever way an MDT is structured, the aim is to improve time to diagnosis and to help plan, coordinate and communicate the best possible care for cancer patients, reducing inequalities and increasing overall effectiveness [1].

## 4.16   Arranging Follow-Up

If a new referral is required to be seen in the outpatient clinic, an appointment is generated from MDT via the neurosurgical administrators. However, this appointment can be one or several weeks away pending urgency, and for a patient and their loved ones, this can be a very difficult time where they feel left in limbo. They may have been discharged home from their local hospital on high-dose dexamethasone, for example, and have no one to turn to for advice and support. The GP often states they are under specialist care, but they have just been discharged home still awaiting specialist review. They don't know if what they are experiencing is normal or not from a symptom management perspective, nor do they know what side effects to look out for or worrying signs of clinical deterioration.

To attempt to alleviate some of these concerns, the key worker within some neurosurgical centres makes direct contact with those patients (and their relatives) due to be seen for neurosurgical review, following on from MDT discussions. This is to partly introduce themselves as their key worker but also to talk them through the next steps and supply them with contact details in the interim should they have any queries or concerns. The key worker explains what to expect from the forthcoming clinic appointment and gauges their prior knowledge of their own situation and ascertains what they have been informed of. Furthermore, the key worker is able to discuss any medication and side effects they may be experiencing but also ascertain if the patient is on any blood thinning agents such as aspirin, warfarin or clopidogrel which will need to be discontinued prior to surgery.

This seemingly small act of reaching out can have significant positive outcomes for the patient. They feel validated and listened to. They have a chance to ask questions and seek clarification probably for the first time since they have been told their head imaging was abnormal. They have been informed about next steps and what to expect in the near future in regard to medication and treatment trajectories. And most importantly, they have been given a direct contact number for their very own key worker who will help them navigate through this very complex system, which can often seem uncoordinated and fragmented.

## 4.17   UK Cancer Waiting Times

Enabling a timely MDT discussion and review of the imaging is only solving part of the overall problem with early diagnosis. The other aspect of prompt MDT discussions is the requirement for the patient to also be *treated* in a timely manner. There is little point in having swift MDT discussions and subsequent clinic review if the patient with a suspected high-grade malignancy then has to wait several months for surgery. Given those time scales, the tumour will likely have grown to such an extent that overall maximal resection is no longer safe or feasible, or the patient may even have died whilst waiting for surgery.

To try and alleviate some of these issues, the National Institute for Health and Care Excellence (NICE) and the Department of Health developed referral guidelines for suspected cancers which essentially state that no one should have to wait for treatment for more than 31 days since a decision to treat the cancer was made [2–4]. The decision to treat is normally the date the patient is seen in clinic, and the risks, benefits, intended outcomes of surgery and alternative options are explained to and discussed with the patient [4].

Within neuro-oncology, for example, this would mean a neurosurgeon has 31 days to operate on a patient once they have been seen in clinic and consented for surgical resection. There are of course caveats and exceptions to these time frames, so the below flow chart is for illustrative purposes only (Fig. 4.1).

## 4.18   Conclusion

This chapter has highlighted the importance of positive teamwork with a patient-centred approach to help obtain the best long-term outcomes for neuro-oncology patients. Guidelines and frameworks have been put into place to help guide the

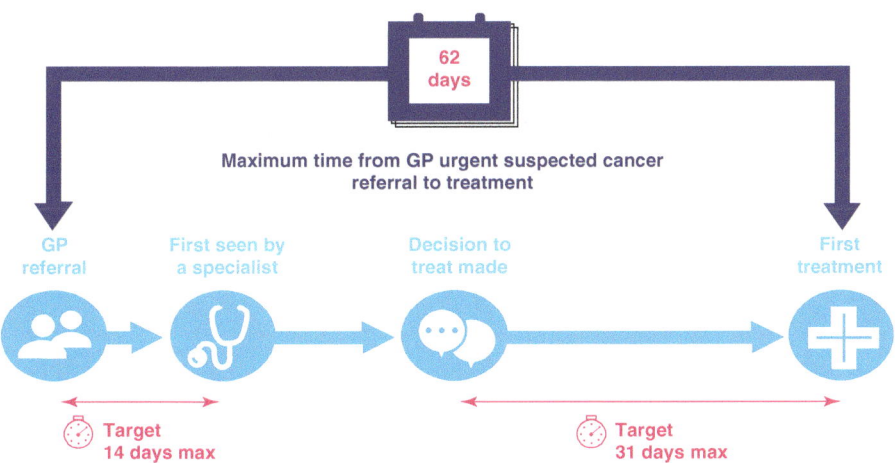

**Fig. 4.1**   Cancer waiting times as published by Cancer Research UK (CRUK) [7]

MDT members into some form of structure in regard to timelines, but ultimately the clinical teams are the ones responsible for the operating time frames and how/when the patients are informed of the surgical plans, pathology results and onward treatment plans with oncology.

Within specific centres, services have been streamlined so that there are minimal delays between first MDT discussions and the patients being seen. From a patient's perspective, this is met with positive views as it also means the patient can be proactively involved in timely decisions involving them and they do not feel like the clinical teams have been in receipt of vital diagnostic information pertaining to them for over a week without sharing these discussions and thought processes with them.

Good, effective communication and teamwork are pivotal to this process, and an effective MDT is an invaluable tool for the neuro-oncology services in today's National Health Service.

## References

1. Taylor C, Munro A, Glynne-Jones R, et al. Multidisciplinary team working in cancer: what is the evidence? Br Med J. 2010;340:c951. Accessed on 12 Jan 2018
2. National Institute for Health and Care Excellence. Guidance on cancer services – improving outcomes for people with brain and other CNS tumours. In: The Manual. London: National Institute for Health and Care Excellence; 2006. Chapter 2.
3. https://www.nhs.uk/conditions/malignant-brain-tumour/. Accessed on 4 Dec 2017.
4. Department of Health (NHS). Equity and excellence: liberating the NHS. London: The Stationery Office; 2010.
5. Louis DN, Perry A, Reifenberger G, et al. The 2016 World Health Organization classification of tumors of the central nervous system: a summary. Acta Neuropathol. 2016;131:803–20.
6. https://www.canceralliance.co.uk/. Accessed on 12 Jan 2018.
7. Cancer Research UK (CRUK) https://scienceblog.cancerresearchuk.org/2015/11/12/unacceptable-cancer-waiting-times-are-testing-patients-patience/. Accessed on 24 Jul 2018.

# Medical Management of Adult Glioma

5

## Robin Grant

**Abstract**

Initial medical management of glioma will depend on distinguishing symptoms related to the direct effects of the tumour, from those that are secondary to the stress or recurrence of a pre-existing psychological illness, and symptoms that are related to medication. The cause of symptoms may vary with time, e.g. headache from raised intracranial pressure to post-craniotomy headache or migraine; therefore the history should be revisited regularly to ensure the most effective treatment is prescribed. Prevention of perioperative complications, e.g. deep vein thrombosis and pulmonary embolus or post-operative seizures, may complicate the management. Care must be taken to minimise medication that may interact with future treatment or produce neurological side effects.

During oncological therapies medical management may involve reducing unnecessary treatment and consolidating support and advice, e.g. on management of epilepsy, treatment of mood disorders and diagnosis and management of ongoing or new symptoms such as headache, seizures, spasticity, bladder problems and fatigue. Neuro-rehabilitation and neurocognitive rehabilitation should be established as early as possible after initial surgery.

Late effects of treatment become an issue in long-term survivors depending on the radiation therapy dose and volume. Late effects may produce episodic disturbances related to vascular, epileptic or metabolic disturbances or a progressive neurocognitive and physical decline that usually requires more complex packages of supportive and palliative care. Endocrine effects from radiation on the pituitary gland are reversible. In late stages of illness, good symptom management is the difference between a peaceful death and a stressful memory that will live with the family forever.

R. Grant (✉)
Edinburgh Centre for Neuro-Oncology, Western General Hospital, Edinburgh, UK
e-mail: robin.grant@nhslothian.scot.nhs.uk

© Springer Nature Switzerland AG 2019
I. Oberg (ed.), *Management of Adult Glioma in Nursing Practice*,
https://doi.org/10.1007/978-3-319-76747-5_5

**Keywords**
Preoperative management · Dexamethasone · Anti-epileptic drugs · Neurological disability · Mood disorder · Late effects

**Learning Outcomes**
- Be able to recognise some of the initial presenting symptoms a glioma patient may exhibit (including clinical signs of raised intracranial pressure) and how to manage them effectively.
- Learn how to recognise and manage potential side effects of medical treatment.
- Understand the crucial role dexamethasone has in treating clinical signs of raised intracranial pressure.
- Gain a deeper understanding of the various types of seizures associated with adult gliomas and their recommended treatment.
- Understand how to monitor for and manage late effects of glioma treatments (surgical and oncological).

## 5.1    Introduction

Adult glioma presents with a wide variety of neurological symptoms. It is always possible to provide good medical symptomatic and supportive therapy irrespective of whether the tumour can be treated. Medical management depends on the correct diagnosis of symptoms, which is not always straightforward as causes can vary at different time points during the illness trajectory. A good clinical history and on occasion a good eyewitness account are of paramount importance as well as an understanding of neurological therapies and knowledge of side effects of treatment.

This chapter will therefore be divided into five sections:

- *Early presenting symptom management ("acute management")*
- *Chronic neurological disability ("continuing disability")*
- *Episodic neurological late effects ("neurological attacks")*
- *Persistent neurological late effects ("neurological deterioration")*
- *Reversible endocrine late effects ("pituitary insufficiency")*

## 5.2    Early Presenting Symptom Management ("Acute Management")

Patients with glioma will present with either symptoms of stimulation of the brain (seizures), damage to the brain (e.g. hemiparesis) or as a result of pressure related to the mass of the tumour (e.g. headache) or a combination of these (Fig. 5.1). Patients with symptoms clearly attributable to the brain, e.g. unilateral weakness,

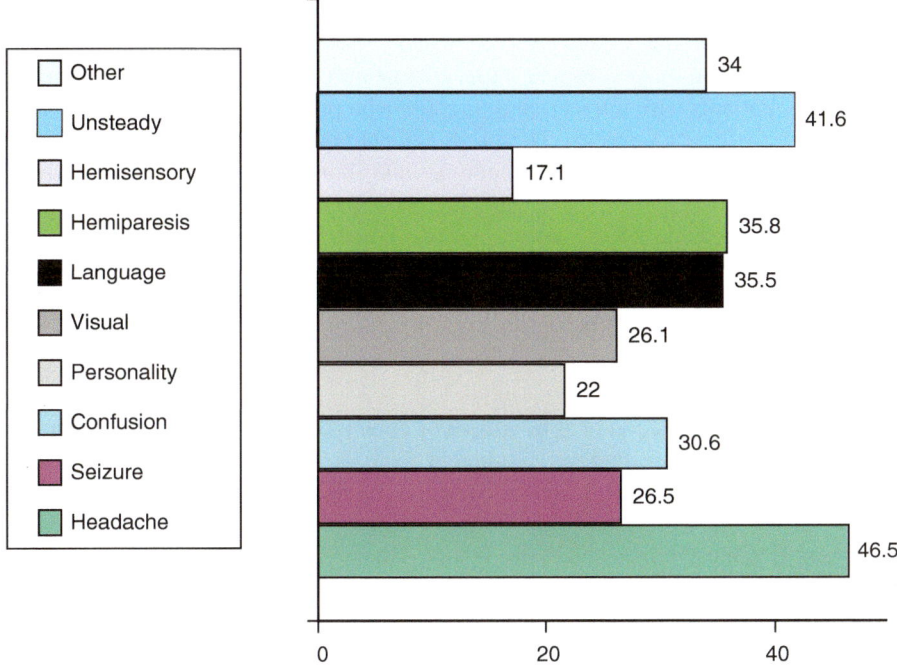

**Fig. 5.1** Presenting symptoms at first hospital visit in 310 people with suspected glioma

numbness, dysphasia or seizures, usually present quickly. Patients with frontal and temporal lobe involvement often have "subtle" symptoms, which may have been put down to life's stresses and present late. While headaches are common, the "red flag" features of raised intracranial pressure (worse on coughing straining; changes with posture (standing); morning headache) only occur in about 10% of cases. Headaches tend to escalate in frequency and severity. Obscuration of vision on standing, postural visual flashes or sparkles, tinnitus or faints with headache are worrying for raised intracranial pressure. Ask about subtle changes in personality, behaviour and mood or problems with cognition (ability to multitask, plan, etc.) and memory in if patients with headache suspicious of raised intracranial pressure.

Twenty-five percent of people admitted with a brain tumour do not have legal capacity to give informed consent for surgery [1]. Of the remaining 75% of patients, half will have an Addenbrooke's Cognitive Examination (ACE) score of ≤88/100, which represents a significant cognitive difficulty. These deficits are frequently not apparent until cognitive screening is tested. Mental capacity issues will be dealt with in a separate chapter. It is therefore important that if there are cognitive difficulties, history taking and treatment explanations should occur when a carer is present, as many patients will be bewildered.

## 5.2.1   Raised Intracranial Pressure and Focal Neurological Signs

Headaches are the most common initial first symptom and at hospital presentation (Fig. 5.1). Patients with intracerebral tumours who present with headaches are more likely to have larger tumours. The brain parenchyma does not contain pain nerve endings, but blood vessels, dural membranes and choroid plexus do, and distortion of these may cause local headaches when the mass is of a sufficient size or in the presence of hydrocephalus. The presence of papilloedema (optic nerve head swelling) confirms raised intracranial pressure (ICP), but the absence of papilloedema does not exclude significant raised ICP. Less than 15% of patients will have papilloedema at presentation (Fig. 5.2) [2]. Headaches are often resistant to simple painkillers.

### 5.2.1.1 Dexamethasone
Dexamethasone is the medical treatment of choice for headache of raised intracranial pressure or where there is significant focal or cognitive deficit. Patients will respond usually well to a low dose of dexamethasone, e.g. 4 mg/day, unless there is brain herniation, where the brain stem is pushed downward through the foramen magnum ("coning"), or where there is major mass effect. In these situations larger oral or intravenous doses of dexamethasone may be required. A randomised controlled trial (RCT) on the use of dexamethasone in brain tumours showed that dexamethasone 4 mg/day results in the same degree of improvement as a dose of 16 mg/day after 1 week of treatment in patients without signs of impending herniation [3]. The headache of coning or "tonsillar herniation" is maximal in the neck and occiput and may be associated with neck stiffness and painful extensor spasms of the spine and limbs, which may mimic a generalised tonic seizure. Where there is severe

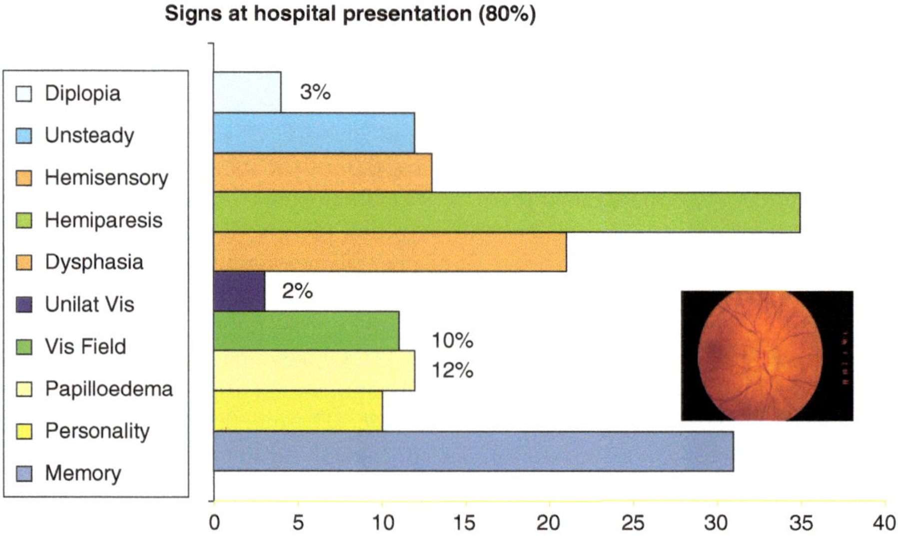

**Fig. 5.2** Presenting signs at first hospital visit in 310 people with suspected glioma (20% have no signs—usually seizure presentation)

neurological impairment, or where herniation of the brain is suspected (e.g. drowsiness and cervical or occipital pain, with downward shift visible on the MRI scan), dexamethasone 8 mg intravenously should be given and repeated every 4 h. The patient should be nursed in a head-up position. If the patient does not respond to dexamethasone and surgery is planned, then mannitol 1 g/kg total dose may be required. This can be given as 100 ml of 20% solution (20 g) over 15 min followed by the remainder over 45 min.

After surgical resection, dexamethasone should be reduced gradually and withdrawn. Withdrawal can be associated with joint pain or muscle aches, anorexia, nausea, vomiting or diarrhoea, which might suggest an intracerebral complication or progression and may lead to dose re-escalation. It is usually sufficient to scan the patient to exclude significant mass effect or intracerebral haematoma/infection, exclude post-operative systemic infection, hypoxia or metabolic disturbance and reassure the patient while encouraging a gradual taper of dexamethasone.

It is worth remembering that 10–15% of the population have migraine and patients with migraine/tension headache may have had the scan for "reassurance". In this situation, tumours are sometimes found incidentally, and are nothing to do with headache symptoms. Evaluation of headache characteristics should always be done in conjunction with the imaging appearances. Steroids are not helpful for migraine/tension headache.

### 5.2.1.2 Proton Pump Inhibitor

A proton pump inhibitor (omeprazole 20 mg or lansoprazole 30 mg) orally per day is commonly started around the same time as dexamethasone to prevent gastric symptoms. Nevertheless, there is no good evidence to suggest this is required unless the patient has a past history of gastric ulcer, is also taking a non-steroidal anti-inflammatory drug or is symptomatic from gastr-oesophageal reflux disorder.

### 5.2.1.3 Anti-emetic

For nausea and vomiting, injections of prochlorperazine 12.5 mg i.m. or cyclizine 100–150 mg subcutaneously over 24 h via a syringe driver is usually effective.

### 5.2.1.4 Analgesia

Management of headache will consist of dexamethasone and step 1 or step 2 for pain relief. Dexamethasone is usually effective at relieving headache within 24–48 h. Non-steroidal anti-inflammatory drugs (NSAIDs) should be avoided in the perioperative period, as this is associated with increased risk of bleeding.

**Step 1**—For mild pain oral paracetamol 1 g four times a day if body weight >50 kg and there is no renal impairment, glutathione deficiency, chronic alcoholism or hepatic impairment.

**Step 2**—For pain, unresponsive to step 1, this would include a weak opioid plus paracetamol. Opioids would include co-codamol (codeine/paracetamol) oral 30/500 mg 1–2 tablets four times daily (max 8 tablets in 24 h), codeine oral 30–60 mg four times daily (max 240 mg/day), or dihydrocodeine oral 30 mg four times daily (max 120 mg/day). Elderly patients with less good cognitive reserve, with multiple comorbidities or taking multiple drugs may experience confusion or constipation requiring laxatives, to prevent the need for straining which will increase ICP, e.g. a faecal softener such as lactulose or a stimulant laxative like senna.

### 5.2.1.5 Anti-epileptic Drugs (AEDs)

Seizures are due to episodic electrochemical excitatory discharges from cortical neurons, producing involuntary "positive phenomena" from one specific area of the brain (focal seizure). Sometimes, focal seizures develop into a generalised attack (tonic-clonic seizure). Most patients with focal epilepsy due to a tumour will get some warning of the attack although brief. Excitation of neurons would cause "positive" symptoms such as hallucinations, jerking and tingling/burning which suggest excessive stimulation of neurones, rather than loss of function "negative" symptoms:

- Temporal cortex—hallucinations of taste, smell, rising sensation from stomach, déjà vu often associated with loss of awareness, lip smacking and fumbling. Sometimes fear and panic.
- Frontal cortex—jerking in limbs on one side with fast spread of jerking up/down that side (Jacksonian march—motor strip) or "speech arrest" with cessation of speech during conversation with occasional utterances or eye deviation and head turn to one side.
- Parietal cortex—tingling and burning on one side with fast spread of sensation up/down that side.
- Occipital cortex—formed (e.g. a dog/person) or non-formed (odd object) visual hallucination often coloured in one visual field.
- Prefrontal cortex—unusual attacks, sometimes involving movement on both sides (fencing-like), strange behaviour and pelvic thrusting, often with some disturbance of awareness. These are often misdiagnosed as "pseudo-seizures". Patients may retain consciousness despite having limb movement on both sides, unlike tonic-clonic seizures.

Important points to consider when taking an attack history from a witness are:

- Are they short-lived, stereotyped (similar) and non-situational (random)?
- Are they "positive" phenomena—jerking, burning, hallucination, etc.?
- Do symptoms correlate with topographical localisation of the tumour?

Prophylactic AEDs pre- and post-operatively are sometimes prescribed despite lack of high-quality evidence of effectiveness and known side effects [4, 5]. Previous randomised controlled trials have used older-generation drugs with poor side effect profiles that interact with other drugs given in the early treatment stage. A well-designed randomised controlled trial of newer AEDs, e.g. levetiracetam versus control, in patients with glioma is needed.

Management of epilepsy should always include referral to an epilepsy specialist nurse or neurologist for advice on reducing risk of further attacks (have a good sleep, don't miss meals, take AED medication regularly); better understanding of what a seizure is; avoiding dangerous situations (driving, heights, power tools, swimming, bathing, rock climbing, nursing babies, etc.); keeping safe during a seizure, carer first aid advice, and explanation of what to do in the event of a seizure and when to call emergency services esp. prolonged or recurrent seizures (if generalised jerking continues for more than 5 min or there are recurrent attacks in quick succession); education on when and how to give buccal, nasal or rectal benzodiazepines; advice about avoiding sudden unexpected death from epilepsy (SUDEP); work-related advice regarding seizures; and general advice about what benefits the patient may be entitled to. The legislation regarding work and driving will vary from country to country and, in the USA, state to state. UK driving regulations can be found in www.dvla.gov.uk.

Anti-epileptic drugs will be started after a single seizure as the likelihood of further seizures in the presence of a glioma is high. The AED chosen will depend on the urgency for treatment (e.g. status epilepticus), speed of achieving seizure control (e.g. prior to a surgery), potential side effects (e.g. rash, haematological toxicity) or likelihood of drug-drug interactions (e.g. with chemotherapy or immunotherapy). For tonic-clonic status epilepticus, lorazepam 0.1 mg/kg by intravenous injection at a rate of <2 mg/min followed by phenytoin 15–20 mg/kg intravenously at a rate no more than 50 ml/minute many be necessary. Status epilepticus is a medical emergency, and management guidelines are available [6].

Ideally epilepsy should be treated with a single anti-epileptic drug agent at the lowest effective dose. Combination therapy may be necessary but is commonly associated with complex drug interactions and increased frequency of side effects. The side effect profile of common AEDs is shown in Table 5.1. The newer AEDs may be better tolerated and have fewer drug interactions and fewer cognitive side effects. Certain anti-epileptic agents (enzyme-inducing AEDs) may alter the bioavailability of chemotherapy. Whether this has any significant effect on the survival or outcome is still uncertain. At present, in Europe and the USA, there is a shift to use levetiracetam because of its lack of interactions with chemotherapy; low liability to rash, unlike carbamazepine, phenytoin and lamotrigine; and low frequency of weight gain unlike valproate (Table 5.1). Fatigue can occur, especially at high doses, and there has been no comparable data with other AEDs in glioma. Dexamethasone reduces levels of enzyme-inducing anti-epileptic drugs (e.g. phenytoin, carbamazepine and phenobarbitone).

Maximal surgical resection in some low-grade neoplasms can cure epilepsy or reduce seizure frequency. Uncontrolled prospective studies suggest that fractionated radiotherapy and radiosurgery can reduce seizure frequency in 54% of patients with brain tumours with intractable epilepsy. Temozolomide may reduce the seizure frequency in intractable epilepsy.

### 5.2.1.6 Anti-Platelet and Anticoagulation Therapy

Anti-platelet therapy should be withdrawn for 1–2 weeks before surgery if at all possible because of the increased risk of bleeding from the resection cavity. However, there is a risk of deep vein thrombosis (DVT) and pulmonary embolus (PE) in patients with gliomas. This has been estimated as about 25% at 1 year and 30% at 2 years in prospective studies [7]. Risk factors include older age, glioblastoma histology and three or more chronic comorbidities within 2 months of neurosurgery. Pulmonary embolus is rare if the DVT is treated by anticoagulation therapy.

**Table 5.1** Cautions, toxicity and side effects of anti-epileptic drugs (AEDs)

| | |
|---|---|
| Carbamazepine | *Cautions*: Hepatic, renal and cardiac disease, glaucoma |
| | *Toxicity*: Diplopia, dizziness, confusion, ataxia, tremor |
| | *Side effects*: Early severe blood disorders and leucopenia, rash, hypersensitivity reaction, agitation, jaundice, renal failure, depression, psychosis, alopecia, hyponatraemia, osteomalacia |
| Lamotrigine | *Cautions*: Hepatic and renal disease |
| | *Toxicity*: Diplopia, dizziness, confusion and ataxia |
| | *Side effects*: Early severe blood disorders and aplastic anaemia and leucopenia. Rash, hypersensitivity reaction, flu-like illness, worsening seizures, agitation, dizziness, drowsiness, insomnia, headache, agitation |
| Levetiracetam | *Cautions*: Hepatic and renal disease |
| | *Toxicity*: Drowsiness, tiredness and dizziness |
| | *Side effects*: Drowsiness, tiredness and dizziness. Rarely amnesia, psychiatric symptoms (e.g. anger), insomnia, headache, rash, anaemia (folate deficiency) |
| Phenytoin | *Cautions*: Hepatic disease |
| | *Toxicity*: Diplopia, dizziness, confusion, ataxia, tremor |
| | *Side effects*: Early severe blood disorders and leucopenia. Rash, agitation jaundice, SLE, hypersensitivity reaction, depression, psychosis, gum hypertrophy, peripheral neuropathy, megaloblastic anaemia, osteomalacia |
| Topiramate | *Cautions*: Hepatic disease and renal disease. May cause secondary acute angle-closure glaucoma in myopes in the first month |
| | *Toxicity*: Diplopia, dizziness, confusion, ataxia, tremor |
| | *Side effects*: Rash, agitation, leucopenia, jaundice, weight loss, paraesthesia, memory, fatigue, speech problems, depression, psychosis |
| Valproate | *Cautions*: Liver disease, clotting disorders, pancreatitis |
| | *Toxicity*: Tremor, diplopia, dizziness, confusion, ataxia |
| | *Side effects*: Leucopenia, alopecia, weight gain, gastrointestinal side effects, memory problems, dementia, gynaecomastia |

However, anticoagulants such as enoxaparin perioperatively carry too high a risk of intracranial bleeding and is to be avoided [8]. A multimodality approach to prophylaxis includes using compression stockings and pneumatic intermittent compression boots during and after operation and encouraging early ambulation. DVT prophylaxis may be considered 24 hours after surgery if the balance of DVT risks outweighs the risks associated with low molecular weight heparin [9]. Aspirin and non-steroidal anti-inflammatory drugs should be avoided when taking low molecular weight heparin or warfarin as they will increase the risk of bleeding.

## 5.3    Chronic Neurological Disability ("Continuing Disability")

### 5.3.1    Post-operative Headaches

Post-operative headache is frequently a source of concern for patients and carers. A good headache history should therefore be taken, especially where the headaches are slow to settle after resection of the tumour. The timing of onset, site, character, frequency, severity, temporal development, relieving factors and aggravating factors, associated features (nausea, vomiting) and focal symptoms and signs (e.g. visual field, optic disc swelling or weakness) should be sought. The headache type may shift from one of raised ICP to one of post-craniotomy pain, migraine or medication overuse headache. All headaches are worse when there is a background of poor sleep, missed regular meals and anxiety. These areas always need to be addressed.

*Craniotomy pain.* After craniotomy, it is common for patients to complain of local tenderness at the craniotomy site, which may persist for weeks or months. These headaches are not helped by dexamethasone. Craniotomy pain occurs as a consequence of injury to the cutaneous nerves that supply sensation to the scalp, and the underlying tissues, or from manipulation of the dura mater. Post-craniotomy pain occurs most commonly after subtemporal and suboccipital approaches [10]. Most patients report superficial tenderness and pain that is classically pounding or pulsating, similar to migraine or tension headaches. Less commonly, it is a continuous and constant pain. Pain may respond to anti-migrainous medication and prophylactic beta blockers or amitriptyline. Occasionally there may be an intermittent sharp stabbing character from scar neuromas that is momentary but frequently recurrent [11]. If the pain is particularly severe, gabapentin, pregabalin or amitriptyline may be helpful—as may be an injection of local anaesthetic. Complaints of a sensation of water running down that side of the scalp or other dysaesthetic sensations are common.

*Postsurgical migraines* are not uncommon. They are unilateral or bilateral episodic throbbing headache lasting for hours associated with nausea and photophobia. There is often a past history of episodic headache or known migraine. Management should be initiated if headaches are frequent or severe. These include:

1. *Lifestyle advice* about regular meals; avoiding excess alcoholic, carbonated or caffeinated drinks; tackling insomnia and fatigue by taking regular exercise and advice on factors managing stress; and avoiding triggers (glare, stress, foods, drink).
2. *Avoid overuse of analgesic* or frequent triptans and medication that may provoke migraine (e.g. oral contraceptive pill).
3. *Acute treatments*—soluble aspirin 900 mg +/− metoclopramide or paracetamol 1 g or non-steroidal anti-inflammatory drugs (NSAIDs) such as ibuprofen 400 mg if bleeding risks are considered to be low. Triptans are considered if attacks are not controlled by simple analgesia. Sumatriptan 100 mg, almotriptan 12.5 mg, other triptans or subcutaneous sumatriptan 6 mg can be helpful if taken early. Opioid analgesia should be avoided as this can aggravate cognitive symptoms, constipation and confusion.
4. *Preventative treatment*—beta blockers (e.g. propranolol) and anti-epileptic (topiramate/valproate) or tricyclic antidepressants at low dose (e.g. amitriptyline) for 3–4 months may be helpful.

*Medication overuse headache* is defined as a headache which is present for 15 days or more per month and which has developed or worsened while taking regular symptomatic medication, in the absence of another intra-cranial cause for headache, e.g. tumour mass, subdural haematoma. Medication overuse headache can develop with any type of primary headache but most commonly develops with migraine. It should be considered when triptans, ergots, opioids or combination analgesics are being used for 10 days or more per month. Simple analgesics or triptans can be stopped abruptly; however, when caused by opioids and combination analgesics, patients should be warned that there is the potential for withdrawal symptoms. Some patients may wish to consider gradual reduction of medication over 2 weeks before stopping. Withdrawal symptoms may be helped by anti-emetics, tricyclics, short-term naproxen or steroid taper.

### 5.3.2 Neurological Rehabilitation

Neuro-rehabilitation aims at enabling patients to reach and maintain their optimal physical, sensory, intellectual, psychological and social functional levels.

A systematic review of trials of individually targeted multidisciplinary rehabilitation in patients with glioma supports a mean 36% improvement in functional independence [12]. Frequency of improvement is similar to stroke and head injury [13]. There is some positive evidence to support use of early physical training, massage therapy and ambulatory rehabilitation may improve functional outcome, reduce stress and improve quality of life in patients with glioma [12]. Speech and language therapy are required for patients with dysphasia, dysarthria and dysphonia and dysphagia. Physiotherapy is required for hemiparesis and gait problems and occupational therapy to assess independence and reduce risk of falls. Advice regarding mobility, pressure sore, spasticity and deep vein thrombosis prevention is important. High-intensity ambulatory (outpatient) multidisciplinary rehabilitation reduces short- and long-term motor disability (continence, mobility and locomotion, cognition), when compared with standard outpatient care [14]. Anti-spasticity agents are usually not required in the early perioperative stages since weakness is more prominent than spasticity and dexamethasone can help both weakness and spasticity. Management of weakness and spasticity will be covered in the chapter on Allied Health Professionals.

### 5.3.3 Cognitive Rehabilitation

Eighty percent of patients with a glioma will have some abnormalities on cognitive testing when assessed preoperatively. This is particularly so for attention and memory. Neuro-cognition may be affected by the tumour, its treatment, associated medication, mood, fatigue and insomnia, and assessment needs to consider these facets in addition rather than neuro-cognition in isolation. Exercise; neurocognitive training; neurocognitive behavioural therapy; medications to treat fatigue, behaviour, memory and mood; and discontinuation of drugs that may be associated with neurocognitive side effects (e.g. anti-epileptic drugs) may all help in the management of neurocognitive impairments [15]. Multi-faceted cognitive rehabilitation produces significant effects for early subjective cognitive functioning and its perceived burden but not for the objective neuropsychological outcomes or for any of the other self-report measures [16]. At 6 months the intervention group demonstrated statistically significant differences in neuropsychological tests of attention and verbal memory and reported less mental fatigue. There is limited evidence for the benefit for modafinil [17], methylphenidate [18] and donepezil [19].

## 5.3.4 Psychological and Psychiatric Problems

### 5.3.4.1 Anger
Anger, loss of emotional control and change in behaviour are commonly reported at diagnosis or after surgery. Personality change may affect up to 60% of patients [20]. Damage to dorsolateral prefrontal areas is associated with impaired executive functioning, orbitofrontal damage may cause disinhibition and impulsiveness, and lesions in the medial-frontal areas may result in apathy. Behavioural change, including anger, occurs in 10–15% of patients taking levetiracetam and in a similar percentage of patients taking dexamethasone. Patient education and referral to neuropsychology and/or neuropsychiatry, if needed, are recommended [21].

### 5.3.4.2 Anxiety
Anxiety occurs in 5–30% of patients prior to operation. It is more common in women and in those with a past or family history of psychiatric disorder. There are no randomised controlled trials of different treatment approaches in the neuropsychiatric management of patients with brain or CNS tumours. The advice on management of anxiety in glioma therefore is at the level of recommendations for best practice from a consensus group of experts.

Short-term highly focused forms of psychotherapy, such as cognitive behavioural therapy (CBT), supportive therapies and group therapies are effective in the treatment of panic disorder, phobias, social anxiety disorder and generalised anxiety disorder. CBT is as effective as antidepressants for mild depression, and 50–60% of patients are in remission by 3–8 months compared with only approximately 25% treated with placebo [22].

### 5.3.4.3 Depression
The 6-month prevalence rate for clinical depression after glioma diagnosis is about 20% [20]. National and international guidelines suggest that major depressive disorder in patients with a chronic physical condition should, where possible, be treated with a combination of antidepressants (e.g. selective serotonin reuptake inhibitors, serotonin norepinephrine reuptake inhibitors) and a high-intensity psychological treatment, e.g. CBT or multimodal psychosocial intervention. There are no randomised controlled trials examining drug treatment of clinically depressed patients with a glioma [20]. There is preliminary evidence to suggest a possible beneficial role for massage therapy or acceptance and commitment therapy (ACT).

### 5.3.4.4 Delirium and Psychosis

Delirium and psychosis can be difficult to manage. Good nursing care with frequent reassurance and rapport is essential. In order to reduce anxiety and disorientation, familiar nursing, regular reassurance, de-escalation and reorientation can provide relief. Dexamethasone or AEDs can induce psychosis. Steroid psychosis generally arises at, or shortly after, onset of corticosteroid treatment, and a higher dose increases the risk. Withdrawal of medications that may cause delirium/psychosis is indicated. Psychosis can also occur after seizures or may be associated with depression or mania. Advice from the psychiatric team about non-pharmacological and pharmacological interventions is important. A low-dose antipsychotic, such as haloperidol, may be given as required rather than long-term regular prescription, and if there is no benefit after a few days, specialist psychiatric advice should be sought.

### 5.3.4.5 Hallucinations

There are many possible causes from hallucinations. Short-lived stereotyped, non-threatening hallucinations would suggest epileptic seizures, and AEDs should be started appropriately. Hallucinations in the context of severe visual impairment may be part of visual release phenomena (Charles Bonnet Syndrome) [23]. Hallucinations of Charles Bonnet Syndrome may last for seconds or minutes but are often recurrent throughout the day and may be difficult to distinguish from seizures, but are rarely stereotyped and they only occur in patients with severe visual impairment. Sufferers understand that the hallucinations are not real and antipsychotics are ineffective and not necessary. Patients generally just require reassurance.

Hallucinations in the context of clouded consciousness or with memory problems can be due to delirium or psychosis, and persecutory delusions make management challenging. Distressing hallucinations that are persistent and part of a psychosis do require pharmacological management with antipsychotics, e.g. haloperidol. Olanzapine and risperidone have also been shown to counteract hallucinations in dementia.

### 5.3.5   Fatigue

Fatigue occurs in between 25% and 90% of patients with primary brain tumours at any stages of care. Fatigue may be due to *primary causes*, affecting the brain, e.g. tumour, irradiation and injury; *secondary causes*, e.g. psychological, sleep disturbance and pain; *comorbid conditions*, e.g. underactive pituitary, infection and malnutrition; or *medication* such as AEDs or analgesics [24]. Pituitary dysfunction and physical impairment may also contribute to fatigue. Management of fatigue should include removal of drugs that may be associated with fatigue; advice about sleep and healthy living, diet and physical exercise; and, if present, management of anxiety or depression through talking therapies, CBT, mindfulness or antidepressants. A Cochrane systematic review [25] found only one of nine randomised controlled trial [26] that included only patients with high levels of fatigue. The other eight trials studied prevention and recruited patients who may or may not have had fatigue at entry. Although negative for fatigue generally, a post hoc analysis of one study showed improved QoL and reduced fatigue with armodafinil for the subgroup with severe fatigue at study entry [27]. If fatigue is part of a major depressive episode, an antidepressant should be considered first. If fatigue is not associated with low mood but is accompanied by excessive daytime sleepiness, then drugs to promote wakefulness (e.g. methylphenidate, modafinil/armodafinil) may be helpful. Adverse reactions to drugs that promote wakefulness include mania, delusions, hallucinations, suicidal ideation and aggression.

## 5.3.6 Sleep Disturbance

Sleep disturbances encompass disorders of initiating and maintaining sleep (insomnia), excessive somnolence (ES) and dysfunctions associated with sleep stages or partial arousals (parasomnias). In general, lifestyle changes should be advised as part of any sleep disturbance: avoiding stimulants in the evening (e.g. caffeine, tobacco and alcohol), stopping smoking, taking regular exercise and having good sleeping habits, e.g. going to bed and rising at the same time every day, not napping during the day or taking time to relax before going to bed.

### 5.3.6.1 Insomnia

Insomnia around the time of diagnosis is often multifactorial—partly situational (e.g. unfamiliar surroundings, hospital bed and noisy environment) and partly anxiety and medication related. Dexamethasone promotes wakefulness and when given orally should be given in the morning only. Anxiety is associated with initial insomnia and frequent wakening. Insomnia may also be associated with pre-existing conditions such as obstructive sleep apnoea syndrome or hypoventilation syndromes, either as a result of tumour in the brain stem or as effect of radiation on the brain stem producing palatal weakness. With sleep apnoea, there can be morning headaches, papilloedema and somnolence during the day, simulating raised ICP. If obstructive sleep apnoea or other sleep-disordered breathing can be confirmed through sleep studies, continuous positive airway pressure (CPAP) therapy may be helpful. Where problems getting to sleep are associated with other symptoms, e.g. cramps in legs or myoclonus and leg spasms, other conditions such as restless legs syndrome and spasticity should be considered. Some medications, including antinausea drugs, antipsychotic drugs, certain antidepressants and sedating antihistamines, may worsen symptoms of restless legs syndrome. Withdrawal of the offending medication and consideration of prescription of a dopamine agonist (e.g. ropinirole or pramipexole) for restless legs would be justified.

*Excessive daytime sleepiness (or somnolence).* Excessive somnolence is sometimes termed hypersomnia and may be due to circadian rhythm problems with insomnia or as a result of other causes of insomnia, e.g. sleep apnoea, but consideration should be given to the side effects of sedative medications such as benzodiazepines or other types of medication like AEDs, painkillers, tricyclic antidepressants and selective serotonin reuptake inhibitors (SSRIs or antipsychotics). Mood disorders are often associated with somnolence in addition to other mood-related symptoms.

*Parasomnia.* Parasomnias are disturbances associated with sleep, sleep stages or partial arousal. Nightmares, nocturnal seizures and other sleep-related disorders may occur in glioma patients. Nightmares usually occur within the first 2 h after sleep, and often begin with a scream, followed by signs of distress such as sweating, rapid breathing and heart rate and seemingly random body movements. Carers report difficulty wakening the patient during these episodes; however, normal sleep seems to return spontaneously within a few minutes. These can sometimes be misdiagnosed as nocturnal seizures. Nightmares may be precipitated by withdrawal of sedative drugs or alcohol and are usually remembered. Bruxism (grinding of teeth) during sleep can also sometimes be misdiagnosed as seizures and may be associated with other parasomnias and movements simulating seizures and often are associated with morning headaches and temporomandibular joint dysfunction.

## 5.4 Episodic Neurological Late Effects ("Neurological Attacks")

Not all "neurological attacks" in glioma are epileptic seizures.

### 5.4.1 Seizures

An important manifestation and diagnostic point are that focal seizures are generally short-lived, stereotyped and non-situational and occur with "positive" phenomena. A good eyewitness account is crucial. If the patient or carer mentions episodes that just last seconds to minutes, always have the same pattern and can come on anytime and not provoked by a particular situation, then this suggests epileptic seizures. Seizures produce "positive" phenomena (see Sect. 5.2.1.5) such as *hallucinations* of taste, smell, rising sensation from stomach, déjà vu (temporal lobe), *jerking* (motor cortex in frontal lobe), *tingling*, *burning* (parietal cortex) and *visual hallucination* (occipital cortex). Seizures will correlate with topographical localisation of the tumour, i.e. right-sided focal jerking of the leg will be due to involvement of the left motor cortex in the leg area. Rarely seizures in the temporal lobe may cause "ictal bradycardia syndrome" where the heart rate slows or stops and is accompanied by fainting or cardiac arrest. In that situation both AED and a cardiac pacemaker may be required.

### 5.4.2 Syncopal Non-epileptic Attacks

Syncope is the sudden transient self-limited loss of consciousness and physical collapse with relatively rapid onset due to transient global cerebral hypo-perfusion to the brain. It is sometimes characterised by symptoms that mimic epilepsy including brief focal or generalised muscle twitching (myoclonic jerks), tonic spasms, tremor and syncopal convulsion. It is important to differentiate them from epilepsy as they do not respond to anti-epileptic drugs and may be made worse by sodium channel blockers (e.g. carbamazepine and phenytoin). The situational nature of attacks such as standing and stressful situations (with coughing or straining) may be a pointer to diagnosis. Pre-syncopal symptoms include light-headedness, blurred or tunnel vision, feeling faint, feeling nauseous, vomiting, sweating, ringing in ears, palpitations, panic and confusion. Metabolic causes (e.g. hypoglycaemia) and drug causes of syncope should be also sought (antihypertensives, antidepressants, strong painkillers, etc.). Pre-syncope is best managed by advice of how to avoid syncope and exclusion of drug or cardiac causes and reassurance and education for vasovagal syncope, possibly tilt training and isometric counterpressure (leg crossing, hand grip and arm tensing) [28]. Cardiac syncope due to arrhythmia (tachycardia or bradycardia) and low blood pressure can come on with little or no prodrome other than occasional palpitation. A good cardiac examination is necessary including lying and standing blood pressures. Cerebral syncope is associated with raised intracranial pressure and often occurs on standing. Loss of consciousness is brief and amnesia is a common feature. The attacks may occur despite dexamethasone. The addition of acetazolamide may sometimes stop symptoms.

### 5.4.3 Dissociative Non-epileptic Attacks

Dissociative seizures can be defined as psychologically mediated episodes of altered awareness and/or behaviour that may mimic epilepsy. They are also sometimes known as functional or psychogenic seizures. They are not uncommon in patients with glioma and are more commonly found in females. Attacks are frightening and panic disorder can mimic either complex partial epilepsy or tonic-clonic epilepsy. The patient may be scared of consequences of the attack, e.g. choking, a heart attack, dying or losing control. The attacks are often situational, e.g. crowded places and supermarkets. Patients may complain of tachycardia, perspiration, hyperventilation, peripheral paraesthesia, carpopedal spasm and a dry mouth prior to or during an attack. *Derealisation* (unreality concerning the environment) and *depersonalisation* (unreality concerning the self) are often features during attacks. Depersonalisation can also accompany sleep deprivation, migraine, seizures, obsessive-compulsive disorder and stress/anxiety. In psychiatric disorder these phenomena are usually of relatively gradual onset, prolonged duration (>2 min) and accompanied by fear and other psychiatric symptoms. In psychosis there may be dissociative attacks with hallucinations. The movements are thrashing, more commonly asynchronous, semi-purposeful or undulating in nature rather than tonic or clonic. Often there are pelvic movements or back arching with side-to-side head shaking. There can be tongue biting, but it is more commonly at the tip than at the sides. There may be ictal crying, prolonged hypotonia, closed mouth and eyelids in tonic phase or vocalisations during tonic-clonic phase. The patient often resists eye opening and the pupillary light reflex is normal. There may be lack of cyanosis and postictal reorientation is rapid. The attacks are a manifestation of psychological distress and therefore may occur in association with a cancer diagnoses. Management is education and understanding of the underlying reasons for attacks. Early identification of patients with anxiety and panic and appropriate counselling (information clearly given, reassurance, message of hope, advice about side effects of medication, a contact telephone number to call if anxious, e.g. neuro-oncology nurse) may be highly effective in reducing the likelihood of further panic attacks. Attacks often settle, but if not, then cognitive behaviour therapy (CBT), counselling, psychotherapy or antidepressants may be helpful.

### 5.4.4  Migraine

During the aura of migraine or during the headache phase, there may be focal, cognitive and emotional features. Prolonged or severe cognitive dysfunction can sometimes occur with mild headache. Auras are usually "negative phenomena"—blurring of vision, numbness and weakness—and spread of symptoms is slow unilaterally or sometimes bilaterally. Cognitive and behavioural features of mental slowing and sometimes depersonalisation may be difficult to distinguish from temporal lobe seizures or panic/dissociative attacks.

Where the attacks are followed or associated with migraine-type headache, the diagnosis is often clear; however headaches can follow seizures. In "migraine equivalent" there is just aura and no headache phase, and the diagnosis is even trickier. Management of migraine includes prevention by influencing lifestyle factors (better sleep, eat regularly, manage stress), along with treatment of acute attack. If attacks are frequent, e.g. more than 1–2 days per week, then prophylaxis may help. Prophylaxis may include beta blockers such as propranolol; anti-epileptic medication, such as topiramate; or antidepressant medication, such as amitriptyline, any of which may help reduce headache frequency.

### 5.4.5  Transient Ischaemic Attacks

Transient ischaemic attacks (TIAs) can occur as a late effect of cranial radiation on cerebral vessels. They are caused by temporary disruption to the blood supply to the part of the brain. Attacks are focal, have a sudden onset and usually have no spread of symptoms. Symptoms are negative phenomena (weakness, numbness, dysphasia, visual field loss or unilateral visual loss), lasting usually a prolonged time but by definition less than 24 h. Management is with aspirin or clopidogrel or rarely consideration of interventional neuroradiology.

### 5.4.6  Stroke-Like Migraine Associated with Radiotherapy (SMART Attacks)

SMART attacks are a late effect of radiotherapy, usually 10–20 years after treatment for cerebral tumour, and therefore more common in childhood brain tumours and in low-grade glioma where survival may be prolonged. The symptoms may present slowly, over some minutes, and the spread of negative phenomena (e.g. numbness, weakness, dysphasia or visual aura) may simulate migraine. The symptoms may be associated with seizures, and then the differential diagnosis includes prolonged Todd's paresis (post-ictal temporary weakness). Symptoms may take several days or weeks to recover. There is often a conspicuous headache characteristic of migraine. MRI with gadolinium shows reversible cortical enhancement often with swelling or patchy enhancement within the lobe involved. The scans are similar to those found with prolonged or ongoing focal seizures. There is no evidence of stroke or tumour progression. Sometimes the recovery is incomplete. There is no proven effective treatment, but aspirin with a statin or even antihypertensive agent is usually prescribed where there has been prolonged hemiparesis. AED is prescribed if there was any jerking during an attack. Some clinicians start steroids especially if there is cortical swelling or if there is a concern about progression [29].

## 5.5 Persistent Neurological Late Effects ("Neurological Deterioration")

Slow progressive neurological brain damage may be the result of demyelination, microvascular changes and degeneration. Management will depend on the severity of the disability and may require expertise in use of anti-spasticity agents, neurogenic bladder/urinary, progressive cognitive decline, mood and personality/behaviour change and neurological fatigue.

### 5.5.1 Cognitive Impairment and Dementia

Late effects of radiotherapy are associated with a gradual decline in cognition, with impairments often in verbal fluency and memory. This slowly progresses to a radiation-induced dementia. Dementia may be associated with unsteadiness, a tendency to fall when turning or fall backwards when rising from a chair as a result of apraxia of gait and incontinence of urine. Apraxia is where strength, sensation and cerebellar and extrapyramidal function are normal on testing, but when the patient tries to do a task, e.g. walking, they have difficulty performing it, e.g. initiating gait, as often their feet seem stuck to the ground or may be short stepped. Apraxia is usually due to damage to the frontal lobes or corpus callosum or left parietal lobe. The patient may also have bladder problems with urge of micturition and ultimately may be incontinent. The clinical picture may resemble normal pressure hydrocephalus or Parkinsonism. Management is supportive, and patients often require more supervision and help when mobilising.

Strategies to prompt recollection and reminding of important tasks—such as using diaries or calendars in paper form or on mobile phone—can be effective. Assistive, adaptive and rehabilitative technologies to help maintain the independence and safety are becoming standard. Grab bars and handrails may assist safety. Involvement of professionals assisting with daily tasks may maintain the patient in their own home independently and in the community. Psychological treatments to help improve memory, problem-solving and language ability can be tried, but compliance and engagement can be difficult. Where cognitive impairment is associated with excessive sleepiness, methylphenidate and other cognitive enhancers may be tried, but they increase the risk of seizures. Cholinesterase inhibitors (for Alzheimer's disease), such as rivastigmine, donepezil, galantamine or memantine, can be tried but often with little clear benefit. Bladder symptoms can be managed by a condom catheter in males or incontinence pads, during the day and night. Ultimately, an indwelling catheter may be required to assist nursing and maintain skin hygiene.

### 5.5.2  Parkinsonism/Parkinson's Disease

Years after radiation involving the basal ganglia, patients can develop Parkinsonism. This is when there is reduced dopamine in the substantia nigra in the basal ganglia secondary to radiation therapy. A dopamine transporter (DAT) scan can be helpful to demonstrate reduced uptake in clinically difficult cases. Usually rigidity (stiffness) and bradykinesia (slowness of movement, e.g. finger tapping) are more pronounced than rest tremor. Drugs such as antipsychotic agents (chlorpromazine, haloperidol), some antidepressants, long-term antinauseant usage (e.g. prochlorperazine) or sodium valproate (AED) can also cause Parkinsonism. Any offending drug should be withdrawn, and if there is no benefit, then dopamine replacement, e.g. co-beneldopa or co-careldopa, or dopamine agonists, e.g. ropinirole, can be tried. Clearly, because patients with malignant brain tumours tend to be elderly, patients may have unrelated idiopathic Parkinson's disease, which will be responsive to medication in most cases.

#### 5.5.2.1 Spasticity
Spasticity is increased muscle tone, as a manifestation of an upper motor neuron injury, physiologically defined as a velocity-dependent increase in muscle tone caused by the increased excitability of the muscle stretch reflex. When the patient has reached a plateau after recovery from hemiparesis and spasticity is problematic, anti-spasticity medication may be required. Spasticity should limit performance and not have satisfactory response to physiotherapy. If there are night-time or daytime spasms, painful jerks or clonus which may interfere with sleep, anti-spasticity agents (e.g. baclofen, tizanidine and gabapentin) may be effective at reducing symptoms and improving function and quality of gait. This may be counterbalanced by potential side effects, e.g. drowsiness, weakness, dizziness, headache, nausea or vomiting, and can sometimes reduce seizure threshold. Therapy with *baclofen* should be administered cautiously in patients with *seizures*. Abrupt baclofen withdrawal may be associated with seizures, hallucinations, fever and rebound spasticity and rigidity.

## 5.6  Reversible Endocrine Late Effects ("Pituitary Insufficiency")

Surveillance for late endocrine effects after childhood CNS cancer treatment or in long-term survivors of glioma following treatment with radiotherapy is important, especially when the tumour is situated in the frontal and temporal lobes where the pituitary gland is within the radiation field. This usually starts to become a problem several years after treatment; therefore it is more commonly seen in low-grade glioma. Growth hormone is usually the first hormone to be involved, and this clearly is more of a problem following treatment of childhood CNS cancers. In adults central adiposity, decreased lean muscle mass, fatigue and change in mood are common. Regular annual surveillance of pituitary hormones (growth hormone, sex hormones, thyroid function and cortisol) is required for early diagnosis. Early referral to an endocrinologist to advise on replacement of pituitary hormones and optimisation of physical, cognitive and psychosocial health is important.

## 5.7 Conclusion

The management of patients with intrinsic brain tumours in the early perioperative and post-operative period can be challenging. As can be seen from this chapter, there are important diagnostic and management dilemmas, and having an experienced multidisciplinary team, knowledgeable about neuro-oncological, general medical and drug-related complications, is important. Neuro-oncology specialist nurses are in an ideal position to bridge the gap between primary care physician, neurologist and neurosurgeon, as well as to act as an initial point of contact for the patient or primary care physician following diagnosis. Increasingly, it is perceived that a multidisciplinary team approach to care is superior to the single clinician approach.

## References

1. Kerrigan S, Erridge SE, Liaquat I, et al. Mental incapacity in patients undergoing neuro-oncologic treatment: a cross-sectional study. Neurology. 2014;83(6):537–41.
2. Grant R. Overview: brain tumour diagnosis and management/Royal College of Physician Guidelines. J Neurol Neurosurg Psychiatry. 2004;75(Suppl 2):18–23.
3. Vecht CJ, Hovestadt A, Verbiest HB, van Vliet JJ, van Putten WL. Dose-effect relationship of dexamethasone on Karnofsky performance in metastatic brain tumors: a randomized study of doses of 4, 8, and 16 mg per day. Neurology. 1994;44:675–80.
4. Weston J, Greenhalgh J, Marson AG. Antiepileptic drugs as prophylaxis for post-craniotomy seizures. Cochrane Database Syst Rev. 2015;(3):CD007286.
5. Tremont-Lukats IW, Armstrong T, Gilbert MR. Antiepileptic drugs for preventing seizures in people with brain tumors. Cochrane Database Syst Rev. 2008;(2):CD004424.
6. Walker M. Status epilepticus: an evidence based guide. BMJ. 2005;331(7518):673–7.
7. Simanek R, Vormittag R, Hassler M, et al. Venous thromboembolism and survival in patients with high-grade glioma. Neuro Oncol. 2007;9:89–95.
8. Dickinson LD, Miller LD, Patel CP, Gupta SK. Enoxaparin increases the incidence of post-operative intracranial haemorrhage when initiated pre-operatively for deep vein thrombosis in patients with brain tumours. Neurosurgery. 1998;43:1074–81.
9. Perry JR, Julian JA, Laperriere NJ, et al. PRODIGE: a randomised placebo controlled trial of dalteparin low molecular weight heparin thromboprophylaxis in patients with newly diagnosed malignant glioma. J Thromb Haemost. 2010;8(9):1959–65.

10. De Benedittis G, Lorenzetti A, Migliore M, Spagnoli D, Tiberio F, Villani RM. Postoperative pain in neurosurgery: a pilot study in brain surgery. Neurosurgery. 1996;38(3):466–9.
11. Kaur A, Selwa L, Fromes G, Ross DA. Persistent headache after supratentorial craniotomy. Neurosurgery. 2000;47:633–6.
12. Piil K, Juhler M, Jakobsen J, Jarden M. Controlled rehabilitative and supportive care intervention trials in patients with high-grade gliomas and their caregivers: a systematic review. BMJ Support Palliat Care. 2016;6(1):27–34.
13. Bartolo M, Zucchella C, Pace A, et al. Early rehabilitation after surgery improves functional outcome in inpatients with brain tumours. J Neurooncol. 2012;107(3):537–44.
14. Khan F, Amatya B, Ng L, Drummond K, Galea M. Multidisciplinary rehabilitation after primary brain tumour treatment. Cochrane Database Syst Rev. 2015;(8):CD009509.
15. Day J, Gillespie DC, Rooney AG, et al. Neurocognitive deficits and neurocognitive rehabilitation in adult brain tumors. Curr Treat Options Neurol. 2016;18(5):22–32.
16. Gehring K, Sitskoorn MM, Gundy CM, et al. Cognitive rehabilitation in patients with gliomas: a randomized, controlled trial. J Clin Oncol. 2009;27(22):3712–22.
17. Gehring K, Patwardhan SY, Collins R, et al. A randomized trial on the efficacy of methylphenidate and modafinil for improving cognitive functioning and symptoms in patients with a primary brain tumor. J Neurooncol. 2012;107(1):165–74.
18. Meyers CA, Weitzner MA, Valentine AD, Levin VA. Methylphenidate therapy improves cognition, mood, and function of brain tumor patients. J Clin Oncol. 1998;16(7):2522–7.
19. Shaw EG, Rosdhal R, D'Agostino RB Jr, et al. Phase II study of donepezil in irradiated brain tumor patients: effect on cognitive function, mood, and quality of life. J Clin Oncol. 2006;24(9):1415–20.
20. Rooney AG, Brown PD, Reijneveld JC, et al. Depression in glioma: a primer for clinicians and researchers. J Neurol Neurosurg Psychiatry. 2014;85:230–5.
21. Chambers SK, Grassi L, Hyde MK, Holland J, Dunn J. Integrating psychosocial care into neuro-oncology: challenges and strategies. Front Oncol. 2015;5:4.
22. DeRubeis RJ, Siegle GJ, Hollon SD. Cognitive therapy vs. medications for depression: treatment outcomes and neural mechanisms. Nat Rev Neurosci. 2008;9(10):788–96.
23. Burke W. The neural basis of Charles Bonnet hallucinations: a hypothesis. J Neurol Neurosurg Psychiatry. 2002;73:535–41.
24. Armstrong TS, Cron SG, Bolanos EV, et al. Risk factors for fatigue severity in primary brain tumor patients. Cancer. 2010;116(11):2707–15.
25. Day J, Yust-Katz S, Cachia D, Wefel J, Katz LH, Tremont I, Bulbeck H, Armstrong T, Rooney AG. Interventions for the management of fatigue in adults with a primary brain tumour. Cochrane Database Syst Rev. 2016;(4):CD011376. https://doi.org/10.1002/14651858. CD011376.pub2.
26. Boele FW, Douw L, de Groot M, et al. The effect of modafinil on fatigue, cognitive functioning, and mood in primary brain tumor patients: a multicenter randomized controlled trial. Neuro Oncol. 2013;15(10):1420–8.
27. Page BR, Shaw EG, Lu L, et al. Phase II double-blind placebo-controlled randomized study of armodafinil for brain radiation-induced fatigue. Neuro Oncol. 2015;17(10):1393–401.
28. Brignole M, Alboni P, Benditt D, Bergfeldt L, Blanc JJ, Bloch Thomsen PE, van Dijk JG, Fitzpatrick A, Hohnloser S, Janousek J, et al. Guidelines on management (diagnosis and treatment) of syncope. Eur Heart J. 2001;22(15):1256–306.
29. Farid K, Meissner WG, Samier-Foubert A, et al. Normal cerebrovascular reactivity in stroke-like migraine attacks after radiation therapy syndrome. Clin Nucl Med. 2010;35(8):583–5.

# Glioma Surgery

6

## Joanna Ashby and Colin Watts

**Abstract**

Neurosurgical intervention is essential for the safe and effective management of adult gliomas. Increasing evidence suggesting that for both low- and high-grade gliomas, maximal cytoreduction is associated with an increased overall survival. Beyond conventional neurosurgical principles, there are a variety of techniques that have been refined over the last decade to maximise the efficiency of the neurosurgeon and post-operative management. Functional magnetic resonance imaging (fMRI) and diffusion tensor imaging (DTI) are two non-invasive techniques used to localise eloquent motor and language anatomy and higher cognitive pathways to inform decision-making and preoperative surgical planning. Novel intraoperative techniques include neuronavigation, cortical and subcortical mapping, high-frequency ultrasonography, Raman spectroscopy, fluorescence-guided surgery and locally delivered therapies such as carmustine. These therapies are valuable tools which act to reduce post-operative neurological deficits therefore reducing the overall tumour burden on the patient by improving quality of life. Operating on elderly patients with gliomas, as well as those with recurrent disease, is still controversial but is becoming more common due to advances in adjunct technologies. In summary this collection of management strategies has aided the neurosurgeon in achieving optimal surgical cytoreduction in the management of adult glioma.

J. Ashby
University of Glasgow, Glasgow, UK

C. Watts (✉)
Division of Neurosurgery, University of Cambridge, Cambridge, UK

Neurosurgery, University of Birmingham, Birmingham, UK

Birmingham Brain Cancer Program, University of Birmingham, Birmingham, UK

Institute of Cancer and Genomic Sciences, University of Birmingham, Birmingham, UK

College of Medical and Dental Sciences, University of Birmingham, Birmingham, UK
e-mail: C.Watts.2@bham.ac.uk

© Springer Nature Switzerland AG 2019
I. Oberg (ed.), *Management of Adult Glioma in Nursing Practice*,
https://doi.org/10.1007/978-3-319-76747-5_6

**Keywords**
Surgery · Glioma · High-grade glioma (HGG) · Neuronavigation · Direct cortical
stimulation · Intraoperative magnetic resonance imaging (iMRI) · Functional
MRI (fMRI) · Extent of resection · Overall survival · Progression-free survival

**Learning Outcomes**
• Gain insight into the varying surgical techniques available, alongside the rationale for using them, depending on the size and anatomical location of the
  glioma.
• Understand the risks, benefits and intended outcomes of various surgical options
  and techniques.
• Understand how safe maximal resection helps improve progression-free
  survival.
• Gain deeper insight into treatment for recurrent gliomas and treatment for the
  elderly patient with a glioma.

## 6.1    Introduction

The first step in the management of adult glioma is specialised multidisciplinary
evaluation with the primary aim of determining whether the patient is appropriate
for surgery, in addition to planning for possible radiotherapy and chemotherapy.
During this evaluation, particular attention is paid to the patients' performance status and neurological function. If the patient is eligible for neurosurgical intervention, the first goal of surgery is to provide a histological diagnosis of the tumour.
Patients undergo biopsy, debulking surgery or maximal resection depending on the
patient condition and tumour location. Whenever possible, maximal cytoreduction
of the tumour without causing post-operative neurological deficit is the surgical
objective because the extent of tumour resection has prognostic value. In the case of
microsurgical resection not being feasible, molecular genetic analyses are performed with the use of a stereotactic biopsy as these can influence treatment strategies. These include establishing $O^6$-methylguanine-DNA methyltransferase
(MGMT) methylation status, loss of heterozygosity in 1p/19q and isocitrate dehy-
drogenase-1 (IDH-1) status [1], explored in more detail in Chap. 7.
     Over the past decade, there has been a large focus on novel surgical approaches
to improve long-term outcomes in glioma surgery, and evidence to support the benefit of maximal extent of resection is growing. Such advances in the armamentarium
of the neuro-oncological surgeon allow for safer, more aggressive surgery to maximise tumour resection whilst minimising post-operative neurological deficit. Such
advances in surgical adjuncts that improve patient outcome include advanced neuronavigation, intraoperative magnetic resonance imaging (iMRI), high-frequency
ultrasonography, fluorescence-guided microsurgery using intraoperative fluorescence, functional mapping of motor and language pathways and locally delivered
therapies. Operating on elderly patients with gliomas as well as those patients with

recurrent disease is still controversial but is becoming more common due to these emerging novel strategies. In this chapter we discuss these emerging techniques and their impact on the future of glioma surgery.

### 6.1.1   Low-Grade Gliomas

Low-grade gliomas (LGGs) are a heterogeneous group of tumours—that is, with distinct morphological and phenotypic profiles. They account for 15% of all adult brain tumours and their incidence bares no ethnic or national preponderance. Depending on the tumour, the WHO grade is assigned and ranges from grade I to grade IV with the higher the number, the more aggressive the tumour type [2]. These diffuse, infiltrating tumours can have astrocytic, oligodendroglial, ependymal or mixed cellular histologies, where the most common histological subtypes are the fibrillary, protoplasmic and gemistocytic variants. Median overall survival for LGG patients is 6.5–8 years [3], and survival estimates for these patients range from 3 to 20 years [4]. As there is substantial heterogeneity in the behaviour and course of progression for these lesions, there is also controversy surrounding the most appropriate management strategy for these patients. However, after adjusting for all factors, extent of resection has been proven to be a significant predictor of overall survival for these patients and acted as a good indicator for progression-free survival [5].

The management of these tumours can largely revolve around observation, surgical intervention, biopsy and resection. Although a purely observational management plan for patients with clinical and imaging evidence of LGGs is rare, some practitioners still advocate this highly conservative approach, often if tumours are deep-seated or in eloquent areas. There is however little evidence to support this treatment strategy and current consensus guidelines do not support this approach. Rather they emphasise the importance of establishing an integrated molecular diagnosis. Stereotactic biopsy and open surgical resection are the two main surgical strategies, with the goals including establishing a diagnosis, treating neurological symptoms and decompressing mass effect and cytoreduction, where the only agreed-upon standard for adult supratentorial non-optic-pathway LGGs involves establishing a diagnosis before active surgical intervention [1].

### 6.1.2   High-Grade Gliomas

High-grade gliomas (HGGs) are a heterogeneous group of brain tumours with devastatingly poor prognoses. Their incidence is approximately 5 per 100,000 population in Europe and the USA with peak incidence occurring in the fifth and sixth decades of life [6]. According to the updated World Health Organisation (WHO) classification system, gliomas are classified into low grade (grades I and II) and high grade (III and IV). The most aggressive type of grade IV glioma is the glioblastoma (GBM). It carries the poorest prognosis and is characterised by high mitotic activity, hypoxia and necrosis, in addition to cellular polymorphism and microvascular proliferation [2]. The neuroanatomy, physiology and pathology are explored in more detail in the earlier chapters.

Optimal treatment for patients with high-grade glioma is maximal safe resection followed by radiotherapy and temozolomide (TMZ) chemotherapy, followed by TMZ monotherapy, also referred to as the Stupp protocol [7]. Patients with good performance status who undergo this treatment protocol have a median survival of approximately 14 months. In patients who are MGMT methylated, which is predictive for a good response to TMZ [8], median survival is around 24 months with approximately half of patients surviving 2 years [6]. It is critical to understand these biomarkers when interpreting the surgical outcome data in the neuro-oncological clinical research.

Survival for anaplastic gliomas that are classified as WHO grade III is 6–7 years, which increases to 14 years in the case of 1p19q-deleted oligodendrogliomas which are optimally treated with radiotherapy and procarbazine, lomustine (CCNU) and vincristine (PCV) chemotherapy [4]. These data illustrate improvement in survival as well as the growing importance of biomarker-based management in the management of gliomas [2], which further emphasise the critical importance of good surgery. Mutations of IDH-1/IDH-2 in WHO grade III and IV gliomas are prognostic biomarkers, and promoter methylation of MGMT is prognostic in patients with grade III gliomas who receive radiotherapy with adjuvant chemotherapy [4].

Neurosurgical intervention is the first step in the safe, effective management of HGG [9]. International guidelines advocate safe maximal resection [1]. Due to the diffusely infiltrative nature of these tumours, resection of often challenging as eloquent brain areas that are associated with language, memory and other higher cognitive functions is often adjacent to tumour tissue. Conventional microsurgery is aided by computed tomography and T1-weighted contrast MRI, but alone, these basic imaging tools are an inadequate means of treating these tumours. Additional surgical techniques such as the use of 5-aminolevulinic acid (5-ALA) have been developed to improve the neurosurgical management of these tumours, and there is now growing evidence that these techniques improve patient survival [10].

## 6.1.3 Extent of Resection

The rationale for surgical resection is to facilitate histological diagnosis and enable the safe maximal removal of the tumour. The ultimate aim is complete removal of the tumour without causing post-operative neurological deficits such as hemiparesis. There is a growing body of literature that supports extent of resection as a prognostic factor. However, this remains controversial. The largest and single only quantitative systematic review investigating the association between extent of resection and survival in glioblastoma supports the use of gross total resection for glioblastoma for reducing 1- and 2-year mortality [11]. In this meta-analysis of 37 studies, gross total resection was significantly associated with a lower relative risk for mortality at these time points compared with subtotal resection, and overall a dose-dependent reduction in mortality was seen with increasing extent of resection.

There are many studies that have investigated the effect of extent of resection on patient outcomes in the management of glioma patients over the past decade [12]. The EORTC 26981-22981/National Cancer Institute of Canada Clinical Trials Group CE3 shows patients with GBM who underwent complete resection had a superior survival outcome compared to those who underwent partial resection in their randomised phase III trial [13]. Further studies which have compared outcomes of complete versus partial resection have achieved more statistically robust evidence supporting benefit to patients. To further support this, a recent meta-analysis supported an improvement in overall survival, functional recovery and tumour recurrence rate when extent of resection was increased, with the analysis involving 12,607 patients from 34 studies [14]. However, the important bias inherent in all studies is that patients who undergo total resection are younger, have a good performance status and have their glioma in a non-eloquent area.

These guidelines led to the consensus that maximal resection provides a survival benefit for patients with high-grade gliomas. Extent of resection is the key therapy-dependent prognostic factor, alongside younger age and better performance status as important positive, therapy-intendent prognostic factors across all glioma entities [1]. Furthermore, the integration of advanced imaging techniques including the use of 5-aminolevulinic acid (5-ALA) allows for visualisation of tumour tissue and therefore an enhanced extent of resection margin, thereby minimising the risk of new neurological deficits. Most recent research focuses on maximising glioma resection using these novel neurosurgical techniques and strategies.

## 6.2   Preoperative Planning

The purpose of performing preoperative imaging techniques is to provide detailed information on tumour location, proximity to eloquent structures and location of eloquent anatomy to inform surgical planning in order to maximise surgical resection of the glioma. Although computer tomography (CT) and conventional MRI techniques were initially integral to the preoperative assessment of brain tumour patients, the role of neuroimaging has progressed from the evaluation of structural abnormalities and the identification of tumour-related complications. It is now essential to perform advanced physiology-based imaging methods to assess functional, haemodynamic, metabolic, cellular and cytoarchitectural alternations, such as diffusion-weighted imaging (DWI), proton MR spectroscopy ($^1$H-MR spectroscopy) and perfusion-weighted imaging, explored in more detail below [15].

### 6.2.1   Functional MRI

Functional magnetic resonance imaging (fMRI) is a non-invasive imaging technique that facilitates the localisation of eloquent areas, namely, those correlating to motor and language function, and has been shown to be significantly superior to analysis of structural MRI [16]. Therefore fMRI-based pre-surgical risk assessment is associated with a superior post-operative clinical outcome with regard to patient quality of life and neurological deficits occurring as a result of neurosurgical intervention. fMRI detects perfusion-related changes that are coupled with neuronal activity using the blood oxygen level-dependent (BOLD) signal. It is a reliable technique in localising the motor cortex but less reliable with regard to language mapping when compared to direct cortical stimulation [17]. In high-grade glioma (HGG), fMRI is limited by proliferation, new blood vessel formation and infiltration of the tumour, which results in the removal of areas of functional cortex that either constitute the tumour or are found in adjacent tissue. Therefore, using fMRI as the sole preoperative planning tool in the safe resection of HGG is not an option.

## 6.2.2  Diffusion Tensor Imaging

Diffusion tensor imaging (DTI) is another non-invasive imaging technique that enables the graphical reconstruction of the white matter pathways in the brain and spinal cord. It is sensitive to the directional diffusion of water molecules along the tracts and has been shown to be an effective tool in the delineation of the glioma tumour margin [18]. In combination, fMRI and DTI are useful tools that have been proven to positively inform preoperative neurosurgical decision-making, surgical approach and extent of resection. In a single prospective, randomised control study of 238 consecutive patients with pyramidal tract gliomas, utilising DTI-integrated neuronavigation with 3D MRI data, reduced post-operative motor deficits and increased overall survival in patients with high-grade gliomas compared to control [19].

## 6.3  Intraoperative Techniques

Intraoperative planning ranges from the common neuronavigation to functional mapping of the cortex and subcortical structures, to more novel surgical adjuncts including ultrasound, intraoperative MRI, Raman spectroscopy and fluorescence-guided techniques.

## 6.3.1  Neuronavigation

Neuronavigation provides a personalised surgical map that the neurosurgeon can use to facilitate a maximal resection through the intraoperative identification of the tumour's location. Neuronavigation has become ubiquitous in neurosurgical operating theatres around the world. It has led to reduction in size of the craniotomy and has aided the anatomical orientation with regard to tumour resection. However, despite these important advances in glioma surgery, its inherent limitation is intraoperative inaccuracy due to leakage of cerebrospinal fluid (CSF) causing brain shift when the dura is opened, during surgery [20].

## 6.3.2  Awake Cortical and Subcortical Mapping

Direct cortical stimulation was first performed in 1931 by Foerster and later developed by Penfield in 1937. Intraoperative cortical and subcortical stimulation is the gold standard technique for the identification of eloquent areas and functional pathways in preoperative surgical planning. The technique involves direct stimulation by contact of electrodes with brain tissue to identify and avoid functional brain areas. This may lead to improved quality of life by preserving sensory, motor, language and cognitive functions. The location of eloquent speech and language areas shows high inter-patient variability, owing to a number of factors, including tumour mass effect, shifting or infiltrating anatomical pathways and functional reorganisation through plasticity [21]. Therefore, cortical and subcortical stimulation during awake surgery allows for direct real-time anatomico-functional correlation by focusing on lesion location and the relationships between functional networks to guide surgery. The contrast-enhancing tumour may be hard to define, and complete removal is difficult, even for the experienced neurosurgeon. Furthermore, contrast enhancement doesn't entirely identify the tumour margin as some tumour cells may lie outside the contrast-enhancing areas. High-grade gliomas (HGGs) commonly recur with 2 cm of the defined tumour margin [22]. It is therefore crucial to balance the goal of maximal resection with an assessment of the risk of neurological deficit during preoperative planning.

## 6.3.3  Ultrasound

Intraoperative ultrasound provides real-time feedback on tumour location during surgery and therefore attempts to reduce the effect of brain shift during surgery [23]. Real-time intraoperative imaging has advantages over preoperatively derived images because of brain shift during surgery, and new features could develop. Intraoperative ultrasound aids tumour localisation, extent of resection evaluation, feeding or draining vessel identification in vascular tumours and with the assessment of the patency of venous sinuses. However, as haemorrhage and oedema limit the use of intraoperative ultrasound, further technical improvements are required before it is used as a mainstream technical adjunct in glioma surgery [24].

## 6.3.4  Intraoperative MRI

Intraoperative magnetic resonance imaging (iMRI) is another relatively recent technique that improves surgical accuracy by offering an updated neuronavigational map during surgery. Like ultrasound, it also eliminates the effect of brain shift. The first study on the effect of iMRI on the extent of resection in glioma surgery showed that using iMRI leads to a significantly higher rate of complete tumour resection compared to control, an increase in progression-free survival and no difference in the rate of new post-operative neurological deficits between groups [25]. In this randomised controlled trial, 58 patients with tumours amenable to radiologically complete resection were enrolled; tumour resection was guided by ultra-low-field intraoperative MRI (0.15 T) in 29 patients, and conventional neuronavigation was used in the remaining 29 patients. This was the first study to provide level I evidence to support iMRI-guided neurosurgery for glioma treatment. At best, level II evidence is available in the support of using iMRI in the surgical management of GBM [26]. This systematic review analysed 12 studies investigating the effectiveness of iMRI-guided surgery for GBM compared to neuronavigation-guided resection with respect to the extent of resection, quality of life and survival. It concluded that iMRI-guided surgery was more effective as it significantly increases the extent of resection, enhances quality of life and prolongs survival in patients with GBM. However, limitations included patient variability, overlapping data, attribution bias, subjective assessment of extent of tumour resection, the use of different field strengths, the variable use of contrast agent and inconsistencies in reported quality of life and survival data. The widespread use of iMRI has been limited by it being time-consuming and expensive.

### 6.3.5   Raman Spectroscopy

Raman spectroscopy is a laser-based technique that uses non-destructive molecular characterisation to aid with the identification of residual tumour. The 'Raman effect' occurs when light changes the tissue chemistry and results in the inelastic scattering of a photon. It is this scattered light that is used for in vivo biopsy and margin assessment. The Raman spectrum is recorded as a 'fingerprint' based on the molecular constituents of white matter and tumour necrosis, identified by methyl-docasehexaenoate (methyl DHA) and phenylalanine, respectively. In a prospective observational study of 40 patients, Raman spectroscopy coupled with 3D-ultrasound has been shown to distinguish LGG from normal brain tissue with a sensitivity and specificity greater than 95% [27].

### 6.3.6   Fluorescence-Guided Surgery

Intraoperative fluorescence is an exciting technique that is becoming a standard part of the surgical management of gliomas, worldwide. 5-Aminolevulinic acid (5-ALA) is a non-fluorescent amino acid precursor in the biosynthesis pathway of haem. It is administered at 20 mg/kg orally as a drink approximately 4 h before surgery and accumulates in the cancer cells where it leads to accumulation of the fluorophore protoporphyrin IX (PPIX). This is a fluorophore (it gives off light when excited by light of a different wavelength allowing real-time intraoperative visualisation of the tumour using a specially adapted microscope). This technique is valuable in maximising the extent of resection in high-grade glioma surgery and is the only adjunct that has been validated in a randomised controlled trial [12]. This phase III trial involving 322 patients assessed the effects of 5-ALA-guided surgery in the management of malignant gliomas on the resection margins of early post-operative MRI and progression-free survival. There was a clinical benefit for patients, where 65%

of patients in the 5-ALA group received complete contrasting-enhancing removal of the tumour, compared to 35% in the white-light microscopy group. In addition, at 6 months, patients in the 5-ALA group had a 50% improvement in progression-free survival (41% versus 21.1%). There are many studies that have investigated the value of 5-ALA in glioma surgery with or without the additional use of complementary novel technologies [9]. 5-ALA has been shown to increase the extent of resection, provide a greater resection when combined with other intraoperative adjuncts and improve outcomes through the improved avoidance of eloquent brain areas during tumour resection. Side effects are limited, but sensitisation to ultraviolet light means patients must avoid direct sunlight for 24 h after administration.

A recent systematic review and meta-analysis assessing accuracy, extent of tumour resection, safety and survival of the use of 5-ALA in patients reported an overall sensitivity of 0.87 (95% confidence interval, CI, 0.81–0.92) and specificity of 0.89 (95% CI, 0.79–0.94) with respect to the diagnostic accuracy of 5-ALA [28]. This evidence illustrates an observed improved extent of resection and higher 6-month progression-free survival which confirms the value of 5-ALA-assisted surgery in glioma surgery. In summary, 5-ALA-guided surgery is an increasingly common, easy-to-use, cost-effective adjunct that has been shown to improve the extent of tumour resection and long-term outcomes in glioma patients.

### 6.3.7 Locally Delivered Therapies

The formation of a cavity following tumour resection by craniotomy allows for the delivery of local therapies that would otherwise not be practical due to the selective delivery of systemic treatments across the blood-brain barrier. Bischloroethylnitrosourea (BCNU: carmustine) is a chemotherapeutic agent that directly diffuses into the tumour cavity following surgery avoiding systemic toxicity and bypassing the blood-brain barrier. Using carmustine wafers in the management of malignant gliomas is safe and can be effective but remains controversial and is not recommended in current guidelines [1, 29]. Their use is associated with increased wound breakdown and infection rates. If this occurs any leaking fluids must be managed as chemotherapy-contaminated with appropriate barrier nursing, safety precautions, disposal of dressings, etc. Carmustine wafers have been shown to be clinically efficacious in malignant glioma management in a phase III prospective randomised controlled trial involving 240 patients randomised to BCNU wafer versus placebo wafer, followed by radiotherapy. A phase III randomised control trial refers to a trial in which a new treatment that has worked well for patients in a phase II clinical trial is now compared with the current gold standard treatment, in which people are assigned to different groups randomly. A survival advantage of 13.9 months versus 11.6 months (95% CI 0.52–0.96; $p = 0.03$) was conferred by BCNU wafers compared to placebo, with a further survival advantage of 14.8 months versus 12.6 months ($p = 0.01$) in those who underwent a complete resection versus incomplete resection. An important limitation is the inclusion of patients with grade III gliomas, as further analysis in their follow-up study reporting the long-term outcomes of these patients showed that BCNU wafers did not confer a survival advantage when grade III gliomas were excluded [30]. A prospective study is required to answer this question definitively but is unlikely. Carmustine wafers and 5-ALA therapy are illustrated in Fig. 6.1 [31].

## 6.4 Recurrent Malignant Glioma

Although recurrent malignant gliomas have long been considered inoperable, advances in neurosurgical innovations and anaesthesiology have meant that they are increasingly amenable to surgical invention. A systematic review summarising evidence on the role of repeat surgery in recurrent malignant gliomas established evidence-based recommendations for this group of patients when there had previously been no consensus [32]. Repeat cytoreduction in locally recurrent or progressive gliomas provided a survival outcome between 6 and 17 months, and age <50 years, KPS 60 or above and tumour location in non-functional brain all support improved overall survival. Although there have been numerous retrospective studies discussing the role of reoperation for these patients, there have been no prospective randomised control trials due to the inherent limitation of these studies, so recommendations are level III at best [9]. The use of 5-ALA has shown to reliably identify tumour tissue in recurrent malignant glioma and may therefore play an important role as a positive predictor of survival with regard to the reoperation and maximal resection of these tumours.

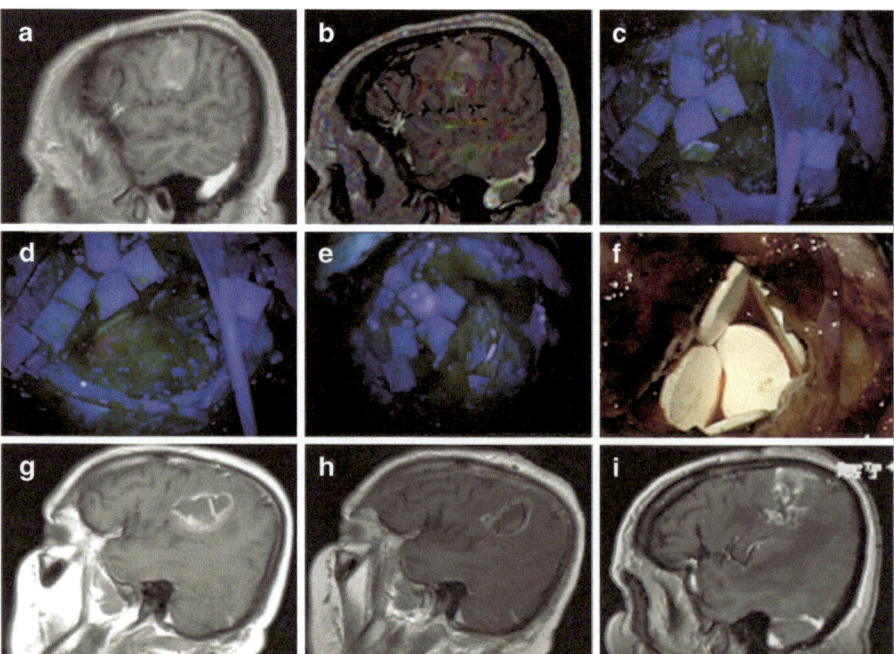

**Fig. 6.1** Patient undergoing 5-ALA-guided glioblastoma resection in eloquent area. (**f**) BCNU wafers are positioned in the surgical cavity [31]

## 6.5 Elderly

With an ageing population, there is a need to identify optimal surgical management strategies for gliomas in the elderly, as people over the age of 65 are now the largest group of patients to be diagnosed with high-grade gliomas [33]. Age is a well-known prognostic factor, where survival is inversely linked to age at diagnosis. Although few studies have assessed the role of surgery, chemotherapy and radio-therapy for gliomas in the elderly [34], prospective data suggest novel adjuncts, including 5-ALA, improve outcomes [35]. In this study, the use of 5-ALA in an elderly cohort was safe compared to younger patients, and the use of temozolomide and radiotherapy improved survival. Therefore, based on this evidence and retro-spective data, elderly patients with good performance status should be offered optimal surgical resection, temozolomide if MGMT-positive and radiotherapy if MGMT-negative [34]. This is further illustrated in Fig. 6.2 with a Kaplan-Meier curve showing survival according to MGMT methylation and postsurgical treatment in elderly patients with newly diagnosed glioblastoma [36].

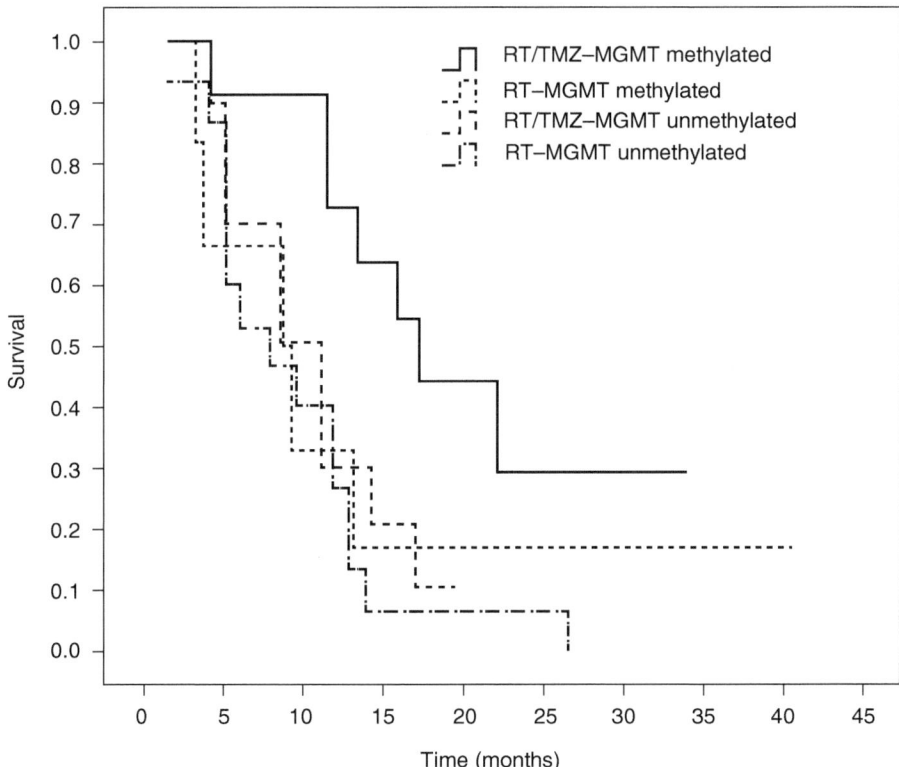

**Fig. 6.2** Survival according to MGMT methylation and postsurgical treatment of glioblastoma in the elderly [36]

## 6.6 Conclusions

There is mounting evidence to support that more extensive surgical resection favours overall survival in the management of adult gliomas. The benefits of extensive resection must be weighed against the risk of incurring neurological deficits. Performing tumour resection in the awake patient and using intraoperative stimulation mapping techniques are associated with fewer neurological deficits and greater extent of resection. The use of speech and language mapping must be emphasised in the preoperative planning paradigm, in addition to the consideration and inclusion of emerging novel technological adjuncts, such as iMRI, intraoperative ultrasound, fluorescence-guided surgery and locally delivered therapies.

## References

1. Weller M, Bent MV, Tonn JC, Stupp R, Preusser M, Cohen-Jonathan-Moyal E, et al. European Association for Neuro-Oncology (EANO) guideline on the diagnosis and treatment of adult astrocytic and oligodendroglial gliomas. Lancet Oncol. 2017;18(6):e315. https://doi.org/10.1016/s1470-2045(17)30194-8.
2. Louis DN, Perry A, Reifenberger G, Deimling AV, Figarella-Branger D, Cavenee WK, et al. The 2016 World Health Organization classification of tumors of the central nervous system: a summary. Acta Neuropathol. 2016;131(6):803–20. https://doi.org/10.1007/s00401-016-1545-1.
3. Johannesen TB, Langmark F, Lote K. Progress in long-term survival in adult patients with supratentorial low-grade gliomas: a population-based study of 993 patients in whom tumors were diagnosed between 1970 and 1993. J Neurosurg. 2003;99:854–62.
4. Van Den Bent MJ, Brandes AA, Taphoorn MJ, et al. Adjuvant procarbazine, lomustine, and vincristine chemo-therapy in newly diagnosed anaplastic oligodendroglioma: long-term follow-up of EORTC brain tumor group study 26951. J Clin Oncol. 2013;31:344–50.
5. Smith JS, Chang EF, Lamborn KR, et al. Role of extent of resection in the long-term outcome of low-grade hemispheric gliomas. J Clin Oncol. 2008;26:1338–45.
6. Stupp R, Brada M, Van Den Bent MJ, et al. High-grade glioma: ESMO clinical practice guidelines for diagnosis, treatment and follow-up. Ann Oncol. 2014;25(Suppl 3):iii93–iii101.
7. Stupp R, Mason WP, Van Den Bent MJ, et al. Radiotherapy plus concomitant and adjuvant temozolomide for glioblastoma. N Engl J Med. 2005;352:987–96.
8. Hegi ME, Diserens AC, Gorlia T, et al. MGMT gene silencing and benefit from temozolomide in glioblastoma. N Engl J Med. 2005;352:997–1003.
9. Watts C, Sanai N. Handbook of clinical neurology: Chapter 4 Surgical approaches for the gliomas. 3rd ed. Amsterdam: Elsevier; 2016.
10. Stummer W, Meinel T, Ewelt C, et al. Prospective cohort study of radiotherapy with concomitant and adjuvant temozolomide chemotherapy for glioblastoma patients with no or minimal residual enhancing tumor load after surgery. J Neurooncol. 2012;108:89–97.
11. Brown TJ, Brennan MC, Li M, Church EW, Brandmeir NJ, Rakszawski KL, Glantz M. Association of the extent of resection with survival in glioblastoma. JAMA Oncol. 2016;2(11):1460. https://doi.org/10.1001/jamaoncol.2016.1373.
12. Stummer W, Pichlmeier U, Meinel T, et al. Fluorescence-guided surgery with 5-aminolevulinic acid for resection of malignant glioma: a randomised controlled multicentre phase III trial. Lancet Oncol. 2006;7:392–401.
13. Stupp R, Hegi ME, Mason WP, et al. Effects of radio- therapy with concomitant and adjuvant temozolomide versus radiotherapy alone on survival in glioblastoma in a randomised phase III study: 5-year analysis of the EORTC-NCIC trial. Lancet Oncol. 2009;10:459–66.

14. Almenawer SA, Badhiwala JH, Alhazzani W, et al. Biopsy versus partial gross total resection in older patients with high-grade glioma: a systematic review and meta-analysis. Neuro Oncol. 2015;17:868–81.
15. Bähr O, Steinbach JP, Weller M. Brain tumor imaging. Med Radiol. 2015;3:8–23. https://doi.org/10.1007/174_2015_1072.
16. Pernet CR, Gorgolewski KJ, Job D, Rodriguez D, Whittle I, Wardlaw J. A structural and functional magnetic resonance imaging dataset of brain tumour patients. Sci Data. 2016;3:160003. https://doi.org/10.1038/sdata.2016.3.
17. Petrella JR, Shah LM, Harris KM, et al. Preoperative functional MR imaging localization of language and motor areas: effect on therapeutic decision making in patients with potentially resectable brain tumors. Radiology. 2006;240:793–802.
18. Price SJ, Jena R, Burnet NG, et al. Improved delineation of glioma margins and regions of infiltration with the use of diffusion tensor imaging: an image-guided biopsy study. AJNR Am J Neuroradiol. 2006;27:1969–74.
19. Wu JS, Zhou LF, Tang WJ, et al. Clinical evaluation and follow-up outcome of diffusion tensor imaging-based functional neuronavigation: a prospective, controlled study in patients with gliomas involving pyramidal tracts. Neurosurgery. 2007;61:935–48. discussion 948–9
20. Reinges MH, Nguyen HH, Krings T, et al. Course of brain shift during microsurgical resection of supratentorial cerebral lesions: limits of conventional neuronavigation. Acta Neurochir. 2004;146:369–77. discussion 377
21. Duffau H, Capelle L. May surgery in eloquent areas induce brain plasticity? Neuroimage. 2000;11((5):S271.
22. Hou LC, Veeravagu A, Hsu AR, et al. Recurrent glioblastoma multiforme: a review of natural history and management options. Neurosurg Focus. 2006;20:E5.
23. Unsgard G, Solheim O, Lindseth F, et al. Intra-operative imaging with 3D ultrasound in neurosurgery. Acta Neurochir Suppl. 2011;109:181–6.
24. Solheim O, Selbekk T, Jakola AS, et al. Ultrasound-guided operations in unselected high-grade gliomas – overall results, impact of image quality and patient selection. Acta Neurochir. 2010;152:1873–86.
25. Senft C, Bink A, Franz K, et al. Intraoperative MRI guidance and extent of resection in glioma surgery: a randomised, controlled trial. Lancet Oncol. 2011;12:997–1003.
26. Kubben PL, Ter Meulen KJ, Schijns OE, et al. Intraoperative MRI-guided resection of glioblastoma multiforme: a systematic review. Lancet Oncol. 2011;12:1062–70.
27. Vaqas B, et al. OS3.6 Optical biopsies in neurosurgery: raman spectroscopy for the real-time identification of tumours during surgery. Neuro Oncol. 2016;18(suppl_4):iv8.
28. Zhao S, Wu J, Wang C, et al. Intraoperative fluorescence-guided resection of high-grade malignant gliomas using 5-aminolevulinic acid-induced porphyrins: a systematic review and meta-analysis of prospective studies. PLoS One. 2013;8:e63682.
29. Brem H, Piantadosi S, Burger PC, et al. Placebo-controlled trial of safety and efficacy of intraoperative controlled delivery by biodegradable polymers of chemotherapy for recurrent gliomas. The Polymer-brain Tumor Treatment Group. Lancet. 1995;345:1008–12.
30. Westphal M, Ram Z, Riddle V, et al. Gliadel wafer in initial surgery for malignant glioma: long-term follow-up of a multicenter controlled trial. Acta Neurochir. 2006;148:269–75. discussion 275
31. Della Puppa A, Lombardi G, Rossetto M, Rustemi O, Berti F, Cecchin D, et al. Outcome of patients affected by newly diagnosed glioblastoma undergoing surgery assisted by 5-aminolevulinic acid guided resection followed by BCNU wafers implantation: a 3-year follow-up. J Neurooncol. 2016;131(2):331–40.
32. Ryken TC, Kalkanis SN, Buatti JM, et al. The role of cytoreductive surgery in the management of progressive glioblastoma: a systematic review and evidence-based clinical practice guideline. J Neurooncol. 2014;118:479–88.
33. Weller M, Platten M, Roth P, et al. Geriatric neuro-oncology: from mythology to biology. Curr Opin Neurol. 2011;24:599–604.

34. Scott JG, Suh JH, Elson P, et al. Aggressive treatment is appropriate for glioblastoma multiforme patients 70 years old or older: a retrospective review of 206 cases. Neuro Oncol. 2011;13:428–36.
35. Stummer W, Nestler U, Stockhammer F, et al. Favorable outcome in the elderly cohort treated by concomitant temozolomide radiochemotherapy in a multi- centric phase II safety study of 5-ALA. J Neurooncol. 2011;103:361–70.
36. Franceschi E, Depenni R, Paccapelo A, Ermani M, Faedi M, Sturiale C, et al. Which elderly newly diagnosed glioblastoma patients can benefit from radiotherapy and temozolomide? A PERNO prospective study. J Neurooncol. 2016;128(1):157–62.

# The Classification of Adult Gliomas

**7**

Kieren S. J. Allinson

**Abstract**

The current classification and grading of gliomas is based on the 2016 World Health Organisation (WHO) system. The WHO 2016 system is the first attempt to classify gliomas by integrating well-established molecular information with the histological features in order to arrive at an integrated diagnosis. The vast majority of adult gliomas grow in a diffuse manner, infiltrating grey and white matter and creating a tumour mass that is inseparable from the surrounding brain tissue and very difficult to surgically remove. When we talk about adult gliomas, we are generally talking about diffuse gliomas. Diffuse gliomas are broadly divided into astrocytoma and oligodendroglioma and graded as II, III or IV. How these are divided and classified into tumour grades and subtypes is explored further in this chapter.

**Keywords**

Glioma classification · WHO grading · Tumour necrosis · Glioblastoma · Gliomas

**Learning Outcomes**
- Understand the basis of the WHO system for classifying and grading adult gliomas.
- Understand the histological differences between low grade and high grade glioma and how increasing tumour grade correlates with a worse prognosis.
- Understand how histological and molecular features can predict individual tumour behaviour and dictate oncological treatment options.

K. S. J. Allinson (✉)
Department of Histopathology, Division B, Addenbrooke's Hospital, CUHFT, Cambridge, UK
e-mail: kieren.allinson@addenbrookes.nhs.uk

© Springer Nature Switzerland AG 2019
I. Oberg (ed.), *Management of Adult Glioma in Nursing Practice*,
https://doi.org/10.1007/978-3-319-76747-5_7

## 7.1     Introduction

The current classification and grading of gliomas is based on the 2016 World Health Organisation (WHO) system [1]. For nearly a century beforehand, the classification of brain tumours was based on the light microscopic appearance of haematoxylin and eosin (H&E)-stained sections and, much more recently, the immunohistochemical expression of various proteins. The WHO 2016 system is the first attempt to classify gliomas by integrating well-established molecular information with the histological features in order to arrive at an integrated diagnosis.

The vast majority of adult gliomas grow in a diffuse manner, infiltrating grey and white matter and creating a tumour mass that is inseparable from the surrounding brain tissue and very difficult to surgically remove. This is in contrast to most other intracranial tumours, such as meningioma, metastatic carcinoma and the special types of astrocytoma, such as pilocytic astrocytoma, that tend to grow as solid tumour masses, pushing the normal brain tissue away rather than diffusely infiltrating into it. When we talk about adult gliomas, we are generally talking about diffuse gliomas. Diffuse gliomas are broadly divided into astrocytoma and oligodendroglioma and graded as II, III or IV. This is discussed in detail in the next section.

## 7.2     The Grading of Gliomas

The histological grading of gliomas is a means of predicting their likely biological behaviour based on their microscopic features. The WHO 2016 classification uses a four-tiered grading system (grade I, II, III and IV) that essentially constitutes a scale of increasing malignancy and worsening prognosis [1]. In clinical practice, gliomas are often considered either low-grade glioma (grades I and II) or high-grade glioma (grades III and IV).

Grade I gliomas generally have low proliferative potential and a non-diffuse growth pattern and may have the possibility of cure with surgical resection alone. Grade I gliomas are usually biologically stable over time, meaning they do not tend to progress to a higher-grade tumour. An example of a grade I glioma is the pilocytic astrocytoma. This is generally a paediatric tumour; however, they do occasionally occur in the adult population [2].

Grade II gliomas (Fig. 7.1a) are usually diffusely infiltrative in nature and hard to resect. They tend to recur despite having a low proliferative activity (i.e. the tumour cells do not divide frequently and the tumour tends to grow slowly). The most common examples are diffuse astrocytoma and oligodendroglioma. Grade II gliomas tend to progress to higher-grade tumours over time. An example of this is a diffuse astrocytoma (grade II) progressing to an anaplastic astrocytoma (grade III) or a glioblastoma (grade IV) or an oligodendroglioma (grade II) progressing to an anaplastic oligodendroglioma (grade III).

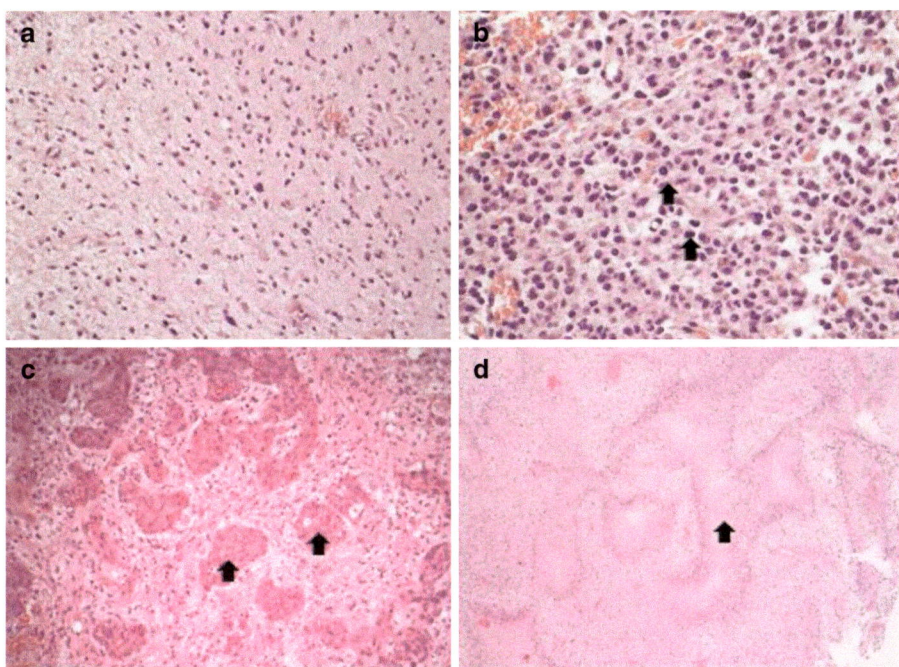

**Fig. 7.1** The histological grading of astrocytoma. (**a**) Diffuse astrocytoma (grade II). The tumour cells bear some resemblance to astrocytes, the principal supporting cell of the CNS. This grade II tumour has a fairly low cellularity and lacks mitotic figures, necrosis and microvascular proliferation. (**b**) Anaplastic astrocytoma (grade III). The cellularity of the tumour is increased in comparison to the grade II tumour depicted in (**a**). Note the presence of mitotic figures (arrows) indicating cell division and therefore tumour cell proliferation. (**c**) Glioblastoma (grade IV). When the blood vessels within the tumour proliferate and grow to form these structures (a couple of with are depicted with arrows), it is referred to as microvascular proliferation. In the context of an astrocytoma, this feature would make the tumour a glioblastoma (grade IV). (**d**) Glioblastoma (grade IV). The other classic feature of glioblastoma is necrosis (arrow) caused by tumour cell death. In glioblastoma, the necrotic areas are often surrounded by a high density of viable tumour cells. This is known as palisading necrosis

Grade III gliomas (Fig. 7.1b) are tumours with clear histological evidence of proliferation, i.e. they have mitotic figures indicating tumour cell division. Examples include anaplastic astrocytoma and anaplastic oligodendroglioma. Note that the latter can also have necrosis and microvascular proliferation and would still be grade III. Oligodendrogliomas cannot be grade IV.

Grade IV gliomas are malignant, mitotically active astrocytomas with either necrosis, microvascular proliferation or both. The vast majority of grade IV gliomas are glioblastoma (Fig. 7.1c, d).

See Table 7.1 for the classification of adult gliomas. The relationship between astrocytoma grade and prognosis is illustrated in Fig. 7.2 [3].

**Table 7.1** Classification of adult gliomas by tumour type and grade

|  | WHO grade | | | |
| Type of glioma | I | II | III | IV |
| --- | --- | --- | --- | --- |
| Astrocytoma | Pilocytic astrocytoma[a] | Diffuse astrocytoma | Anaplastic astrocytoma | Glioblastoma |
| Oligodendroglioma |  | Oligodendroglioma | Anaplastic oligodendroglioma |  |

[a]Note that pilocytic astrocytoma is a rare diagnosis in adults and is not genetically related to the diffuse gliomas

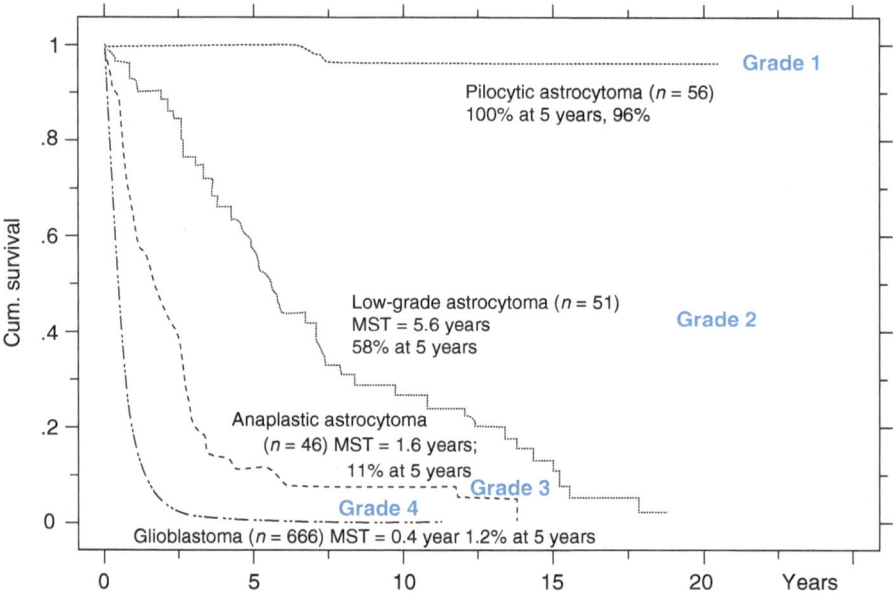

**Fig. 7.2** The relationship between tumour grade and survival in astrocytomas. From *Ohgaki H., et al. Neuropathol Exp Neurol (2005) 64:479–489*

## 7.3    Low-Grade Gliomas

The two most commonly occurring low-grade gliomas in the adult population are diffuse astrocytoma (WHO grade II) and oligodendroglioma (WHO grade II).

When examining a glioma, the pathologist will try to decide whether the glioma is an astrocytoma or an oligodendroglioma. Astrocytomas and oligodendrogliomas are best thought of as being composed of cells that resemble astrocytes and oligodendrocytes, respectively, rather than being derived from these cell types. Current evidence points to the origin of all gliomas from less differentiated precursor cells or central nervous system (CNS) stem cells [4].

Astrocytomas are composed of cells with at least some similarity to astrocytes, the principal supporting cell of the central nervous system. In H&E-stained slides, the cells of an astrocytoma tend to have irregular, dark, elongated—and generally not round—nuclei. The cytoplasm tends to be pink and may form long tapering processes (Fig. 7.1a).

The average age of patients with diffuse astrocytoma is mid-30s. There is a slight male predominance, with a male-to-female ratio of 1.3:1 [5].

Oligodendrogliomas are composed of cells that have a superficial resemblance to oligodendrocytes, the myelinating cell of the CNS. The cells of an oligodendroglioma will tend to have evenly round nuclei and clear cytoplasm to create the so-called 'fried egg' appearance (Fig. 7.3a).

Both of these tumour types are grade II and therefore would not be expected to have much proliferative activity (i.e. they would have very few or perhaps no mitotic figures). They would also not have necrosis or microvascular proliferation.

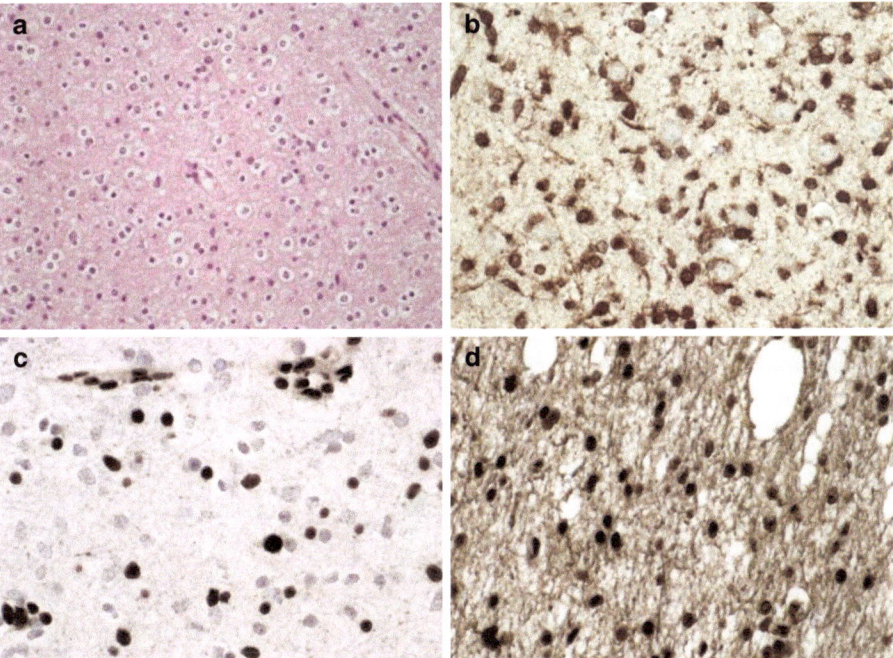

**Fig. 7.3**  Low grade gliomas. (**a**) Oligodendroglioma (grade II). Note the round nuclei with a surrounding clear zone (perinuclear halo) imparting a resemblance to fried eggs. A glioma with this histology would be expected to have an IDH mutation and a 1p/19q co-deletion. (**b**) Mutation specific immunohistochemistry for mutant IDH. The cells of this tumour shows positive staining for the mutation as would be expected in a low grade glioma such as diffuse astrocytoma (this case) and oligodendroglioma. (**c**) ATRX deleted or lost. The tumour cells in this diffuse astrocytoma do not stain with ATRX whereas the intermixed native brain cells do. This staining pattern indicates that this tumour is ATRX deleted. This tumour did not have a 1p/19q codeletion. (**d**) ATRX retained. The tumour cells in this oligodendroglioma show normal staining with ATRX. The tumour also had an IDH mutation and was 1p/19q codeleted

## 7.3.1  The Molecular Pathology of Low-Grade Gliomas

The distinction between an astrocytoma and an oligodendroglioma used to be made solely by microscopic examination of H&E-stained slides. This changed with the publication of the WHO 2016 classification. The diagnosis of an oligodendroglioma now requires the demonstration of a 1p/19q co-deletion (see section below). Furthermore, mixed gliomas, in which the tumour was composed of a mixture of oligodendroglioma and astrocytoma ('oligoastrocytoma'), used to be recognised. It is now thought that, at least on a molecular level, these mixed tumours are actually either pure oligodendrogliomas or pure astrocytomas, depending on the molecular profile, and this mixed category no longer exists [6].

The distinction between oligodendroglioma and diffuse astrocytoma is of clinical importance. It is generally accepted that oligodendroglioma has a better prognosis and a better response to chemotherapy. The median survival time for diffuse astrocytoma is reported to be in the range of 6–8 years but shows a great variation [7]. In contrast, oligodendrogliomas have a better prognosis with a median survival time of 11.6 years [3].

### 7.3.1.1 Isocitrate Dehydrogenase

Isocitrate dehydrogenase (IDH) is an enzyme involved in the Krebs cycle and therefore part of normal cellular metabolism. Two main types (isoforms) are identified and named IDH-1 and IDH-2. The vast majority of low-grade gliomas (of grade II) will have a mutation in the gene coding for IDH-1. A small minority will instead have a mutation in the gene coding for IDH-2 [8]. If a diffuse glioma does not have an IDH mutation, it is called IDH-wildtype. IDH-wildtype low-grade diffuse gliomas are unusual, and they may be expected to behave more like a high-grade glioma, despite having low-grade histological features [9]. Alternatively, the lack of an IDH mutation may indicate that the tumour is actually one of the rare grade I entities that can mimic a grade II glioma such as ganglioglioma, pilocytic astrocytoma or dysembryoplastic neuroepithelial tumour and may therefore have a better prognosis. Either way, failure to demonstrate an IDH mutation in a prima facie oligodendroglioma or diffuse astrocytoma should force a reconsideration of the diagnosis. IDH-1 mutant immunohistochemistry has revolutionised the pathological reporting of brain tumours and will detect the vast majority of IDH-mutated gliomas (Fig. 7.3b).

### 7.3.1.2 1p/19q Co-deletion

This chromosomal abnormality is characterised by the deletion of the short arm of chromosome 1 (1p) and the long arm of chromosome 19 (19q). This molecular alteration can be detected by a variety of methods including fluorescent in situ hybridisation (Fig. 7.4) or comparative genomic hybridisation (CGH). It is detected in oligodendrogliomas and therefore associated with a better prognosis and a better response to chemotherapy [9]. It also indicates a better prognosis in the context of a

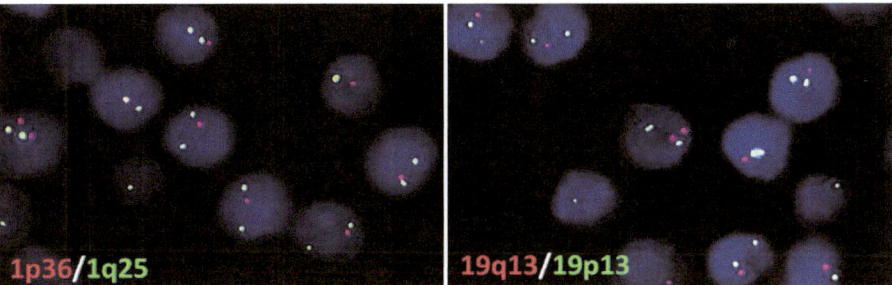

**Fig. 7.4** 1p/19q fluoresent in situ hybridisation (FISH) in an oligodendroglioma. The Vysis 1p36 and 1q25 dual colour probes (left) show 1 copy of the target locus at 1p36 (red signal) and two copies of the reference locus at 1q25 (green signal), and 19q13 and 19p13 probes (right) show one copy of the target locus at 19q13 (red) and two copies of the reference locus at 19p25 (green) in the most tumour nuclei. Note a background normal nucleus shows two copies of both 1p36 and 1q25 (left) and two copies of both 19q13 and 19p13 (right). The FISH results are consistent with the presence of a co-deletion of 1p36/19q13 in the tumour cells (picture courtesy of Dr Hongxiang Liu)

grade III glioma (anaplastic oligodendroglioma). A 1p/19q co-deletion would not be compatible with the diagnosis of glioblastoma.

### 7.3.1.3 ATRX
ATRX mutations are identified in diffuse astrocytomas and are not found in oligodendrogliomas. They can be detected with immunohistochemistry where loss of the normal nuclear staining indicates that the tumour cells have the mutation (see Fig. 7.3c). In the context of an IDH-mutated glioma of grade II or III, ATRX mutations would indicate that the tumour is an astrocytoma and not an oligodendroglioma, would not have a 1p/19q co-deletion and may have a poorer prognosis [9].

### 7.3.1.4 The Molecular Pathology of Oligodendroglioma
The diagnosis of an oligodendroglioma now requires the demonstration of two molecular changes: a mutation in either IDH-1 or (rarely) IDH-2 *and* a 1p/19q co-deletion. A tumour would not be regarded as an oligodendroglioma unless it has both of these genetic changes [1]. Oligodendrogliomas are also likely to have TERT promoter mutations and are very unlikely to have mutations in p53 (Fig. 7.5).

### 7.3.1.5 The Molecular Pathology of Diffuse Astrocytoma
Diffuse astrocytomas, like oligodendrogliomas, would usually have an IDH mutation. In contrast to oligodendrogliomas, they would also be expected to have ATRX and p53 mutations and lack a TERT promoter mutation and a 1p/19q co-deletion [10].

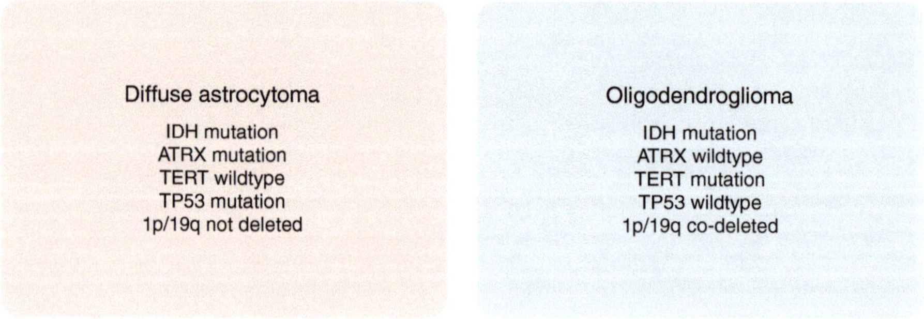

| Diffuse astrocytoma | Oligodendroglioma |
|---|---|
| IDH mutation<br>ATRX mutation<br>TERT wildtype<br>TP53 mutation<br>1p/19q not deleted | IDH mutation<br>ATRX wildtype<br>TERT mutation<br>TP53 wildtype<br>1p/19q co-deleted |

**Fig. 7.5** The molecular pathology of diffuse astrocytoma and oligodendroglioma. Note that the only mutation shared by both is IDH. Note that if an IDH mutated tumour has an ATRX mutation or a TP53 mutation it will not have an 1p/19q co-deletion and vice versa, a low grade glioma with a 1p/19q co-deletion will not have mutation in ATRX or TP53. These two molecular profiles are mutually exclusive, leading to the extinction of the concept of a mixed glioma or oligoastrocytoma

## 7.4 The Grade III (Anaplastic) Diffuse Gliomas

These are anaplastic astrocytoma and anaplastic oligodendroglioma. Both are WHO grade III. They can arise from a lower-grade diffuse glioma (diffuse astrocytoma and oligodendroglioma, respectively) but are also commonly diagnosed without evidence of a less malignant precursor.

### 7.4.1 Anaplastic Astrocytoma

These are diffusely infiltrative astrocytomas with evidence of proliferation (i.e. mitotic figures) but which lack the necrosis and microvascular proliferation that would instead define them as glioblastoma and grade IV [1]. On a molecular level, they tend to have similarities with diffuse astrocytoma (grade II) in that they tend to have an IDH mutation and an ATRX mutation. They will not have a 1p/19q co-deletion [10].

The presence of an IDH mutation is a very important prognostic indicator in grade III gliomas and anaplastic astrocytomas specifically. Historically, median survival for anaplastic astrocytoma has been quoted in the range of 3–5 years. However, a study that looked at outcomes for 562 IDH-mutated anaplastic astrocytomas showed a median survival of 9.3 years [5]. In contrast, IDH-wildtype anaplastic astrocytoma had an outcome similar to that of IDH-wildtype glioblastoma (grade IV) [11]. This is an example of how the molecular features of a tumour can prove more important than the traditional WHO grading system.

### 7.4.2 Anaplastic Oligodendroglioma

These are oligodendrogliomas with malignant features such as brisk mitotic activity, necrosis and microvascular proliferation. Like their grade II counterparts, they will have both an IDH mutation and a 1p/19q co-deletion. Failure to demonstrate these two genetic alterations means that the tumour under consideration is not an anaplastic oligodendroglioma. As well as being necessary for the diagnosis, both of these mutations are associated with a better prognosis and a better response to combined radiotherapy and chemotherapy (see Chap. 15) [12].

## 7.5    Glioblastoma

Glioblastoma is by far the most common glioma in adults and is also the most malignant. They are almost invariably fatal with only very rare exceptions. The traditional name of glioblastoma multiforme (GBM) alludes to the many different appearances that this tumour can have microscopically. They typically occur within the cerebral hemispheres, but they can occur in the brainstem, cerebellum or spinal cord. Glioblastoma is defined as the highest grade of astrocytoma—a grade IV astrocytoma and as such the tumour cells possess astrocytic characteristics. They would also be expected to show evidence of cell proliferation in the form of mitotic figures and have either necrosis, microvascular proliferation or both [1]. In glioblastomas, the necrosis is often lined by a layer of tumour cells and is referred to as palisading necrosis (Fig. 7.1d). Microvascular proliferation is the abnormal growth of small blood vessels within the tumour (Fig. 7.1c) and is another cardinal feature of glioblastoma.

Glioblastoma can be divided broadly into two different types—secondary glioblastoma—which constitute approximately 10% of all glioblastomas and arise from a low-grade precursor (usually a grade II diffuse astrocytoma). In contrast, approximately 90% arise de novo, without a low-grade precursor, and are termed primary glioblastoma. Generally speaking, secondary glioblastomas tend to occur at a younger age of onset, 20s to 40s, and have a better prognosis. The distinction between secondary versus primary glioblastomas is more or less determined by the presence or absence of IDH mutations [1].

In the same fashion that a modern molecular understanding of low-grade glioma has put an end to the diagnosis of the mixed 'oligoastrocytoma', it has also led to the conceptual extinction of mixed high-grade gliomas, and the glioblastoma with oligodendroglial component (GBM-O) no longer exists [13].

## 7.5.1    The Molecular Pathology of Glioblastoma

Two molecular changes have been associated with a longer survival in glioblastoma—IDH mutations and *O6-methylguanine-DNA methyltransferase* (MGMT) promoter methylation (see Figs. 7.6 and 7.7).

### 7.5.1.1 Glioblastoma, IDH-Wildtype

Glioblastomas that do not have mutations in the genes for IDH are termed IDH-wildtype (Fig. 7.6a). These represent approximately 90% of glioblastomas. They have a peak incidence in patients aged 55–85 years (mean, 62 years [14]). Most

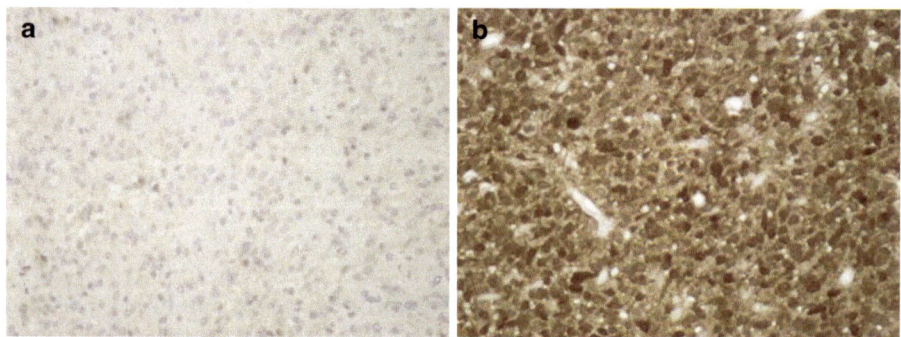

**Fig. 7.6** IDH wildtype and mutant glioblastomas. (**a**) There is no staining for IDH-mutant anti-bodies in this primary glioblastoma (Glioblastoma, IDH-wildtype). This tumour would be expected to have a worse prognosis than the mutated one depicted in 5b. Unfortunately, the IDH-wildtype glioblastoma represents 90% of these tumours. (**b**) There is staining for IDH-mutant antibodies in this secondary glioblastoma (Glioblastoma, IDH-mutant). This tumour would be expected to have a better prognosis than the wildtype one depicted in Fig. 7.5a

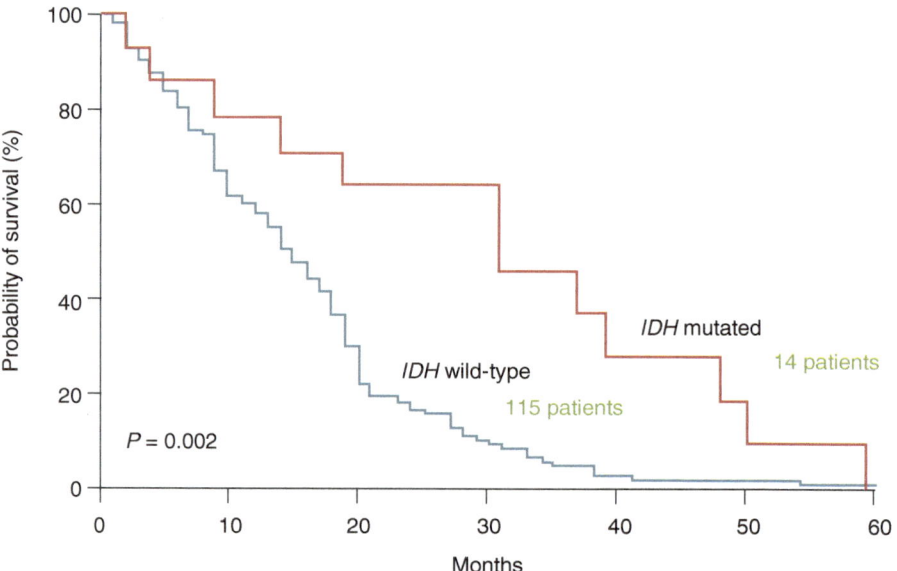

**Fig. 7.7** The difference in survival of IDH-mutated glioblastomas compared with IDH-wildtype glioblastomas. Note a considerably better survival curve those with IDH-mutated tumours. From *Hai Yan et al., New England Journal of Medicine 2009*

patients die within 15–18 months of diagnosis, and less than 5% of patients are still alive after 5 years. The mean overall survival of patients with an IDH-wildtype glioblastoma, having been treated with radiotherapy and chemotherapy, is 11.3 months [15].

### 7.5.1.2 Glioblastoma, IDH-Mutant

Approximately 10% of glioblastomas have mutations in the IDH gene, usually IDH-1 but occasionally IDH-2 (Fig. 7.6b). These tumours develop in patients that are significantly younger (mean, 45 years) [3]. IDH-mutated glioblastomas have a longer survival than IDH-wildtype glioblastomas. The mean overall survival of patients with an IDH-mutated glioblastoma, having been treated with radiotherapy and chemotherapy, is 27.1 months, 2.4 times as long as that of patients with an IDH-wildtype glioblastoma [16].

### 7.5.1.3 Histone-Mutated Gliomas

Mutations in the histone genes have recently been demonstrated in a subset of high-grade gliomas [17]. The histone H3.3 K27M mutation is almost exclusively seen in high-grade gliomas occurring in the midline structures of the central nervous system (basal ganglia, thalamus, brainstem, cerebellum and spinal cord). These are known as diffuse midline gliomas. This new category incorporates most cases that used to be called diffuse intrinsic pontine glioma (DIPG). These tumours may also have ATRX mutations. They tend to occur in children and generally have a very poor prognosis.

### 7.5.1.4 MGMT Promoter Methylation

MGMT is a DNA repair protein. It repairs the damage done to DNA by alkylating chemotherapy agents such as temozolomide. If the promoter region for MGMT is methylated, the gene is 'switched off', and the damage done to tumour cell DNA by temozolomide is repaired less effectively. For this reason, if a glioblastoma is 'MGMT promoter methylated', it will tend to respond more to temozolomide. MGMT promoter methylation is therefore associated with improved survival in patients with glioblastoma when treated with temozolomide. Approximately 50% of glioblastomas are MGMT promoter methylated, but over 90% of long-surviving glioblastoma patients have MGMT promoter methylation [18].

## 7.6   Conclusion

The pathological classification of adult glioma requires determining both the type of glioma (astrocytoma or oligodendroglioma) and the grade of the glioma (generally II, III or IV for adult gliomas). Determining the glioma type requires examining tumour tissue with a microscope and may also involve conducting various molecular tests. The grade is usually still determined solely by the tumour's histological features, but certain molecular properties may indicate a better or worse prognosis or treatment response. In general, the molecular changes associated with a better prognosis in adult glioma of grade II and III are the presence of an IDH mutation and the presence of a 1p/19q co-deletion. For the highest grade of glioma (glioblastoma), the two most important prognostic molecular changes are the presence of an IDH mutation and the presence of MGMT promoter methylation. Even with both these changes, glioblastoma has a poor long-term survival rate. Further research into these tumours will undoubtedly reveal further prognostic biomarkers and hopefully new therapies that will treat, or at least control, these devastating diseases in the future.

## References

1. Louis DN, Perry A, Reifenberger G, et al. The 2016 World Health Organization classification of tumors of the central nervous system: a summary. Acta Neuropathol. 2016;131:803–20.
2. Theeler BJ, Ellezam B, Sadighi ZS, Mehta V, Diep Tran M, Adesina AM, Bruner JM, Puduvalli VK. Adult pilocytic astrocytomas: clinical features and molecular analysis. Neuro Oncol. 2014;16(6):841–7.
3. Ohgaki H, Kleihues P. Population-based studies on incidence, survival rates, and genetic alterations in astrocytic and oligodendroglial gliomas. J Neuropathol Exp Neurol. 2005;64(6):479–89. https://doi.org/10.1093/jnen/64.6.479.
4. Modrek AS, Bayin NS, Placantonakis DG. Brain stem cells as the cell of origin in glioma. World J Stem Cells. 2014;6(1):43–52. https://doi.org/10.4252/wjsc.v6.i1.43.
5. Reuss DE, Mamatjan Y, Schrimpf D, et al. IDH mutant diffuse and anaplastic astrocytomas have similar age at presentation and little difference in survival: a grading problem for WHO. Acta Neuropathol. 2015;129(6):867–73. https://doi.org/10.1007/s00401-015-1438-8.
6. Sahm F, Reuss D, Koelsche C, Capper D, Schittenhelm J, Heim S, Jones DT, Pfister SM, Herold-Mende C, Wick W, Mueller W, Hartmann C, Paulus W, von Deimling A. Farewell to oligoastrocytoma: in situ molecular genetics favor classification as either oligodendroglioma or astrocytoma. Acta Neuropathol. 2014;128(4):551–9. https://doi.org/10.1007/s00401-014-1326.
7. Bourne D, Schiff D. Update on molecular findings, management and outcome in low-grade gliomas. Nat Rev Neurol. 2010;6:695–701.
8. Cohen A, Holmen S, Colman H. IDH1 and IDH2 Mutations in Gliomas. Curr Neurol Neurosci Rep. 2013;13(5):345. https://doi.org/10.1007/s11910-013-0345-4.
9. Leeper HE, Caron AA, Decker PA, Jenkins RB, Lachance DH, Giannini C. IDH mutation, 1p19q codeletion and ATRX loss in WHO grade II gliomas. Oncotarget. 2015;6(30):30295–305.
10. Eckel-Passow JE, Lachance DH, Molinaro AM, Walsh KM, Decker PA, Sicotte H, et al. Glioma groups based on 1p/19q, IDH, and TERT promoter mutations in tumors. N Engl J Med. 2015;372(26):2499–508. https://doi.org/10.1056/NEJMoa1407279.
11. Hartmann C, Hentschel B, Wick W, Capper D, Felsberg J, Simon M, Von Deimling A. Patients with IDH1 wild type anaplastic astrocytomas exhibit worse prognosis than IDH1-mutated glioblastomas, and IDH1 mutation status accounts for the unfavorable prognostic effect of higher age: implications for classification of gliomas. Acta Neuropathol. 2010;120(6):707–18. https://doi.org/10.1007/s00401-010-0781-z.
12. van den Bent M, Brandes A, Taphoorn M, Kros J, Kouwenhoven M, Delattre J, Bernsen HJ, Frenay M, Tijssen C, Grisold W, Sipos L, Enting R, French P, Dinjens W, Vecht C, Allgeier A, Lacombe D, Gorlia T, Hoang-Xuan K. Adjuvant procarbazine, lomustine, and vincristine chemotherapy in newly diagnosed anaplastic oligodendroglioma: long-term follow-up of EORTC brain tumor group study 26951. J Clin Oncol. 2013;31(3):344.
13. Hinrichs BH, Newman S, Appin CL, et al. Farewell to GBM-O: Genomic and transcriptomic profiling of glioblastoma with oligodendroglioma component reveals distinct molecular subgroups. Acta Neuropathol Commun. 2016;4:4. https://doi.org/10.1186/s40478-015-0270-7.
14. Ostrom QT, Gittleman H, Liao P, Rouse C, Chen Y, Dowling J, Wolinsky Y, Kruchko C, Barnholtz-Sloan J. CBTRUS statistical report: primary brain and central nervous system tumors diagnosed in the United States in 2007–2011. Neuro Oncol. 2014;16(Suppl 4):iv1.
15. Purkait S, Mallick S, Sharma V, et al. Prognostic stratification of GBMs using combinatorial assessment of IDH1 mutation, MGMT promoter methylation, and TERT mutation status:

experience from a tertiary care center in India. Transl Oncol. 2016;9(4):371–6. https://doi.org/10.1016/j.tranon.2016.06.005.

16. Nobusawa S, Watanabe T, Kleihues P, Ohgaki H. IDH1 mutations as molecular signature and predictive factor of secondary glioblastomas. Clin Cancer Res. 2009;15(19):6002–7. https://doi.org/10.1158/1078-0432.CCR-09-0715.

17. Schwartzentruber J, et al. Driver mutations in histone H3.3 and chromatin remodelling genes in paediatric glioblastoma. Nature. 2012;482:226–U119.

18. Hegi ME, Diserens AC, Gorlia T, Hamou MF, De Tribolet N, Weller M, et al. MGMT gene silencing and benefit from temozolomide in glioblastoma. N Engl J Med. 2005;352(10): 997–1003. https://doi.org/10.1056/NEJMoa043331.

# Pre- and Post-operative Complications

8

Ingela Oberg

**Abstract**

The predominant factor of undergoing glioma surgery is not one of cure, since this cannot be achieved. The main purpose is to establish a definitive diagnosis and to achieve cytoreduction, in order to stabilise and hopefully improve the neurological deficits and also to enable other treatment options (such as radiotherapy and/or chemotherapy) to be more effective, as they have less residual tumour bulk to deal with.

However, no surgery is without risks, and this is very much the case with neurosurgery, especially when dealing with gliomas that diffusely infiltrate the surrounding brain tissue, destroying specific functions as they grow and causing irreversible damage to the brain. Wound healing impairment, surgical site infections (SSI) and post-operative morbidity are serious problems in neurosurgery, associated with prolonged inpatient stays, increased costs and patient discomfort. Thirty-day readmission rates have become a proxy for quality of care, contributing significantly to high health-care costs. Helping to reduce surgical complications and improve patient's quality of life is pivotal to neurosurgical nursing.

This chapter will therefore explore some of the more common surgical complications associated with glioma surgery (both pre- and post-operatively) and help equip the novice nurse with practical information about how to not only identify surgical problems early but also how to treat them effectively and how to help the patients and their carers cope with long-term side effects and adapt to a new way of living with a life-limiting disease.

I. Oberg (✉)
Department of Neurosurgery, Addenbrooke's Hospital, Cambridge University Hospitals NHS Foundation Trust, Cambridgeshire, UK
e-mail: Ingela.oberg@addenbrookes.nhs.uk

© Springer Nature Switzerland AG 2019
I. Oberg (ed.), *Management of Adult Glioma in Nursing Practice*,
https://doi.org/10.1007/978-3-319-76747-5_8

**Keywords**
Glioma surgery · Neurosurgery · Wound infections · Surgical site infections ·
Brain tumours · Post-operative complications

**Learning Outcomes**
- Be able to identify some of the more common pre-operative complications that glioma patients can develop or present with, and how these are managed.
- Be able to identify and safely manage some of the more common post-operative complications following glioma surgery.
- Be able to identify a rapidly deteriorating neurosurgical patient and know how to escalate and document any concerns accordingly.

## 8.1    Pre- and Post-operative Wound Care

If one was to audit the post-operative wound care advice given to patients upon discharge from each neurosurgical centre in the UK, there would undoubtedly be a vast variation in practice. There are no specific guidelines to adhere to, merely generic recommendations that apply to surgery in general, but not neuro-oncology specifically [1].

What we do know about wound care is that every measure needs to be taken to help minimise risks of infection, both pre- and post-operatively, as any infection in a newly operated glioma patient will prevent or delay the start of concomitant or adjuvant treatment with oncology. *Staphylococcus aureus*, for example, is a very prevalent skin bacterium, which causes no harm whilst on the surface of the skin. If it gets into the surgical wound however, it can quickly establish a foothold and can become a superbug known as MRSA (multiresistant *Staphylococcus aureus*), which in turn can have serious complications for the patients' health and wellbeing [2, 3].

## 8.2    Hair Shaving

Patients frequently ask if they should shave their head prior to (and in preparation for) surgery, as they often have misconceptions around hair removal requirements for neurosurgery. This would be advised against, as razors can cause irritation to the skin surface, resulting in raised, swollen and inflamed hair follicles (known as razor burn), which in turn allow for easier transmission of the skin bacteria into the wound cavity. It is recommended hair shaving for surgical purposes takes place in the operating room with single-use (disposable) clippers to minimise infection risks. Only minimal hair shaving is done, a few centimetres margin around the scar itself [1, 4, 5].

Once surgery has been undertaken, the patient is often returned to the ward setting with a surgical pressure bandage in situ. Depending on the type and complexity of surgery, it is recommended this dressing is taken off within 24–48 h to allow for adequate and accurate wound observations and documentation [1].

Creating a hot, moist environment is a breeding ground for bacteria to establish themselves, so closed surgical wounds are often better left open to air, with simple surgical tape over the sutures should minimal oozing continue. Scarves or headwear can be worn when out and about should the patients feel it is unsightly.

## 8.3   Wound Closure

Closing of surgical wounds is very much down to surgical preference. There are no current guidelines within the UK on which techniques to use for primary or recurrent glioma surgery, and listed below are the varying techniques used for wound closure:

*Nylon sutures*—This is a very commonly used suturing technique, and the sutures are normally removed 7–10 days after surgery by either a general practitioner (GP) practice nurse or by the neurosurgical specialist nurse, which then allows for detailed review of the wound at the same time. For early reoperations requiring reopening of the surgical scar, the sutures would normally stay in for around 14 days to ensure good wound closure [4].

*Vicryl rapide (self-absorbing sutures)*—This is an increasingly common technique to use mainly due to convenience—many glioma patients find it difficult to get to a GP surgery in the early post-operative days due to their inability to drive and/or due to their general clinical condition. With self-dissolving sutures, very little needs to be done from a patient or carers perspective. The wound needs to be kept dry for around 3 days following surgery. Gentle washing with mild (baby) shampoo is recommended as other products may be quite abrasive and may sting as a result, in turn causing the patient to scratch their fragile wound and further increasing the risk of infections.

Self-absorbing sutures need to become wet to dissolve, so after the initial period of keeping it dry, patients are recommended to soak the sutures in the shower and pat the wound dry with a clean towel. Strands of sutures will poke out of the scar as they dissolve, and it is important to advise the patient not to cut or pull them as a result. Normally the sutures completely dissolve within a 3-week period, but they have been known to take up to 6 weeks in some instances [4].

*Staples*—Surgical staples (or clips) are also a very commonly used closing technique. The staples are removed within 7–10 days after surgery depending on factors such as size and location of the scar. They are quick and easy to administer at the time of surgery. They have a lower frequency of keloid scarring and are straight forward to remove with staple removers. Often alternative staples are removed if the scar is large (e.g. a bifrontal craniotomy), with the remaining staples to be removed 3–5 days later [4].

The downside of surgical staples is that the patient has to be discharged home with staple removers as this is not something GP surgeries have in stock due to the specialism involved. Hence, it is often more convenient to remove them as part of their neurosurgical follow-up, allowing for wound observations to be recorded at the same time.

## 8.4    Cerebral Spinal Fluid (CSF) Leak

CSF surrounds the brain and spinal cord (central nervous system) supplying it with vital nutrients. It is a very proteinaceous fluid, laden with (amongst other things) proteins and glucose. As such, it is a very attractive substance for bacteria, as it gorges on the nutrients required to multiply. A CSF infection can therefore be very serious and lead to bacterial meningitis [6]. As a rule of thumb, if any wound leaks CSF, it is a sign that the fluid can seep out, and subsequently, 'bugs' can get it. Most CSF leaks will require hospitalisation to find the leak, repair the defect and monitor the patient for clinical signs of infection.

During surgery, after the craniotomy (removal of a portion of the skull), the dural layers need to be cut in order for the brain to be exposed and the tumour reached. The dural membranes consist of three layers (dura, arachnoid and pia mater—see Chap. 1 for further details)—the dura mater is a watertight layer which seals the CSF inside the central nervous system and prevents it from leaking out [7].

CSF leak is (along with SSI) one of the most prevalent complications following neurosurgery. CSF leaks are more common in endo-nasal approaches, which will require post-operative nasal douching with saline solution. It is also very common following head trauma, where the dura mater has been sheared or torn as a result. However, it is not uncommon in other neurosurgical methods, where the dural layers have been disrupted, such as with glioma resections.

CSF leaks are normally relatively easy to identify. It is a clear fluid that is constantly dripping and running, with tear-like droplets forming at the scar, continually seeping. Depending on the surgical approach, CSF can also drip continually from the nose (rhinorrhoea), but this is less common following glioma surgery. Sometimes the leak only becomes apparent when lying down and the intracranial pressure is elevated. It may dry on the pillow case with a halo effect. To confirm the fluid is indeed CSF, a sample will need to be collected in a sterile specimen pot and send it off to microbiology for beta-2 transferrin testing—this is a protein nearly exclusively found in CSF [6].

Treatment for a CSF leak depends on the severity and location of the leak and the clinical condition of the patient. In some instances, all that may be required is an additional suture—in other cases a lumbar puncture or even a lumbar drain may be required to minimise raised intracranial pressure around the affected area, giving it time to heal spontaneously. In extreme cases reopening of the craniotomy and re-closure of the dura with additional dural seals, fibrin glue or dural replacements may be required [8].

## 8.5    Baseline Observations

Post-operative baseline observations include blood pressure and temperature readings, in conjunction with blood tests such as white cell count and CRP (C-reactive protein, an infection marker). Visual inspection of the wound is also vital—does it look 'angry' and swollen? Is it erythematous (red and inflamed looking) along with worsening swelling? An easy way to establish this is to outline the edges of the swollen area with a skin marker pen and see if the swelling exceeds this boundary line next time it is reviewed. Of note, post-operative swelling is to be expected; post-operative infections are not. Is the wound seeping, and if so, is it normal serous fluid or a mixture of blood/pus? Is it clear water-like fluid that seeps or drips regularly from the wound, more so on lying down? If so, this is often a sign of CSF leakage which requires prompt intervention (see above section for more details). Is the wound very sore or hot to touch? If there is any clinical doubt, also swab the wound and send it to microbiology for testing.

## 8.6   Dehiscence

When a wound opens up partially or fully along the suture line, this is known as dehiscence. This is not very common but can happen if the skin is taught and fragile from treatments such as long-term steroid use, repeated operations to the same area or previous radiotherapy (RT) treatment to the same area—all of which makes the skin fragile [9]. In patients with a glioma on a short-course (accelerated) RT, treatment may commence within 2 weeks of surgery, meaning adequate wound healing may not have ensued, leaving the patient at slightly higher risk of dehiscence occurring [9]. Patients with severe and prolonged wound infections are also at risk of dehiscence—in some instances, involvement of plastic surgery teams may be required to help with skin grafting and tissue expanders to ensure adequate wound closure in very difficult cases.

Mild dehiscence can sometimes be treated by a GP or practice nurse with Steri-Strips or wound glue. However, in most instances, this will require surgical re-closure of the wound, and sutures are left in situ for longer (minimum 14 days) to ensure adequate knitting together of underlying muscles and tissues [4].

## 8.7   Surgical Site Infection (SSI)

Post-operative SSIs following primary glioma surgery are estimated to be in the region of 5%, rising to around 20% for glioma re-resections, following completion of chemotherapy and radiotherapy and prolonged use of steroids [9].

The reason for this large escalation of infection risk is twofold. Firstly, the surgeon needs to cut through the same incision line as previously and reopen the dura, both of which will have developed scar tissue formation and possible dural adhesions. This makes knitting of the fibrous tissues and muscles after second surgery much more fragile. Secondly, the wound will also be brittle as a result of likely dexamethasone usage (dexamethasone suppresses the immune system and is known to delay wound healing and cause thinning of the skin), and previous (possible) radiotherapy treatment, further adding to the risk of infection, abscess and dehiscence [9].

### 8.7.1 Abscess

An abscess can develop anywhere in the brain, but if related to prior surgery, it normally manifests itself within 6–12 weeks in the surgical scar (wound infection), in the underlying bone (osteomyelitis), or it can track along the surgical resection margin and develop deep inside the tumour cavity and/or the surrounding brain tissue (abscess). As most glioma patients will be on high-dose dexamethasone for a period immediately post-operatively, the risk of developing a SSI remains high following glioma surgery [10].

Clinical signs of sepsis (e.g. blood pressure changes, tachycardia and pyrexia) can be difficult to detect if the patient has been on dexamethasone, which can mask infection markers. The only certain way to detect an abscess is via neuroimaging, predominantly a contrast-enhanced CT head, to see if pockets of contrast-enhanced infection are picked up. For infection purposes a CT head is normally quicker to obtain in an emergency situation, and if required, a more detailed MRI head with diffusion-weighted imaging (DWI) to rule out (or in!) the presence of centrally restricted diffusion, confirming an abscess, can be undertaken.

In terms of an intracranial abscess (pre- or post-operatively), this is dealt as a clinical emergency with prompt neurosurgical intervention and aspiration of the abscess to help minimise long-term consequences. If not dealt with promptly, abscesses within the brain can be fatal or lead to non-reversible brain damage [10]. Once pus has been aspirated, this is sent to microbiology for culturing, and the type and duration of antibiotic therapy would normally be commenced on microbiology advice and input. In certain circumstances within the UK, if the patient is otherwise clinically well, long-term intravenous antibiotics (around 6 weeks of duration) can be administered by the outpatient antibiotic therapy (OPAT) teams, enabling the patient to be discharged home from the hospital, receiving treatment in the community setting, freeing up vital hospital capacity.

### 8.7.2 Osteomyelitis

As noted in chapter 6, the *bone flap* (section of the skull) is removed at the time of glioma surgery (craniotomy) - this is sterilised and is ready to be replaced towards the end of surgery, once the tumour has been excised. The skull (like any bone) is a porous substance, much like a honeycomb in its appearance, which means once an infection sets in, it is easy for the infection to establish itself within these porous cavities [7], predominantly as this section of the skull has no blood supply to enable white blood cells to adequtely fight any infection.

An infection in the bone flap itself is extremely difficult to eradicate, leading to a condition known as osteomyelitis. This will require prolonged inpatient stay for around 6 weeks or more of intravenous (IV) administered antibiotics, inevitably delaying the next crucial phase of the patients' planned treatment. In some instances, these additional week's delays are enough time for the glioma to regrow, and treatment trajectories subsequently alter from active treatment to one of palliation.

Preventing prolonged inpatient stay with IV antibiotics is vital for the patient's well-being, medically, mentally and physically, and not least for the national health economy. This includes having a low threshold for a surgical review of the patient, should they have concerns about their wound. In many cases, the clinical nurse specialist (often referred to as a CNS or key worker) will arrange to see the patient as a ward attender or in clinic for a wound consult, rather than sending them to their general practitioner (GP) for review. Ultimately it is a surgical decision if the bone flap needs to be removed, either as a precaution or because it is infected—and that is not a decision a GP can make.

## 8.8   Pseudomeningoceles

This type of wound problem is very commonly found after posterior fossa surgery where the CSF passes through the fourth ventricle and down through the spinal canal. It can be common for fluid to seep through the craniotomy scar and 'pool' under the skin surface, as is demonstrated below (Image 8.1). Treatments of pseudomeningoceles are often managed conservatively with a 'watch-and-wait' approach, unless there are clinical signs of obvious infection. The reason for this is any insertion of a needle to drain fluid will simply allow the fluid to reaccumulate. Furthermore, every time an aspiration is performed, the risk of introducing a nosocomial infection increases. Over time, the fluid should reabsorb gradually, but if it is persistently causing problems with ongoing treatment options (like fitting of RT mask which will be difficult due to altered swelling), or low-pressure headaches, then a surgical conduit or shunt can be considered [11].

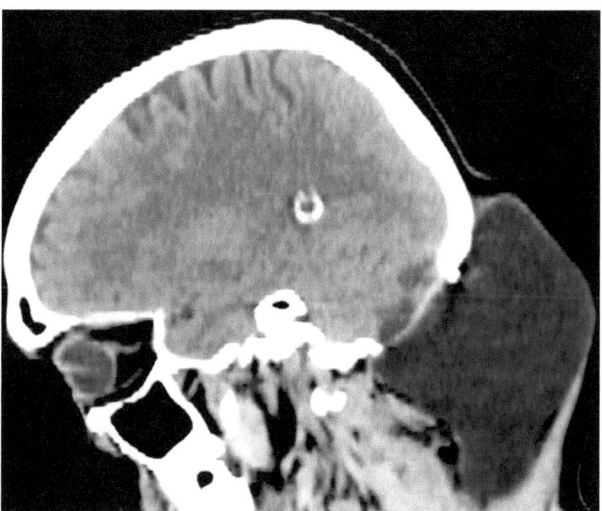

**Image 8.1** Image below shows large post fossa pseudomeningocele on unenhanced CT scan, measuring around 14 cm overlying the suboccipital craniectomy

## 8.9 Evacuation of Acute Haematoma

There are two types of haematomas (blood clots) that can occur as a direct result of head trauma but which are also recognised complications of surgery to the brain: subdural haematoma and extradural haematoma.

*Subdural haematomas* occurring hours or a few days after surgery are referred to as *acute* subdural haematomas. They occur as a result of venous damage, and blood seeps from the damaged vessels, creating a collection (normally in the shape of a thin 'crescent moon') between the skull and the surface of the brain. Sometimes, these bleeds don't manifest themselves until some weeks after surgery, and this is referred to as *subacute* or *chronic* haematoma—they are often treated conservatively unless clinical signs of raised intracranial pressure are manifested.

An *extradural (epidural) haematoma* is a blood clot that forms between the inner surface of the skull and the outer layer of the dura. This is often caused by trauma to the head, with the source of bleeding usually arterial, hence the potential for rapid neurological decline with life-threatening implications and consequences (see image 8.2 below) [7].

Acute subdural haematomas and extradural haematomas (also referred to as epidural bleeds) with clinical signs of raised ICP and neurological deterioration require surgical drainage (either via burr hole or craniotomy) to prevent long-term damage or even death.

Clinical deterioration could involve fluctuating GCS (Glasgow Coma Score—see Chap. 3), acute confusion, hemiparesis and/or speech difficulties. Pupil(s) can become sluggish to light stimulation or even become fixed and dilated (unresponsive). Other symptoms may also involve worsening headaches (not alleviated by analgesics) along with vomiting, neck stiffness and photophobia [7, 12]. It is vital to perform and document regular nursing observations and highlight and escalate any concerns you may have early. A CT head can confirm the presence of either form of haematoma.

## 8.10 Venous Thromboembolism (VTE)

VTE is a disease that includes deep vein thrombosis (DVT) and pulmonary embolisms (PE), occurring in approximately 3% of patients undergoing brain tumour resections, including gliomas [13]. All patients should have a VTE risk assessment completed to identify and minimise risks, and patients should be fully mobilised within 24 h following surgery, where possible. If complete bed rest is indicated, or if the patient is requiring assistance (e.g. hemiparesis), ensure prophylactic regime with relevant anticoagulation is prescribed and signed for, once administered. In many neurosurgical centres, ALL patients receive prophylactic anticoagulation unless contraindicated, to minimise risks of post-operative VTEs. Applying compression stockings for all inpatients is also a must in the UK—they need to be accurately measured to ensure a good fit to aid in capillary and deep venous return [14].

Clinical signs of a PE would include sudden onset of shortness of breath (SOB), low saturations and shallow breathing with a stabbing pain on inhalation. Central chest pain in some patients can mimic signs of a heart attack. Prompt clinical intervention is required, as PEs can be fatal: sit the patient upright with legs down to take pressure off the heart and lungs; check saturations and blood tests for D-dimers; and ensure high-flow oxygen is administered via a facial mask. Ensure the medical team is alerted immediately—an urgent chest X-ray and CT pulmonary angiogram (CTPA) will be required to confirm the presence of clots and to also rule out other causes such as severe chest infection or a collapsed lung [15].

Once a clot (embolism) is confirmed, treatment will vary according to local guidelines and size and number of clots found. If PEs happen prior to surgery, consider having an inferior vena cava (IVC) filter placed via interventional radiology to prevent clots from dislodging and spreading during (or shortly after) surgery. This can be done as a day-case procedure under local anaesthetic. The IVC filters are normally removed post-operatively on an individual basis once the patient has fully recovered, around a month or so after surgery [15].

Signs of DVT include red, swollen calf muscle with redness and tenderness to touch. The calf swelling is normally unilateral and not bilateral and can feel hot to touch [15]. A DVT can happen several weeks after surgery so can be a continued risk, especially if patients go home and take to bed. A leg ultrasound (doppler) can establish the presence of a DVT, and treatment would be as per local guidelines as described above.

## 8.11  Dysphasia

There are two types of dysphasia: expressive and receptive, both of which are very common in patients with a glioma, particularly those who have a tumour in the left fronto-temporal area as this (in most right-handed patients) is the dominant area for the speech and language cortex [16].

'Expressive dysphasia' means a difficulty in *forming* the correct words and creating complete, coherent sentences. Often patients know what they want to say, but the words come out jumbled and can sometimes be completely incomprehensible. 'Receptive dysphasia' means the patient has difficulties in *interpreting* and comprehending the spoken words of other people.

Some patients with dysphasia also suffer from dysphagia, which is a medical term for having difficulties with swallowing. Symptoms can range from mild (dribbling, hoarse voice) to extreme (consistently choking on food). Patients with both dysphasia and dysphagia will need a thorough examination and evaluation by a speech and language technician (SALT) and a dietician to ensure patient safety is maintained and any possible requirements (such as thickened fluids), for continued and adequate nutritional needs, are met.

### 8.11.1  Aphasia

'Aphasia' is a complex communication disorder, meaning the patient is unable to formulate or comprehend language and is unable to read or write [7, 16]. In particular, patients with receptive and aphasic difficulties need to have their capacity assessed and their safeguarding needs taken into consideration (please see Chap. 13 for further details).

For patients with frontal and temporal gliomas in their dominant hemisphere (primarily left sided), surgery is often performed with the patient being awake throughout the procedure in order to fully map and assess their speech functionality during surgery and to minimise risks of developing dysphasia or aphasia as a neurosurgical complication [16].

## 8.12  Hemiparesis/Hemiplegia

Hemiparesis is defined as having a unilateral weakness on one side of the whole body. There is normally some functional ability there, even if mild. For instance, the patient may be able to wiggle their finger or hold someone's hand but not be able to squeeze it. Hemiplegia, however, is a total paralysis of one side of the body with no functional ability. Both can be a temporary or permanent disability.

For glioma patients, treatment would normally comprise of steroid treatment with high-dose dexamethasone (e.g. 8 mg BD). This is to establish whether the symptoms are due to oedema (i.e. pressure-related effects), which would subsequently resolve the symptoms, and function would return to (near) normal. If the symptoms do not improve with dexamethasone, then the tumour has likely infiltrated and permanently damaged this part of the brain and caused irreversible harm. In such instance, the merits and perceived benefits of surgery need to be considered and closely discussed in a multidisciplinary team (MDT) setting and subsequently with the patients and their caregivers.

Physiotherapists (PT) and occupational therapists (OT) need to fully assess the patients to ensure they are safe prior to discharge. In the UK, we would do 'stair assessment' with the physiotherapists to ensure the patients can safely and independently navigate a flight of stairs with minimal assistance to minimise falls risk. A 'kitchen assessment' is also undertaken with the OTs when a glioma patient has a weakness or has a residual impairment, such as confusion, to ensure they are safe and have the right manual handling equipment to enable them to remain independent. This may include equipment such as grab rails in the bath, to a bannister on either side of the stairs, to a commode or raised toilet seat. Referrals to community-based teams are instigated at this point as required.

From a nursing perspective, considerations need to be taken into account to help minimise complications associated with weakness or paralysis. Frequent repositioning to prevent pressure ulcers and elevating the affected limb on pillows to allow for adequate venous return need to be undertaken and documented. Falls risk needs to be done, along with a VTE assessment. Any changes in functionality should be documented and passed on to the relevant teams looking after that patient, either as a sign of ongoing recovery or as a potential and early sign of post-operative complications which in turn may require further investigations.

## 8.13  Posterior Fossa Syndrome

This is sometimes referred to as *cerebellar mutism syndrome* and is a rare surgical complication caused by surgery to the post fossa region. It is more common in children and the developing brain as opposed to adults, but it has been documented frequently enough within the adult population too. Symptoms include speech disturbances, dysphagia, decreased motor movement, facial nerve palsies as well as emotional lability [17]. Speech and language therapy (SALT) input is required for a swallow assessment and to obtain appropriate communication aids. A referral to a clinical neuropsychologist is also required to rule in (or out) psychological aspects that may be contributing to the post fossa syndrome.

From a brain tumour/glioma perspective, full recovery is anticipated as long as there is no evidence of stroke or other compounding factors; however, a time frame is difficult to establish, and the patient would be a suitable candidate for full inpatient neuro-rehabilitation, depending on age, performance status and overall prognosis [17].

## 8.14   Supplementary Motor Area (SMA) Syndrome

SMA is a rare post-operative complication following surgery to the supplementary motor area, predominantly following surgery to the parietal lobe, or the posterior fronal lobe. Patients will exhibit a reduction of spontaneous movement and difficulty in performing voluntary muscle movements on the contralateral side to where surgery was performed, despite normal muscle tone. Main features of SMA include hemi-sensory neglect and apraxia, both of which are explored in more detail below [18].

Patients with SMA are expected to regain their motor functions within weeks to months, on the proviso the sensory-motor area was not permanently damaged at the time of surgery (or directly thereafter); and their neurological symptoms abated preoperatively with dexamethasone treatment, indicating these issues were predominantly oedema related in the first instance.

### 8.14.1  Apraxia

Apraxia (sometimes referred to as dyspraxia if symptoms are mild) is a neurological disorder where the affected person loses the ability to perform certain movements and gestures to command, even though their muscles and muscle tone are normal. Apraxia results from dysfunction of the cerebral hemispheres (in particular the parietal lobe) and can arise from damage to the brain, such as that caused by glioma surgery, especially if the tumour involved the motor or supplementary motor area [18].

Another common example of apraxia would be *speech apraxia*, where the patient has an inability to coordinate the tongue and muscles involved to produce speech, despite there being no abnormality to the muscles involved. Speech apraxia is not to be confused with aphasia however, and although they have similar manifestations whereby the patients have problems with expressing themselves with words, they have very different pathophysiologies behind them. Aphasia means the person has lost the ability to comprehend words themselves, whereas speech apraxia means the person has an articulation disorder and problems in initiating (and performing) the movements involved to create the spoken word.

## 8.14.2 Hemi-sensory Neglect/Inattention

Sensory neglect is where the brain has an impaired ability to perceive objects or stimuli from one side of the body. This can be caused by damage to the brain, such as that caused by a glioma or from surgery. In a healthy brain, both right and left cerebral hemispheres attend to the right spatial awareness, but only the right hemisphere attends to the left side of space. Hence, left-sided inattention is more common and often more severe in patients with hemi-sensory neglect [19].

Manifestations of sensory neglect are normally quite easy to detect. A patient who dresses themselves simply forgets to dress one side of their body, leaving arms outside of sleeves, or forgets socks and slippers on one foot. They will be unable to see a person approaching the bedside from one side, for example, so in order not to scare a patient by suddenly appearing out of nowhere, consider how and where the patient is placed in a ward environment. Stand in front of the patients or along their 'good side' so that they are aware of your presence and can fully interact.

If the neglect is due to SMA, full recovery of the symptoms is to be expected, normally over the course of several weeks. However, it is important to recognise that hemi-sensory neglect can also be a lasting result following a cerebral infarction (stroke), not uncommonly seen following extensive glioma resections. Should this be the case, symptoms are likely to be more enduring and severe with a poor prognostic indicator of future functional independence [19].

## 8.15  Post-operative Stroke

There are two main types of stroke, both commonly seen in patients with gliomas: ischaemic stroke and haemorrhagic stroke. An ischaemic stroke is where a blood clot blocks off the blood flow to that part of the brain, starving it of oxygen and nutrients. *Ischaemia* means reduced blood flow, and if this is compromising oxygenation to that part of the brain, it eventually strokes out [20]. As such, ischaemic strokes can sometimes be a direct consequence of a surgical intervention such as glioma surgery, where blood vessels have been cauterised during surgery (to prevent bleeding in the first place), increasing the risk of developing reduced flow or a clot.

A haemorrhagic stroke (also known as cerebral or intracranial haemorrhages) on the other hand occurs when a blood vessel bursts, bleeding into the surrounding brain tissue. Although the rarer of the two forms of stroke in the general population, this is commonly seen in patients with a glioma, partly due to the breach of the blood-brain barrier (BBB) and partly due to the increased risk of surgery. For a malignant tumour to grow, the BBB needs to be disrupted, allowing for valuable nutrients and oxygen to be diverted to the tumour. Furthermore, disrupting the BBB causes weakened blood vessels, increasing the risk of spontaneous bleeding [20].

Common symptoms of a stroke (whether ischaemic or haemorrhagic) can include any combination of facial asymmetry, slurred speech, unilateral weakness, thunderclap headaches, confusion, difficulty understanding others, loss or blurring of vision and dysphagia. Often, glioma patients present with stroke-like symptoms, and only during investigations and subsequent imaging is the glioma identified [20]. Symptoms can range from very mild to extreme, with the more extreme symptoms likely requiring intensive inpatient rehabilitation in hope angiogenesis may recover some of the functional mobility over time [20]. Treatment of a stroke very much depends on which type of stroke the patient has suffered, and normally the cause of the stroke (if applicable) is treated i.e. high blood pressure, cholesterol, alcohol consumption, etc. to minimise the risk of recurrence [20].

## 8.15.1 Case Report

The below case report is an example of a patient who presented to Addenbrooke's Hospital, Cambridge (UK), following a 3-month history of progressive expressive dysphasia and right-sided visual field loss. His name and age have been changed to protect his identity—he will be referred to as Mr Smith, and he was 60 years old at the time of presentation.

Mr Smith's case was discussed in our neuro-oncology MDT meeting where his imaging was reviewed. His MRI scan showed a left inferior temporal lesion, likely a glioblastoma (GBM). He was seen the following week in outpatients clinic where the consultant neurosurgeon consented him for 5-ALA (fluorescent guided) craniotomy and awake resection of this tumour. Below is an extract from his clinical notes—identifiable information has been removed:

*'R-handed male*
*PMH: HTN*
*Family noticed problems*
*Lots of stress*
*Memory problems*
*Confusion*
*Looking at a mouse unable to name it*
*Unable to get words out*
*Started with little things*
*Progressively worse*
*Forgetful, can't remember which hospital coming today*
*Vision intermittently going*
*Peripheral vision poor – worse above*
*Walking – fine*
*Limbs OK*
*H/A – very mild*
*Dizzy at times*
*Steroids – 8mg bd +PPI*
*Since starting steroids – H/A better*
*O/E: R hemianopia*
*Otherwise N*
*MRI-enhancing tumour L temporal lobe – extends superiorly*
*Medially is white matter fibres*
*TCI awake 5-ALA resection'*

He underwent complete resection of the enhancing portions of his tumour less than 2 weeks later, and post-operative dalteparin (anticoagulant) was commenced after 24 h for prevention of VTE. He was recovering well on the ward, with no focal deficits and only mild dysphasia remained. He was beginning to mobilise with assistance of one, eating and drinking well with only minimal pain. He did have a significant (albeit stable) facial swelling over his left cheek and eye, extending to his temple/ear area. This was very tender and sore to touch.

During the night, some 2 days after surgery, Mr Smith suddenly develops worsening dysphasia, only being able to answer to 'yes' or 'no' questions and becoming very distressed. His GCS drops to 13/15. Documentation is as follows:

*Patient becoming increasingly more dysphasic—(noted around 03:00), dropping GCS to 13/15 because of it, being unable to form more than inappropriate words- ?Re-bleed*

He continued to further drop his Glasgow Coma Scale (GCS) to 12/15, and an urgent CT head demonstrated a resection bed haematoma with an overlying extradural haemorrhage with resultant mass effect and some midline shift (see below Image 8.2). He was taken back to theatre that same night for emergency evacuation of both clots, and made a good post-operative recovery, with his dysphasia improving post-operatively and no noticeable residual limb weakness.

In the interim, his pathology report confirms his tumour to be primary, malignant WHO IV glioblastoma. He and his family were informed of diagnosis and the fact that this is an incurable malignancy with a limited life expectancy.

Mr Smith is subsequently seen by our oncologists who have open and honest discussions with him and his family regarding his prognosis and eventual treatment options. Due to his facial swelling, a radiotherapy mask is unable to be fitted until this is resolved. He is also very frail with episodes of dizziness with difficulties in

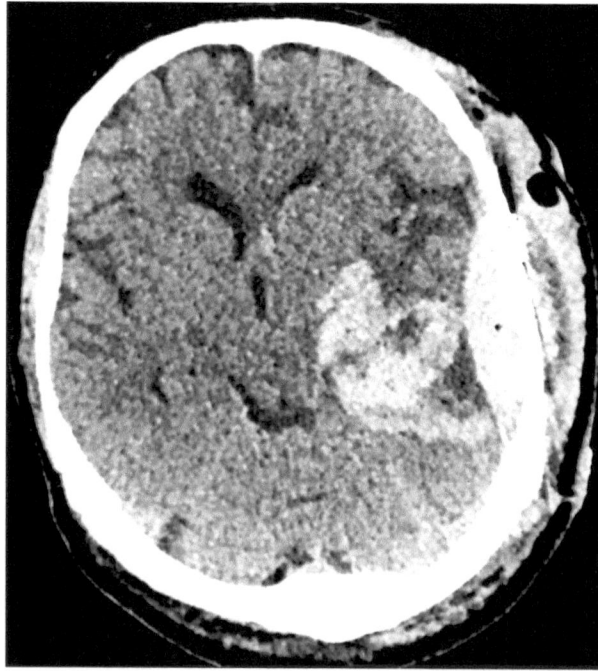

**Image 8.2** CT showing a left fronto-parietal extradural (epidural) haematoma and post-operative haematoma within the left temporal tumour resection cavity, requiring emergency evacuation

walking and has visual disturbances. Mr Smith has also started developing anxiety attacks and does not wish to prolong his life if his symptoms and quality of life will not improve much beyond his current performance status. His symptoms were manageable however, and he was offered concomitant chemotherapy and radiotherapy treatment (ChemoRT) with oncology.

He has full capacity and he eventually decides to decline any further treatments. Mr Smith feels he has been well informed every step of the way and had been anticipating a malignant diagnosis. He and his family have felt empowered to be involved in the decision-making, and he has made fully informed decisions, knowing what his options were, and likely outcomes of each option.

He is placed onto a palliative care pathway with end-of-life care undertaken in the community by specialist nurses and family members looking after his needs. He passes away peacefully at a local hospice some months later, surrounded by loved ones.

*Points to consider*: Close neurological monitoring by the nursing staff identified his declining neurology status quickly, and he was dealt with promptly and efficiently. He recovered well following both neurosurgical procedures. He has a past medical history of hypertension (HTN), and his amlodipine had been withheld immediately after surgery, whilst simultaneously dalteparin had been commenced for VTE prevention purposes. Could this have contributed to his bleed?

Open and honest discussions with continuous patient involvement along his treatment trajectory, anticipating the next steps (including the potential diagnosis and various treatment options), made it easier for the patient to both accept the definitive diagnosis and also to make informed decisions about what was best for him as an individual in regard to treatment options, side effects, benefits and prognosis.

Mr Smith was only 60 years old, and as health-care professionals, it is sometimes hard to accept that patients make decisions we would not have anticipated or necessarily agree with. In the case of Mr Smith, he was offered concomitant ChemoRT treatment, which he subsequently declined.

## 8.16   Seizures

Please see Chap. 5 for in-depth discussion of medical management of seizures and also Chap. 3.

## 8.17   5-ALA Nursing Implications

For high-grade primary brain tumours, a substance called 5-aminolevulinic acid (5-ALA or Gliolan) is taken orally by the patient around 3–5 h prior to surgery. It comes in a powder form for oral solution and is reconstituted with tap water. This clear fluid will help distinguish normal-appearing brain from tumour-infiltrated, diseased brain tissue by lighting up the tumour tissue as pink once it has been exposed to ultraviolet light—see Chap. 6 for more details. In the UK, it is licenced for use for primary (and recurrent), high-grade gliomas and can only be administered if the surgeon feels at least 95% of the tumour can safely be resected [21, 22].

It is administered as a drink (it has been reported to be very bitter tasting!), and each vial contains 1500 mg, dosed at 20 mg/kg. Take an adult male weighing 80 kg as an example, 20 mg/kg × 80 kg = 1600 mg, which is just over one full vial. In reality, this means discarding nearly a full vial of 5-ALA, which is not a trivial amount of money; hence lots of specialist neurosurgical centres now cap doses to a maximum amount of 1500 mg (i.e. one full vial) with good effect. Certainly, in some UK centres, doses have been capped at 1500 mg for patients 75 kg and over—even with 120 kg plus patients, reductions in the fluorescent capabilities of 5-ALA have not been identified when capped.

Administering a drink to the patient a few hours prior to surgery seems straight-forward enough from a nursing perspective. However, 5-ALA do come with some serious side effects which need some careful considerations: it is known to cause hypotension, so following administration, 30-min blood pressure checks need to be undertaken and documented, and any significant trends or alterations must be esca-lated accordingly. It is contraindicated in patients with any type of porphyria and pregnant women [23]. If patients are on regular antihypertensives, these medicines should be highlighted to the doctor to see if they should be omitted on the morning of surgery or even a day prior to surgery. 5-ALA can also cause nausea and vomiting (risking the newly ingested dose to be brought back up), so an antiemetic is rou-tinely administered at the same time [21, 22].

Following surgery, due to the photosensitive properties, the patient may be very sensitive to sunlight exposure, and a rash is a reported side effect. Patients having undergone 5-ALA resection should not be placed next to a window without an ade-quate UV film, and following discharge from hospital, they should avoid direct sunlight or any photosensitising agents for up to 2 weeks following oral administra-tion. Should surgery be delayed, a second dose does not need to be administered, but should surgery be cancelled and rescheduled a few days later, a second dose can safely be administered without ill effect [21, 23].

## 8.18   Carmustine Wafers

These are small, coin-like wafers that contain a cytotoxic chemotherapy agent called carmustine (also known as Gliadel). The aim of these wafers is as an adjunct therapy to surgery, in that chemotherapy wafers are directly placed inside the tumour cavity following near-complete resection of the tumour. As with 5-ALA, over 95% of the tumour needs to be removed for them to be deemed effective, and they also are licenced for use in primary (and recurrent) high-grade gliomas [24].

Once placed inside the tumour cavity, up to eight of these wafers are administered, and the surgical wound is closed as per normal. These wafers then start to dissolve once they come into contact with the CSF or blood in the tumour cavity, over a 6-week period. As the wafers dissolve, they disseminate the chemotherapy into the surrounding brain tissue, with around a 5 cm margin, with the aim of killing off as many of the remnant tumour cells as possible. This is an additional treatment to con-comitant chemotherapy/radiotherapy treatment as described in previous chapters.

As one might imagine, handling and disposing of chemotherapy agents need to be done with care, with the wafers signed out from pharmacy and signed on delivery to theatres. Only qualified staff (normally specialist pharmacists or trained theatre staff) can handle the wafers. A pack of carmustine wafers contains eight individually wrapped wafers. They are stored in a dry freezer at −20 °C and can only be out of the freezer for <6 h prior to being returned again; hence surgery times (and requesting carmustine) need to be done with great precision [25].

Patients who have had carmustine wafers inserted into their tumour cavity need to be made aware of the cytotoxic risks by their medical team. Should they develop a SSI or CSF leak after surgery, this CSF will be contaminated with cytotoxic material which may be hazardous to health [24]. From a nursing perspective, any handling of wound dressings or suture removals needs to be done with double gloving to protect against chemical burns—not so much from a one-off use for a patients' perspective but from repeated exposure to carmustine from several patients you are likely to nurse during your neurosurgical career. Furthermore, the dressings need to be disposed of as per your local policies and procedures for handling substances hazardous to health. If in doubt, please seek advice from your health and safety department. In the UK, we use purple topped chemotherapy bins, indicating these contain cytotoxic materials and need to be collected by hospital porters for incineration. Any materials affected by the CSF leak (such as pillow cases, shirts, pyjamas, etc.) also need to be disposed of safely and incinerated as a result.

## 8.19   Conclusion

Caring for patients with a glioma is a complex process and consideration needs to be given to every aspect of neurosurgical nursing, not least looking after the patient's pre- and post-operative care requirements by helping to minimise any (un)foreseen issues that may lead to preventable delays to their treatment pathway.

As this chapter has demonstrated, there are a myriad of complications with varying degrees of severity that could arise at any stage in the patient's treatment trajectory. These complications may compromise the timing of anticipated surgery; the recovery process immediately after surgery; as well as negatively impacting on adjuvant and concomitant treatment options with oncology, at times necessitating their delay if certain complications such as wound infections arise.

It is hoped this chapter has highlighted some of the more common surgical complications of glioma patients, as well as helping to equip the nurse with practical investigations and nursing interventions to consider when caring for this multifaceted patient cohort.

## References

1. https://www.nice.org.uk/guidance/cg74/evidence/full-guideline-pdf-242005933. Accessed on 03 Jan 2018.
2. Hong B, Winkel A, Ertl P, et al. Bacterial colonisation of suture material after routine neurosurgical procedures: relevance for wound infection. Acta Neurochir. 2018;160:497–503.
3. Skally M, Finn C, O'Brien D, et al. Invasive MRSA infections in neurosurgical patients-a decade of progress. Br J Neurosurg. 2017;31(3):374–8.

4. Cho J, Harrop J, Veznaedaroglu E, et al. Concomitant use of computer image guidance, linear or sigmoid incisions after minimal shave, and liquid wound dressing with 2-octyl cyanoacrylate for tumor craniotomy or craniectomy: analysis of 225 consecutive surgical cases with antecedent historical control at one institution. Neurosurgery. 2003;52:832–40. discussion 840–1
5. Broekman MLD, Van Beijnum J, Peul WC, et al. Neurosurgery and shaving. What is the evidence? A review. J Neurosurg. 2011;115(4):670–8.
6. Nandapalan V, Watson ID, Swift AC. Beta-2-transferrin and cerebrospinal fluid rhinorrhea. Clin Otolaryngol. 1996;21(3):259–64.
7. Hickey J. Overview of neuroanatomy and physiology. In: The clinical practice of neurological and neurosurgical nursing. 7th ed. Philadelphia, PA: Lippincott, Williams and Wilkins; 2013. Chapter 5, 14 and 23.
8. Lepanluoma M, Takala R, Kotkansalo A, et al. Surgical safety checklist is associated with improved operating room safety culture, reduced wound complications, and unplanned readmissions in a pilot study in neurosurgery. Scand J Surg. 2014;103(1):66–72.
9. Krishnan KG, Muller A, Hong B, et al. Complex wound-healing problems in neurosurgical patients: Risk factors, grading and treatment strategy. Acta Neurochir. 2012;154(3):541–53.
10. Sonneville R, Ruimy R, Benzonana N, et al. An update on bacterial brain abscess in immunocompetent patients. Clin Microbiol Infect. 2017;23(9):614–20.
11. Merkler AE, Ch'ang J, Parker WE, et al. The rate of complications after ventriculoperitoneal shunt surgery. World Neurosurg. 2017;98:654–8.
12. Mantia C, Uhlmann EJ, Puligandla M, et al. Predicting the higher rate of intracranial hemorrhage in glioma patients receiving therapeutic enoxaparin. Blood. 2017;129(25):3379–85.
13. Cote DJ, Dubois HM, Karhade AV, et al. Venous thromboembolism in patients undergoing craniotomy for brain tumors: a U.S. nationwide analysis. Semin Thromb Hemost. 2016;42(8):870–6.
14. Wade R, Paton F, Woolacott N. Systematic review of patient preference and adherence to the correct use of graduated compression stockings to prevent deep vein thrombosis in surgical patients. J Adv Nurs. 2017;73(2):336–48.
15. Bhattacharya V, Stansby G, Kesteven P. Prevention and management of venous thromboembolism. 1st ed. London: Imperial College Press; 2015. Chapters 4,7 and 10
16. Duffau H. Mapping the connectome in awake surgery for gliomas: an update. J Neurosurg Sci. 2017;61(6):612–30.
17. Kirk EA, Howard VC, Scott CA. Description of posterior fossa syndrome in children after posterior fossa brain tumor surgery. J Pediat Oncol Nurs. 1995;12(4):181–7.
18. Bannur U, Rajshekhar V. Post operative supplementary motor area syndrome: clinical features and outcomes. Br J Neurosurg. 2000;14(3):204–10.
19. Parton A, Malhotra P, Husain M. Hemispatial neglect. J Neurol Neurosurg Psychiatry. 2004;75:13–21.
20. Teasell R, Bayona N, Salter K, et al. Progress in clinical neurosciences: Stroke recovery and rehabilitation. Can J Neurol Sci. 2006;33(4):357–64.
21. Senders JT, Muskens IS, Schnoor R, et al. Agents for fluorescence-guided glioma surgery: a systematic review of preclinical and clinical results. Acta Neurochir. 2017;159(1):151–67.
22. Ma R, Watts C. Selective 5-aminolevulinic acid-induced protoporphyrin IX fluorescence in Gliomas. Acta Neurochir. 2016;158(10):1935–41.
23. http://www.ema.europa.eu/docs/en_GB/document_library/EPAR_-_Scientific_Discussion/human/000744/WC500021788.pdf. Accessed on 5 Jan 2018.
24. Roux A, Caire F, Guyotat J, et al. Carmustine wafer implantation for high-grade gliomas: evidence-based safety efficacy and practical recommendations from the Neuro-oncology Club of the French Society of Neurosurgery. Neurochirurgie. 2017;63(6):433–43.
25. Sage W, Guilfoyle M, Luney C, et al. Local alkylating chemotherapy applied immediately after 5-ALA guided resection of glioblastoma does not provide additional benefit. J Neurooncol. 2018;136:273–80.

# Neurorehabilitation

9

## Michelangelo Bartolo and Chiara Zucchella

**Abstract**

People affected by brain tumours (BTs) can experience a wide range of symptoms and disabilities, such as reduced mobility, cognitive and psychological problems, difficulties with self-care and relationship and work issues, which can result in reduced ability in daily life activities and in performing (or maintaining) usual family and social roles, with a substantial impact on quality of life.

Neuro-oncological rehabilitation refers to the process of assisting a person who has become disabled as a result of tumour (or therapies) to improve symptoms and maximise functional independence, activity (e.g. walking) and participation (e.g. employment, reintegration into social and domestic life), within the limits of the persisting impairment. As for other diseases/impairments, disabilities caused by BTs can be expressed within the conceptual framework of the International Classification of Functioning, Disability and Health (ICF), which was developed by World Health Organization (WHO) to describe health and the multidimensional health-related concerns of individuals. Symptoms and disabilities may be addressed through a "multidisciplinary rehabilitation" delivered by a team of different healthcare professionals working in an organised manner. Nurses assume a pivotal role for the creation of a supportive environment for rehabilitation as most of nurses' activities represent essential rehabilitative skills. Rehabilitation nurses also provide patients and caregivers with education and emotional support and act as a link between patients and families and the different healthcare settings. The complexity of knowledge and skills required to

M. Bartolo (✉)
Department of Rehabilitation, Neurorehabilitation Unit, HABILITA, Zingonia di Ciserano, Bergamo, Italy
e-mail: michelangelobartolo@habilita.it

C. Zucchella
Neurology Unit, University Hospital of Verona, Verona, Italy

© Springer Nature Switzerland AG 2019
I. Oberg (ed.), *Management of Adult Glioma in Nursing Practice*,
https://doi.org/10.1007/978-3-319-76747-5_9

127

provide such comprehensive care illustrates the need for increasing specialisation in neuro-oncology to strengthen and raise the nurses' professional profile.

**Keywords**
Brain tumours · Neurorehabilitation · Neuro-oncology · Functional outcome · Nurse

## Abbreviations

| | |
|---|---|
| ADL | Activities of daily living |
| ARN | Association of Rehabilitation Nurses |
| BT | Brain tumours |
| CNS | Central nervous system |
| EORTC | European Organisation for Research and Treatment of Cancer |
| GBM | Glioblastoma multiforme |
| HGG | High-grade gliomas |
| HRQOL | Health-related quality of life |
| ICF | International Classification of Functioning, Disability and Health |
| KPS | Karnofsky Performance Status |
| OT | Occupational therapy |
| PNS | Peripheral nervous system |
| QoL | Quality of life |
| WHO | World Health Organization |

## Learning Outcomes

- To understand why neurorehabilitation becomes really important in achieving the highest degree of functional recovery and autonomy for glioma patients.
- To gain knowledge and insight into varying rehabilitation tools and knowing the difference between different concepts and types of neurorehabilitation—be it cognitive, functional or sensory-motor.
- To provide caregivers with support, education and coping strategies.
- To explore the crucial, specific neuro-rehabilitative roles and activities nurses undertake on a daily basis, which represent essential rehabilitative skills.

## 9.1    Introduction

Brain tumours (BTs) represent a heterogeneous group of lesions of the central nervous system (CNS) in which can be recognised primary tumours and brain metastases. While primary tumours present a lower prevalence (it is estimated that 1/5000 adults will suffer from a primary brain tumour), the incidence of brain metastases has recently increased due to the substantial development of oncologic therapies, with a predominance in the sixth and seventh decades of life.

The primary adult tumours include meningiomas, schwannomas, primary CNS lymphomas and gliomas of the cerebral hemispheres (i.e. glioblastoma multiforme, anaplastic astrocytoma, low-grade astrocytoma and oligodendroglioma). In adults, high-grade gliomas (HGG), WHO grade III or grade IV, are the most common primary brain tumours, and glioblastoma multiforme (GBM) is the most frequent glioma.

BTs represent about 2% of the total incidence of cancer that will presumably increase in the future since the life expectancy is outspreading; the overall incidence is the same in males and females, but GBM is more frequent in men, while meningiomas and schwannomas occur more often in women.

Median overall survival in patients with GBM remains poor, 15 months for newly diagnosed GBM and 5–7 months for recurrent/relapsed GBM.

Given the poor prognosis of many BTs, the primary objectives of the therapies are to reduce morbidity and restore or preserve neurologic functions and the ability to perform daily activities as long as possible. Nowadays therapeutic progress in fact is transforming many of these diseases either into chronic processes or that require long-term treatments; however current forms of available treatment (i.e. chemotherapy, radiotherapy, surgery) often determine significant consequences on functioning and quality of life (QoL) of individuals with cancer.

Lastly, as far as public health is concerned, the impact of BTs is significant in spite of their low incidence because they include high direct costs (diagnostic resources, high complexity treatments and rehabilitation) and high unforeseen costs (labour leave, family and social expenditures). A population-based comparison of cancer survivors with matched controls found a substantially increased burden of illness in cancer survivors, manifested in days lost from work, inability to work, poor general health perception and the need for help with daily activities. Furthermore, compared with age-matched controls, cancer survivors reported poorer health outcomes, decreased functioning and higher levels of burden across multiple domains. Interestingly, these decrements were consistent across tumour sites and time since diagnosis [1]. Additionally, these concerns and functional decrements appear to persist across age categories.

These data suggest that cancer patients experience an elevated burden of illness, and this relationship appears to exist irrespective of age, tumour site or time since diagnosis.

## 9.2    Brain Tumours and Disabilities: Rehabilitation Needs

Neuro-oncological patients are prone to a number of neurological symptoms, both sensory-motor and cognitive, due to the primary tumour itself (*mass effect*) or to the side effects of the treatments.

The most common symptoms induced by BTs may include headache, nausea and vomiting and drowsiness during the day and are commonly related to high intracranial pressure, whereas local tumour effects might result in focal neurological problems, such as paresis, ataxia, dysphagia, sensory loss, visual-perceptual deficits,

**Table 9.1** The most common neurological symptoms in primary brain tumours

| | |
|---|---|
| Cognitive deficits | 80% |
| Motor deficits | 78% |
| Fatigue | 40–70% |
| Visual-perceptual deficits | 53% |
| Sexual dysfunction | >50% |
| Sensory loss | 38% |
| Bowel/bladder impairment | 37% |
| Cranial nerve palsy | 29% |
| Dysarthria | 27% |
| Dysphagia | 26% |
| Speech disorders aphasia | 24% |
| Ataxia | 20% |

cognitive deficits and seizures [2] (Table 9.1). Changes in personality and behaviour, as well as mood issues (anxiety and depression), also frequently occur [3].

Also cancer-related fatigue, low energy and weakness are frequent and extremely distressing symptoms among BT patients that may be one of the most challenging barriers to effective rehabilitation [4]. Fatigue is commonly considered to have a multifactorial basis, including several physical and mental factors such as pain, anxiety, deconditioning, sleep problems, anaemia, malnutrition, infection, cognitive disturbance as well as the type of treatment. Therefore, all patients should be evaluated about potential fatigue with treatment, and potential interventions should be considered. Pharmacologic treatments for fatigue can include medications to optimise sleep, mood and pain control, while among non-pharmacologic treatments exercise, behavioural and coping strategies, high-protein diet, adequate hydration and management of anaemia have been proposed.

Symptom severity fluctuates during the course of the disease, and patients may experience a temporary improvement when responding to treatment or a progressive neurological and functional decline as the disease progresses.

Physical and neurological functioning can also be strongly affected by the side effects of treatments. In recent decades, in fact, therapeutic advances in oncology have prolonged the survival of individuals, also those with CNS tumours, even though these individuals are often left with residual neurological deficits [5]. The CNS and peripheral nervous system (PNS) in fact become "target" organs of the therapies, which in turn determine a number of side effects to be considered within the global evaluation of the patient: postsurgical morbidity; acute, subacute and late radiation effects on the normal brain; chemotherapy-induced toxicity; high-dose corticosteroids; and anticonvulsants can all produce adverse effects [4, 6] (Fig. 9.1a–c).

Overall, these symptoms cause functional impairments similar to those seen in patients commonly submitted to rehabilitation programmes [7] and have a considerable impact on patients' daily life, hindering their ability to function independently and to maintain usual family and social roles, influencing ultimately their QoL as well as the QoL of their family members. Relatives bear the burden of care, which disrupts family life. Families experience initial chaos and confusion followed by a heavy burden of care and feelings of helplessness and isolation, with a negative impact on their well-being [8].

At this point the role of rehabilitation becomes really important to favour the highest degree of functional recovery and autonomy for patients and to provide caregivers with support, education and coping strategies.

The plasticity of CNS and its capacity to reorganise itself after damage represent the foundation of any rehabilitative intervention. Since Hebb's suggestion that

**a**

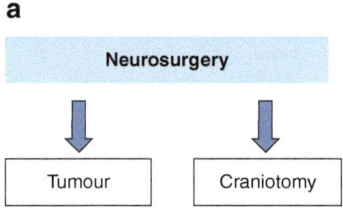

- Management of pain
- Infections treatment
- Bowel and bladder problems management
- Nutrition
- Post-surgery haematoma / perioperative neuropathies
- Other clinical comorbility
- Thromboembolic
- Epileptic treatment

**b**

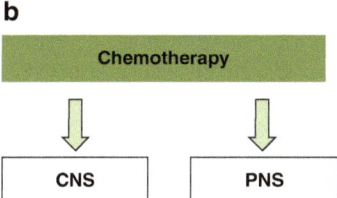

- *Fatigue*
- *Chemofog o chemobrain*
- Constipation
- Headache
- Peripheral neuropathy (e.g.: vinca alkaloids, cisplatin, oxaliplatin, ...)
- Cardiac effects (e.g.: antracicline)

**Fig. 9.1** Main side effects of therapies for brain tumours on central and peripheral nervous system

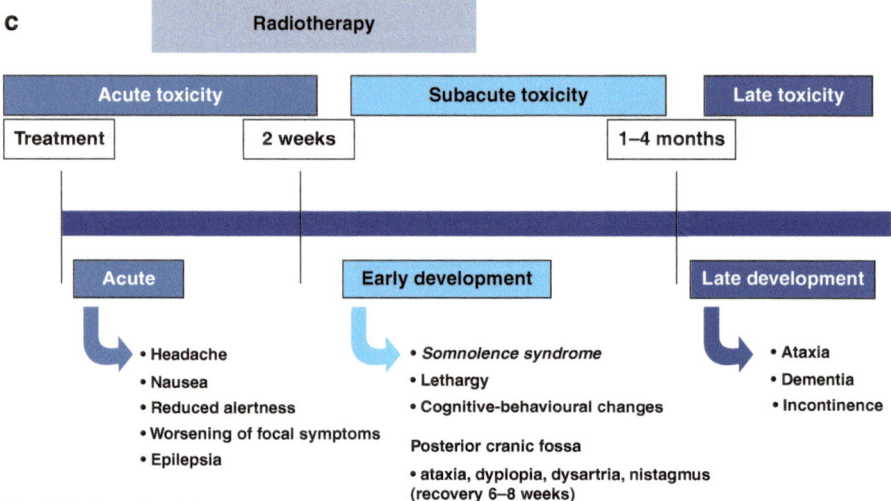

**Fig. 9.1** (continued)

neuronal cortical connections can be remodelled by experience, evidence derived from animal studies and new imaging techniques increased our understanding of neurological recovery and the role of rehabilitation therapies in promoting such recovery [9]. The neurobiological mechanisms of plasticity and spontaneous recovery include cell genesis, functional plasticity and structural adaptations, such as axonal sprouting and synaptogenesis. Overcoming the old dogma that there is a fixed number of neurons in the adult mammalian brain that cannot be replaced when the cells die, the studies in the last century showed that in some areas (olfactory bulb, *gyrus dentatus* of the hippocampal formation, subventricular zone), neurogenesis (regeneration) may occur. Moreover, connections between neurons in the nervous system are continuously being altered depending on environmental and behavioural stimulation and responses to bodily injury. Through axonal sprouting and synaptogenesis, the brain has the ability to form new functional connections after it has experienced a perturbation or injury [10].

The nature and timing of these mechanisms are revealed by the course of motor recovery observed in patients (mainly stroke survivors), most of whom reach their recovery plateau within the first 3–6 months. However, considering some prognostic factors (type of disease, age, lesion site, neurological impairment and performance status), it is widely accepted that improvements can continue for years, through rehabilitation-guided learning-dependent processes.

## 9.2.1 The "Total Pain": A Global Concept

Literature data reported that between 30% and 50% of cancer patients experience significant pain due to disease progression or therapeutic interventions with a prevalence of 90% in advanced stages. Along with other factors, such as young age, recent diagnosis and tumour aggressiveness, pain was significantly associated with a low level of functioning and a reduced QoL.

The neurophysiology of cancer pain is a striking example of the complexity of pain as it involves chemotherapy-induced neuropathic pain; iatrogenic radionecrosis (cell deaths due to radiotherapy effects); postoperative pain; inflammatory, ischaemic and compressive phenomena; and direct tumour invasion of tissues including nerves and plexuses with a neuropathic component [11]. However, it is not purely a physical experience but involves various other components of human functioning, including psychological, social and spiritual components as well as social relationships, and it is often referred to as "total pain" to underline the global nature of pain within a "whole-person" framework [12]. The combination of these elements is believed to result in a comprehensive suffering experience that is individualised and specific to each patient's particular situation. Albeit so widespread, pain remains one of the most difficult diagnostic and therapeutic problems in oncology, and literature evidence suggests that an inadequate assessment is far too common. Some nurses may rely only on their own observation to assess pain, without asking the patients to describe their pain; however, this approach does not allow to adequately evaluate a patient's "total pain" because patient's perspective or spiritual, psychological and social aspects are ignored. Moreover, the complexity of treating patients with "total pain" may be exacerbated by the patients' inability to identify exactly which component is causing pain, as in most cases they may be unaware of the fact that their pain experience results from a combination of factors.

It therefore follows that pain assessment must include aspects that go beyond the mere physical manifestations of pain in order to effectively manage oncological pain and that the treatment of only physical symptoms, without a wider exploration of the other dimensions of the patient's suffering experience, results in an incomplete and often inappropriate pain regimen [13]. Psychological support for patients and families confronted with a life-threatening illness is often overlooked and can be even more undermined when physical pain becomes the main focus of treatment plan. Family meeting including patient, family and health professionals can be an effective tool to overcome these difficulties as all members of the family may be heard and understood; may share feelings, concerns and expectations; and may support one another. Communication represents an essential intervention that allows health professionals to understand patients and family needs to provide appropriate interventions.

## 9.3 Taking Care of the Person with Brain Tumour: The ICF Framework

Owing to improved surveillance and treatment methods, survival rates of cancer have improved over time creating the need to recognise and attend to a variety of concerns unique to cancer survivorship. In order to identify such potential concerns, it may be useful to utilise an overarching framework to guide the provision of care. As for other diseases/impairments, disabilities caused by BTs can be included within the conceptual framework of the International Classification of Functioning, Disability and Health (ICF), which was developed by the World Health Organization to provide a framework to describe health and the multidimensional health-related concerns of individuals [14].

The ICF framework is increasingly being used in the rehabilitation field, but it has been utilised for a diverse array of purposes in the field of oncology, evaluating functioning in persons with cancer, assessment in oncology rehabilitation, assessing the outcome measures and comparing the primary concerns of health professionals with those of their patients.

Briefly, the ICF model shifts the focus of disablement from cause to impact, from disability to health and function and from a static to a dynamic process.

Using a global approach to the person named *biopsychosocial model*, the ICF defines three domains of human function: *body function and structure*, *activity* and *participation* (Fig. 9.2). *Body function and structure* refers to the anatomical and physiological function of the body systems and is categorised into subdomains. Deficits in this domain are defined "impairments" (e.g. muscle weakness, spasticity, restricted joint motion, pain, visual deficits, seizures and poor cardiorespiratory fitness).

The *activity* describes the ability of a person to perform specific tasks such as bathing or showering, dressing and feeding; reductions in the activity domain are named "limitations"

The *participation* domain describes the ability of a person to be involved in life situations. Participation restrictions describe the reduced ability of a person to maintain normal role functions in the person's environment, where different factors can

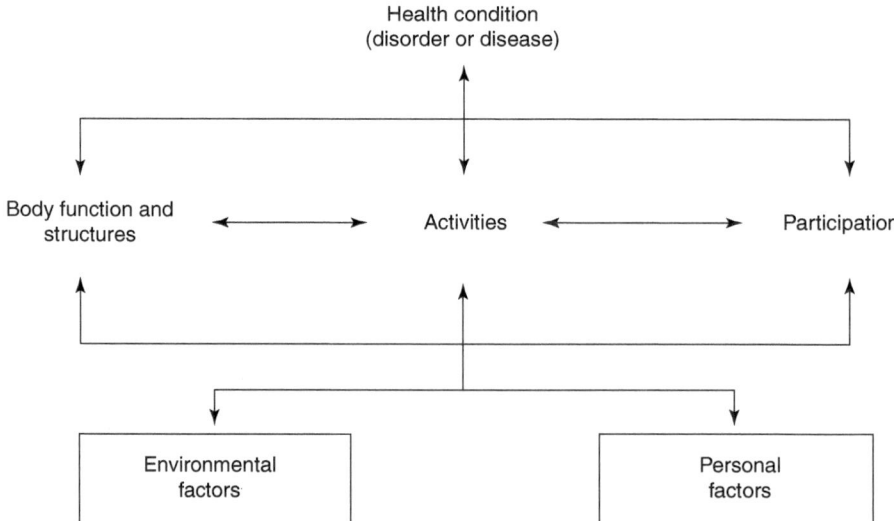

**Fig. 9.2** The International Classification of Functioning, Disability and Health. Reproduced by the beginner's guide developed by the World Health Organization (*downloaded from*: http://www.who.int/classifications/icf/training/icfbeginnersguide.pdf)

act as barriers or facilitators. For BT patient's physical, cognitive and psychological factors may represent barriers to social integration. In the ICF model, health conditions, personal factors and the environment interact dynamically across the three domains of body function to help determine whether disordered function results in disability (e.g. if a cancer treatment, such as chemotherapy, causes the development of peripheral neuropathy and ankle weakness, the patient may have a limited ability to walk "limitation" and may require long-term use of an ankle brace).

The ICF framework seems to be a useful model for describing global function in patients with a cancer diagnosis [15]. In recent years there has been increased use of the ICF in clinical settings, including ICF checklists to identify patient-reported problems in both acute and chronic conditions, and the basis for defining a dedicated core set was described [16]. The development of ICF Core Sets provides clinicians and researchers with comprehensive but concise measurement categories that describe a patient's global function from a biopsychosocial view. Some ICF Core Sets have been developed for patients with head and neck cancer and breast cancer.

The interaction among cancer as a modification of the health condition, impairments in body function and structure, activity limitations and participation restrictions in the context of the person and the environment is relevant to define an effective oncology rehabilitation intervention. Compensatory strategies, adjusting goals and expectations, educating friends and family and accepting support from others, facilitate social reintegration throughout the trajectory of living with brain tumour.

## 9.4 The Multidisciplinary Approach

Rehabilitation was defined as "a problem-solving educational process aimed at reducing disability and handicap (participation) experienced by someone as a result of disease or injury" [17].

For persons affected by BTs, rehabilitation can be challenging because, as previously described, they can present with various combinations of symptoms, such as physical, cognitive, psychosocial, behavioural and environmental issues which can substantially impact their QoL and that need to be addressed through "multidisciplinary rehabilitation". Multidisciplinary rehabilitation programmes assume that besides the anatomical or physiological problem, psychological factors such as fear, anxiety and mood disturbance may amplify symptoms; similarly, social/environmental factors such as physical job demands, workplace and social issues may worsen disability. These insights have led to the design of interventions that address multiple factors, typically involving a combination of physical, psychological, social and/or work-related components, which are delivered by a team of clinicians with different skills [18]. Therefore, multidisciplinary rehabilitation can be defined as the coordinated delivery of multidimensional rehabilitation interventions provided by two or more disciplines (i.e. nursing, physiotherapy, occupational therapy, social work, psychology and other allied health), in conjunction with medical professionals (oncologist, rehabilitation, surgeon, palliative physician), which aims to improve patient symptoms and maximise functional independence and participation (social integration) using a holistic biopsychosocial model of care, as defined by the ICF.

A multidisciplinary approach provides patients with skills needed to manage their own care to improve their coping ability, knowledge base and QoL. It prioritises patient-centred care and focuses on person's functions and disabilities, using a goal-based functionally oriented approach that is time-based. Specifically, in order to engage in effective patient-centred care, personal factors such as an individual's experiences, coping style, self-efficacy, attitudes, values, preferences and knowledge are relevant factors for consideration, and the patients (as well as family or carer) are active participants in the goal setting process. The content, intensity and frequency of therapy in multidisciplinary rehabilitation can vary, as programmes are individualised according to clinical needs (e.g. physical reconditioning, task reacquisition strategies, cognitive and behavioural therapy, vocational and recreational programmes and psychological support).

Although not conclusive and with a "low level" of evidence, preliminary studies seem to support the benefit of multidisciplinary rehabilitation in reducing disability in people with BTs: persons in the multidisciplinary rehabilitation group in fact showed a greater improvement in their functional abilities (e.g. continence, mobility) and cognitive functions compared with standard care [19].

Given these general but essential assumptions, two main aspects make the neuro-oncological rehabilitation particular and need to be underlined: first, the "limitations" due to life expectancy and the imposition upon health professionals to provide flexible clinical choices, with frequent reassessments and adjustments of the rehabilitative projects and programmes [5], and second, the "frailty" of neuro-oncological patients, due to the intrinsic features of the disease and the possibility of intercurrent clinical events, treatment side effects and comorbidities, which can cause sudden changes in the clinical pictures.

Considering these aspects, the model named "simultaneous care", which is deeply multidisciplinary, seems to describe the best approach to neuro-oncological patients. This approach not only ensures the "continuity of care" (adherence to treatment protocols—in terms of both dose intensity and the dosing interval) but also introduces the supportive care (control the side effects related to treatment and manage comorbidities related to malignancy) and palliative care (prevention and the relief from suffering) at the same time as anticancer therapies are administered (simultaneous care) [20].

## 9.5  Sensory-Motor Rehabilitation

The health benefits of regular physical exercise have been recognised for centuries, and structured exercise training is considered critical for primary and secondary disease prevention in multiple clinical settings. However, for neuro-oncological patients until recently, clinicians were either not aware of rehabilitation services or do not believe in the benefits of rehabilitation or just were uncomfortable providing such care for a progressive disease with poor prognosis. Only in the last decades has rehabilitation gained acceptance as a potential adjunct therapy for cancer patients.

Cancer rehabilitation attempts to maximise patients' ability to function, to promote their independence and to help them to adapt to their condition, improving their QoL, no matter how long or short the timescale. Rehabilitation is recommended throughout the course of the disease with different aims according to patient's needs; indeed, because of diverse clinical picture and varying levels of disability, an individualised approach is always warranted. In the early phase, the intervention aims to restore function [7], while in more advanced stages, rehabilitation is an important part of palliative care with the aim of preventing complications, controlling symptoms and maintaining patients' independence and QoL.

When planning the rehabilitative intervention, specificity of medical treatment, complication of surgery and side effects of irradiation and chemotherapy such as fatigue have to be taken into consideration; side effects of corticosteroids and anticonvulsants are also relevant, because their chronic use can be associated with myopathy, osteoporosis, behavioural changes and psychiatric disorders that can all influence the rehabilitation process [21]. Oncologic and other treatments may also impact the timing of physical therapy interventions, which should be performed in a phase of patient's peak performance [5].

To date, about a hundred studies have been performed investigating the effects of structured exercise training in cancer population. Although studies were considered with "low level" of evidence [19], papers that specifically addressed the effects of rehabilitation in neuro-oncological patients demonstrated that BT patients, after inpatient rehabilitation, achieve functional improvements comparable to stroke or traumatic brain injury patients, irrespective of the tumour type, location and concomitant tumour treatment [5–7]. Meta-analyses and systematic reviews reported that structured exercise training is a safe and well-tolerated therapeutic strategy associated with significant improvements in a broad range of cancer-related toxicities including physical, fatigue, exercise capacity and improved quality of life. As a result, a number of exercise guidelines for cancer patients have been published.

In brain cancer trials, "established" clinical outcomes are usually represented by progression-free survival or overall survival that considers tumour control and containment of treatment side effects. In rehabilitation, objective assessment of patient function and performance is generally preferred.

Performance status is widely used at baseline because of its prognostic value, but there is relatively little emphasis on functional status as an outcome, although changes in performance may indicate the effect of a rehabilitative intervention as well as the presence of clinical progression.

There are two commonly used outcome measures of overall rehabilitation functional outcomes: the Barthel Index, the simpler tool that focused on basic mobility function and personal activities of daily living, and the Functional Independence Measure (FIM®) that other than motor function and activities of daily living also includes cognition-communication. Although other tools can be used to measure multiple aspects of physical functioning in cancer patients, these tools are accepted in the literature as useful to describe overall patients' functioning.

In the neuro-oncological literature, the Karnofsky Performance Scale (KPS), Fig. 9.3, is the most widely used outcome measure that allows patients to be classified as to their functional impairment. The lower the Karnofsky score, the worse the survival for most serious illnesses. However, this scale presents important drawbacks, among which the most relevant concern is the fact that it was not specifically designed as an assessment for people with brain disease and therefore is oriented towards physical illness, rather than the effects of brain impairment (the concept of dependence, e.g. does not take account of the difficulties typical of people with cognitive impairment).

A further weakness of the KPS is that the lower levels of function are partly defined by dependence on medical support in hospital (an adaptation has been proposed that is appropriate for patients living at home). Given the limitations of the KPS as an outcome for brain tumour studies, at present there is a gap in the tools available for brain tumour studies, and there is a need for consensus over whether it is sensible to try to adapt the existing instrument, or whether it would be better to adopt another approach. The overarching aim is to achieve an international consensus on the core outcome set in neuro-oncology, also considering the patient-related counterpart.

Finally, in recent years, interest is growing in determining whether the benefits of exercise therapy may extend beyond symptom control to modulate cancer-specific outcomes (i.e. cancer progression and metastasis). Accordingly, over the past several years, research tried to shed light on the potential association between physical exercise, objective measures of exercise capacity/functional capacity and prognosis following a cancer diagnosis as well as the cellular and molecular mechanisms underlying these associations. Knowledge of the effects and underlying mechanisms will be critical to inform hypothesis-driven clinical trials and ensure the optimal safety and efficacy of exercise in cancer control.

| Karnofsky performance status scale | | |
|---|---|---|
| Able to carry on normal activity and to work; no special care needed | 100 | Normal no complaints; no evidence of disease |
| | 90 | Able to carry on normal activity; minor signs or symptoms of disease |
| | 80 | Normal activity with effort; some signs or symptoms of disease |
| Unable to work; able to live at home and care for most personal needs; varying amounts of assistance needed | 70 | Cares for self; unable to carry on normal activity or to do active work |
| | 60 | Requires occasional assistance but is able to care for most of his personal needs |
| | 50 | Requires considerable assistance and frequent medical care |
| Unable to care for self; requires equivalent of institutional or hospital care; disease may be progressing rapidly | 40 | Disabled; requires special care and assistance |
| | 30 | Severely disabled; hospital admission is indicated although death not imminent |
| | 20 | Very sick; hospital admission necessary; active supportive treatment necessary |
| | 10 | Moribund; fatal processes progressing rapidly |
| | 0 | Dead |

**Fig. 9.3** Karnofsky Performance Status Scale

## 9.6 Neuropsychological Issues: Cognitive Rehabilitation and Psychological Support

### 9.6.1 Cognitive Rehabilitation

Cognitive deficits in neuro-oncological patients may be found in one or more cognitive domains, such as executive functioning, language and memory, with the prevalence ranging from 29% to 90% according to different tumour types; patients often report short-term memory and attention deficits as well as problems in word-finding and in carrying out complex tasks [22, 23]. In turn cognitive deficits can have major consequences on patients QoL, return to work or autonomy, as well as on patients' ability to make informed decisions related to their own treatment and care.

Factors affecting cognitive functioning can be related to the patient (e.g. age, education, psychological distress), the tumour (grade, location, biological features, etc.) and to the treatments (chemo-/radiotherapy, surgery). Mechanical effects of the tumour mass inducing ischaemic changes in the surrounding tissue, cell death by tumour-released excitotoxins and alterations in synaptic transmission can produce direct neuronal damages in the region of the tumour, as well as more widespread alteration of brain connectivity that harms cognitive functioning. *Chemobrain* or *chemofog* is the term used to describe cognitive side effects of chemotherapy that manifest as a decline in memory, concentration and executive functions; also, the early- and late-delayed radiotherapy effects on cognition have been widely described [22].

As focal and more evident neurological deficits may often cover cognitive impairments, a comprehensive and sensitive neuropsychological evaluation is necessary to detect possible deficits; conversely, standard screening tests aimed at cognitive decline are often useless because they lack sensitivity and domain-specific information. Cognitive status was found to be a stronger prognostic factor for survival than physical state, as assessed by the Karnofsky Performance Scale and reliable also as an index of tumour progression. A lot of studies also reported a negative prognostic value of cognitive impairment on recovery, while a significant positive correlation between mental status at admission and functional outcome after rehabilitation treatment was found in other studies [24].

As pharmacologic interventions have not proven effective yet in the treatment of cognitive deficits in patients with gliomas, cognitive rehabilitation could represent a therapeutic option aiming at relieving patients' cognitive deficits, improving the individual abilities to perform cognitive tasks, by retraining previously learned skills and/or teaching compensatory strategies, with the ultimate goal of fostering a positive adaptation of the patients to their environment.

Literature evidence in this field is still scarce, but preliminary evidence suggest that cognitive rehabilitation has a beneficial effect on cognitive performance and mental fatigue [24, 25]. Studies addressing the cognitive functioning of neuro-oncological patients by use of specific neuropsychological tools could prove to be very interesting, particularly in view of the evidence of effectiveness of neuropsychological rehabilitation reported in national and international guidelines on the management of stroke.

In the context of a multidisciplinary approach, cognitive rehabilitation can be combined with occupational therapy (OT) aimed at facilitating engagement in meaningful everyday activities and maintaining or improving patients' independence in performing the activities of daily living (ADL), through the use of a variety of techniques and tools (see Chap. 16 on AHP input for details).

Goals are defined in collaboration with the patients to identify the activities most important to their QoL. Usually training focuses on improving the patients' functional capacity, body, activity and participation level by adapting activities, regaining or developing activity abilities and/or rebuilding and developing patient skills for preserving functional independence and avoiding the necessity for care from others [26].

Even if OT has the potential to limit and reverse cancer-related disability, it still remains severely underused in BT patients. Barriers to a wider utilisation of OTs are represented by the poor awareness of OT by the health professionals, lack of knowledge of whom OT would benefit and the practical accessibility to the service.

As more cancer rehabilitation programmes are developed and the scope of OT becomes better understood, accessing an occupational therapist will become more standard practice. Occupational therapists treat each patient holistically and use creative solutions to improve the overall cognitive and functional capacity of patients, making the occupational therapist a critical member of the multidisciplinary team.

## 9.6.2  Psychological Support

Feelings of anxiety, depression and future uncertainty were shown to be highly prevalent among BT patients as psychological reactions to the disease and to the treatments. Patients with HGG report higher levels of panic, depression, anxiety and fear of death than patients affected by low-grade gliomas. Besides being a response to stress, psychiatric symptoms may also depend on tumour location, patient's premorbid psychiatric status and cognitive impairment. Due to the dramatic emotional sequelae of having a BT, it is important that patients are routinely screened for psychological distress to implement adequate support intervention to improve their psychological well-being.

Psycho-oncology as an integral part of oncology has become internationally recognised, though it has not always been implemented as standard care. The primary aim of psycho-oncological management is to retain and optimise the subjective QoL of cancer patients throughout the illness trajectory, providing existential support to facilitate adjustment to diagnosis, treatment and end-of-life issues. Literature evidences suggest that many people appreciate the opportunity to discuss existential fears and concerns early in the illness rather than support only being offered towards the end of life. This is particularly relevant considering that disease progression can greatly compromise people's cognitive and communication skills.

The effectiveness of psycho-oncological support (that ranges from psychoeducative measures to psychotherapeutic interventions) has been shown in various studies, both in group and individual therapies.

Professionally or peer-led support groups may provide patients with cancer with a sense of community, unconditional acceptance and information about the disease that they would not experience elsewhere. In addition, support groups have in different settings repeatedly been shown to increase the well-being of the patient. They may also facilitate the patient's relationship with family and friends by relieving the burden of care and providing a safe place for the expression of emotions [27].

## 9.7    Family Care

Several studies have documented the considerable burden and distress that caregivers may face as a result of providing care without being trained or prepared for this role, with substantial physical, social and psychological consequences [28].

Caring for BT people in fact may be particularly challenging because of the rapid progression of the disease; the presence of cognitive impairment and behavioural changes; the fast, physical deterioration; the changes in family life that require the caregivers to take on new roles and responsibilities; as well as the uncertainty of the future. In a short time, a high level of assistance with personal daily living tasks, problem-solving and decision-making is often needed. In turn, caregivers' psychological and behavioural responses to caregiving may impact on their own emotional and physical health and may also influence the quality of care delivered to the patient at home as well as the decision to institutionalise patients.

Intervention research suggests that educational programmes and cognitive-behavioural therapy may relieve neuro-oncology caregiver distress and that identifying and addressing concerns early may lead to better carer health outcomes. Recommendations from literature include having educational programmes for caregivers to prepare them for changes in their loved one and to increase understanding of treatment processes, teaching caregivers stress reduction techniques and coping strategies, involving caregivers more in communication and having family consultations in the crisis phase. In spite of this, the evaluation of family caregivers' support needs is often neglected while focusing primarily on the patient, resulting in informal and undocumented needs assessment. As evidenced in the literature, the most prevalent caregiver needs soon after diagnosis usually regard "getting information about the illness and its evolution" and "dealing with fears and worries", while at follow-up visits the needs usually shift on "getting a break from caring", "practical help in the home" and "equipment to help care" as well as "managing patient's symptoms" [28].

Professional support in assessing and meeting the unique support and palliative care needs of family caregivers of BT persons is imperative to enable them to continue their caregiving activities, easing their burden and maintaining the best possible level of patients' well-being.

## 9.8    QoL and Palliative Rehabilitation

Despite multimodal treatment, the vast majority of BT patients cannot be cured and have a poor prognosis. Therefore, the benefits of therapies, in terms of prolonged survival or delay of progression, have to be carefully weighed against the side effects of the treatments, which may adversely influence the patient's functioning and well-being during his/her remaining life span. For these patients the attainment of an acceptable quality of life is at least as important as the duration of survival.

Health-related QoL (HRQOL) is a multidimensional concept that includes physical, emotional, cognitive, social and spiritual aspects that are believed to be influenced by a person's experience, beliefs, expectations and perceptions. Although some concerns regarding HRQOL appear to be universal (e.g., emotional distress and/or impaired functional status), many others are uniquely determined and depend on the presence of factors that may initially appear unrelated to the disease process.

As QoL reflects the patient's subjective evaluation of important and personal aspects of his/her well-being, HRQOL measures should be patient-reported, even if proxy-reported are still used when patient evaluation is no longer feasible.

In recent decades, with the debate on whether the survival endpoint alone can provide sufficient evidence of the superiority of one treatment modality over another, HRQOL has become an increasingly important endpoint in cancer studies, next to outcome measures such as overall survival, progression-free survival and time to tumour progression, and the American Society of Clinical Oncology has suggested that QoL measurements should be primary endpoint in any phase III study.

Measuring a complex aspect of the person, such as QoL, is by no means easy and a lot of instruments were developed over the course of years.

One frequently used HRQOL tool used for cancer patients is the European Organisation for Research and Treatment of Cancer (EORTC) QLQ-C30. This questionnaire contains 30 items organised into five functional scales: three symptom scales, one global health and quality of life scale and several single symptom items. The EORTC QLQ-C30 is often used in conjunction with the brain tumour-specific questionnaire, the EORTC QLQ-BN20. This questionnaire, developed for and validated by BT patients, consists of 20 items subdivided into four multi-item scales on future uncertainty, motor dysfunction, communication deficits and visual disorders.

Although HRQOL is important in all stages of the disease, it is of utmost importance in the end-of-life phase, when the main goals of palliative care are to offer adequate symptom control, to maintain the QoL of the patients and their caregivers through the relief of suffering, to provide psychological support to spiritual needs of patients and families and to facilitate a calm and dignified way of dying, without inappropriate prolongation of life.

In end-of-life phase, medical concerns are often in regard to non-treatment decisions (withholding or withdrawing) around therapies given for the alleviation of symptoms. However, often in advanced stages of the disease, patients manifest cognitive deficits, confusion and disorders of consciousness that may reduce their competence and ability to participate in such critical decisions, leaving the whole responsibility on caregivers.

Hence, as patients' participation in end-of-life decision-making is only possible at a relatively early stage in the disease course, advance care planning should be considered to reach a consensus about possible end-of-life decisions, in order to obtain a consensus, respecting both patients and caregivers' values and warding patients' autonomy [29].

## 9.9 Nurses' Role in Rehabilitation

Until recently, the figure of nurses in rehabilitation has often been considered marginal as if their only role was to "prepare" patients for rehabilitation and much of nurses' care remained invisible, receiving relatively scant attention in the literature.

Actually, most of nurses' activities represent essential rehabilitative skills, used by rehabilitation nurses every day such as easing pain, mobilising, healing pressure areas or caring for wounds, providing adequate nutrition and hydration, administering medications and caring for sleep, rest and stimulation. Although the ultimate goal of rehabilitation is to enable patients to live as independently as possible, rehabilitation nurses may also be required to assist patients with everyday tasks as well, such as bathing and dressing, personal hygiene and continence.

As suffering from a disability or having a loved one who suffers from a disability can be very confusing and frustrating at times, rehabilitation nurses are also asked to provide patients and caregivers with education and emotional support in addition to their other roles. Of particular significance is the creation of a supportive environment for rehabilitation to occur. Unless such needs are fully met and built into an educational rehabilitation programme, all other activities are ineffective.

In addition to their clinical role, rehabilitation nurses also have an important administrative function, effectively acting as case managers, especially in acute care and acute rehabilitation settings. In this role, nurses must advocate for patients and families, representing their concerns regarding care both within and outside the clinical setting; moreover, nurses may provide a link between patients and families and the hospital. Patients and relatives often describe the role of the nurse specialists as one of active companionship throughout the disease, appreciating in particular qualities as availability, proactive and flexible support, professionalism and personal tone. The close contact with families allows nurses to identify caregivers whom are at risk of negative emotional and physical reactions to providing care and to plan appropriate and effective interventions to meet their needs. In fact, nurses are an essential resource to caregivers to assist with bringing out care demands as well as identifying resources that can decrease distress of meeting care demands. Nurses are often responsible for both teaching family and caregivers tasks of care and disease and symptom management, as well as being responsible for identifying factors that may place caregivers at risk for negative consequences and intervening with the caregiver as necessary. Other topics frequently addressed by nurses include reinforcing information already given or providing additional information about treatment and side effects, changing of appointments, symptom advice and test results. The case manager must review each patient individually to establish what treatments and services are appropriate. This role is bound to become increasingly important in the context of the ever-increasing need to achieve better management of resources and shorter hospitalisations.

After discharge the district or community nurse has the potential to play a central part in community rehabilitation provision, by making assessments, referring on to other members of the multi-professional team, advocating for and liaising with other services, helping people to adapt, teaching and motivating patients and carers, supporting and involving families and providing technical care. A number of challenges to community-based nursing roles were apparent, including feelings of exclusion, lack of recognition, a lack of time for rehabilitation and paucity of referrals for rehabilitation by clinicians. Greater clarity and recognition is needed of the community-based nursing contribution to rehabilitation, and there is a need to ensure that community nursing assessments contribute to patients' rehabilitation goals and the promotion of independent living.

Specifically, in the field of neuro-oncology, the introduction of nurse specialist was strongly advocated; nurses who are interested in neuro-oncological rehabilitation are concerned with changes and functional abilities, rather than the disease process, and with how to improve the remaining time, rather than with how many months an individual has left to live.

The complexity of knowledge and skills required to provide such comprehensive care to neuro-oncological patients illustrates the need for increasing specialisation within the health professions. Although nursing is purportedly about meeting the needs of all, the development of an understanding of patients with disabilities is one area that is generally not given specific attention in undergraduate nursing curricula. Only a third of nurses felt, with hindsight, that their preregistration education had provided them with adequate skills and knowledge for their role in rehabilitation; furthermore, nurses have expressed the need to have access to more education and training focused on rehabilitation per se and associated clinical skills, in order to strengthen and raise the profile of their professional role. In this regard, recent studies supported this view [30], and surely *The Specialty Practice of Rehabilitation Nursing: A Core Curriculum, 7th Edition*, published by the Association of Rehabilitation Nurses (2015), represents a key text in this area.

## References

1. Yabroff KR, Lawrence WF, Clauser S, Davis WW, Brown ML. Burden of illness in cancer survivors: findings from a population-based national sample. J Natl Cancer Inst. 2004;96(17):1322–30.
2. Mukand JA, Blackinton DD, Crincoli MG, Lee JJ, Santos BB. Incidence of neurologic deficits and rehabilitation of patients with brain tumors. Am J Phys Med Rehabil. 2001;80:346–50.

3. Boele FW, Klein M, Reijneveld JC, Verdonck-de Leeuw IM, Heimans JJ. Symptom management and quality of life in glioma patients. CNS Oncol. 2014;3(1):37–47.
4. Asher A, Fu JB, Bailey C, Hughes JK. Fatigue among patients with brain tumors. CNS Oncol. 2016;5(2):91–100.
5. Kirshblum S, O'Dell MW, Ho C, Barr K. Rehabilitation of persons with central nervous system tumors. Cancer. 2001;92:1029–38.
6. Vargo M. Brain tumor rehabilitation. Am J Phys Med Rehabil. 2011;90(Suppl):S50–62.
7. Bartolo M, Zucchella C, Pace A, Lanzetta G, Vecchione C, Bartolo M, et al. Early rehabilitation after surgery improves functional outcome in inpatients with brain tumours. J Neurooncol. 2012;107(3):537–44.
8. Sherwood PR, Given BA, Donovan H, Baum A, Given CW, Bender CM, et al. Guiding research in family care: a new approach to oncology caregiving. Psychooncology. 2008;17(10):986–96.
9. Teasell R, Bayona N, Salter K, Hellings C, Bitensky J. Progress in clinical neurosciences: Stroke recovery and rehabilitation. Can J Neurol Sci. 2006;33(4):357–64.
10. Fuchs E, Flügge G. Adult neuroplasticity: more than 40 years of research. Neural Plast. 2014;2014:541870.
11. Schmidt BL, Hamamoto DT, Simone DA, Wilcox GL. Mechanism of cancer pain. Mol Interv. 2010;10(3):164–78.
12. Saunders C. Introduction: history and challenge. In: Saunders C, Sykes N, editors. The management of terminal malignant disease. London: Hodder and Stoughton; 1993. p. 1–14.
13. Bartolo M, Chiò A, Ferrari S, Tassorelli C, Tamburin S, Avenali M, et al. Assessing and treating pain in movement disorders, amyotrophic lateral sclerosis, severe acquired brain injury, disorders of consciousness, dementia, oncology and neuroinfectivology. Evidence and recommendations from the Italian Consensus Conference on Pain in Neurorehabilitation. Eur J Phys Rehabil Med. 2016;52(6):841–54.
14. World Health Organization. International classification of functioning, disability, and health (ICF). Geneva: WHO; 2001.
15. Stucki G, Melvin J. The international classification of functioning, disability and health: a unifying model for the conceptual description of physical and rehabilitation medicine. J Rehabil Med. 2007;39:286–92.
16. Khan F, Amatya B. Use of the international classification of functioning, disability and health (ICF) to describe patient-reported disability in primary brain tumour in an Australian community cohort. J Rehabil Med. 2013;45(5):434–45.
17. Wade DT. Stroke: rehabilitation and long-term care. Lancet. 1992;339(8796):791–3.
18. Langbecker D, Yates P. Primary brain tumor patients' supportive care needs and multidisciplinary rehabilitation, community and psychosocial support services: awareness, referral and utilization. J Neurooncol. 2016;127(1):91–102.
19. Khan F, Amatya B, Ng L, Drummond K, Galea M. Multidisciplinary rehabilitation after primary brain tumour treatment. Cochrane Database Syst Rev. 2015;(8):CD009509.
20. Meyers FJ, Linder J. Simultaneous care: Disease treatment and palliative care throughout illness. J Clin Oncol. 2003;21:1412–5.
21. Pace A, Metro G, Fabi A. Supportive care in neurooncology. Curr Opin Oncol. 2010;22:621–6.
22. Taphoorn MJ, Klein M. Cognitive deficits in adult patients with brain tumours. Lancet Neurol. 2004;3:159–68.
23. Zucchella C, Bartolo M, Di Lorenzo C, Villani V, Pace A. Cognitive impairment in primary brain tumors outpatients: a prospective cross-sectional survey. J Neurooncol. 2013;112(3):455–60.
24. Zucchella C, Capone A, Codella V, De Nunzio AM, Vecchione C, Sandrini G, et al. Cognitive rehabilitation for early post-surgery inpatients affected by primary brain tumor: a randomized, controlled trial. J Neurooncol. 2013;114(1):93–100.
25. Gehring K, Sitskoorn MM, Gundy CM, Sikkes SA, Klein M, Postma TJ, et al. Cognitive rehabilitation in patients with gliomas: a randomized, controlled trial. J Clin Oncol. 2009;27(22):3712–22.
26. Chan V, Xiong C, Colantonio A. Patients with brain tumors: who receives postacute occupational therapy services? Am J Occup Ther. 2015;69(2):1–6.

27. Ford E, Catt S, Chalmers A, Fallowfield L. Systematic review of supportive care needs in patients with primary malignant brain tumors. Neuro Oncol. 2012;14:392–404.
28. Sherwood PR, Cwiklik M, Donovan HS. Neurooncology family caregiving: review and directions for future research. CNS Oncol. 2016;5(1):4.
29. Koekkoek JA, Chang S, Taphoorn MJ. Palliative care at the end-of-life in glioma patients. Handb Clin Neurol. 2016;134:315–26.
30. Bartolo M, Zucchella C, Pace A, De Nunzio AM, Serrao M, Sandrini G, et al. Improving neurooncological patients care: basic and practical concepts for nurse specialist in neurorehabilitation. J Exp Clin Cancer Res. 2012;1:82.

Isabella Robbins

**Abstract**

My story of being diagnosed with a low-grade glioma includes the social, psychological, emotional and physical challenges of living with a primary brain tumour. Each of these challenges can be seen in isolation, except each has an impact on the others. My life changed dramatically after the diagnosis on the 20 March 2008. After my diagnosis, surgery and a period of stability, this situation has changed. Seven years on, the start of epilepsy and the tumour recurring have overwhelmingly changed my condition. The tumour growing and becoming inoperable has resulted in having radical radiotherapy. The next phase is the control of symptoms. Through this I have learnt about life and myself. Most of all I have learnt to seize the day.

**Keywords**

Low-grade glioma · Epilepsy · Radiotherapy · Management of symptoms · Living with a brain tumour · Fatigue

**Learning Outcomes**
- To gain first-hand insight and knowledge of a patient's journey and intimate experiences of living with a low-grade glioma.
- To understand and have deeper insight into the impact such a diagnosis has on every aspect of their life and how they manage day-to-day life in the knowledge that their life expectancy will be greatly diminished.

I. Robbins (✉)
Department of Neurosurgery, Addenbrooke's Hospital, Cambridge University Hospitals NHS Foundation Trust, Cambridgeshire, UK
e-mail: ingela.oberg@addenbrookes.nhs.uk

© Springer Nature Switzerland AG 2019                                        147
I. Oberg (ed.), *Management of Adult Glioma in Nursing Practice*,
https://doi.org/10.1007/978-3-319-76747-5_10

- To hear first-hand about issues and matters of importance from a patient's per- spective that may not otherwise be overtly obvious to the health-care professional.

## 10.1 Introduction

This is a story of living with a brain tumour for the past 9 years or, rather, becoming familiar with its symptoms and its impact on my family and me. In order to tell this story with clarity, I have taken a chronological approach whilst simultaneously extracting some key themes that have challenged me, frightened me and endorsed my belief in love and kindness.

At the age of 46, I was diagnosed with a very large WHO grade II astrocytoma in my right temporal lobe. I am married and have three daughters. At the point of diag- nosis, they were 12, 14 and 16 years old. I qualified as a general nurse in 1983 work- ing primarily in haematology. After 17 years of nursing, I decided to study sociology, which subsequently led to funding for a master's degree, shortly followed by a doc- toral exam (PhD). My intention in higher education had been to apply sociology to my nursing knowledge and pursue a career using these new skills—the diagnosis changed all that. However, writing this chapter has become a way of giving some- thing back and extracting something positive out of a brain tumour.

When I talk about my brain tumour, it is never with respect, but I have an almost reverence for my brain; I'd like to think our brains are not only full of vital func- tions, cells and synapses but that it also houses our minds, our souls and the essence of who we are. This is a recurring theme for me. Religious representation aside, Michelangelo's 'Creation of Adam', for me, represents life and its connections to people. Michelangelo was an artist/anatomist, and it has been argued that his 'Creation of Adam' is a depiction of the human brain (https://en.wikipedia.org/wiki/ The_Creation_of_Adam) [1, 2].

## 10.2 A Diagnosis

### 10.2.1 The Best Decision I Ever Made

I think perhaps most people remember the point at which they received a devastat- ing diagnosis. It becomes etched in your memory and ownership of that diagnosis begins: for me, *my* brain tumour. Nine years on, I can still remember the intricate detail of events leading up to the diagnosis.

During the preceding 2 years, I had become increasingly tired. As a 44-year-old woman with three teenagers, trying to complete a PhD and managing a busy house- hold, most people said it was my age. The General Practitione (GP) thought it was my busy life and that my painful legs were post-viral syndrome. The head-splitting headaches were put down to hormonal changes—depression was diagnosed and anti-depressants prescribed.

In March 2008 I was struggling to submit my final PhD thesis. I fell asleep every afternoon, unable to concentrate or keep my eyes open. My eyesight was deteriorating. I already wore glasses for shortsightedness, but this was different, rather like looking through a mist. I could no longer put it down to the context of my life, so I arranged to see an optician—the best decision I ever made.

## 10.2.2  Seeing What We Don't Expect to See

The first thing the optician asked me was 'What are you doing here? It's only a year since your last check'. She took my history of headaches, painful eyes that felt like they were bruised and constant tiredness. She examined my eyes and asked the technicians to do a visual field test. I'd never had this done before and didn't realise I was missing the sight in the left upper quadrant of each eye (quadrantanopia). The optician explained this to me, but offered no hint of the significance. From that point onwards, I started to see the everyday behaviour of people we take for granted changing, and it greatly unsettled me. The optician asked me to wait and offered me a cup of tea! An optician had never offered me that before. She emphasised that the letter she had written *must* be dropped off to my general practitioner (GP) immediately, which I did.

My phone rang at 09.30 the next morning with the GP asking me to attend surgery as soon as possible. That also had never happened before. As an independent woman, I had always done my own thing with medical issues (apart from baby scans and caesarian sections). However, this was different. Without asking, my husband came with me. There was an unsaid urgency. My GP briefly checked my field of vision, and the reassuring look of understanding I was expecting didn't come. Instead, indecision crossed his face. Eye casualty was called, and I was asked to go straight there.

For the next 4 h, I had various lights shone into my eyes, getting nowhere. The senior doctor was frustrated in trying to understand my symptoms, or lack of. Finally, late afternoon, he decided a CT scan of my head was needed. My husband went home to check the three girls were ok. Our oldest daughter was studying for her final school exams.

## 10.2.3  Truth Telling

My oldest daughter called me on my mobile to say the hospital had called and wanted to *speak to dad* but that he was on his way back to the hospital. Something was wrong. I was worried now. It was late afternoon, but the doctors and nurses were rushing around, something about 'we'll use that room and sister (nurse) can you come in too'. My husband arrived back, and we quickly exchanged stories of the last hour. We were ushered into the consulting room. I asked the doctor to be honest with me. He said in the gentlest way that I had a large brain tumour. In an apologetic tone, he said he didn't know anything about them, and an admission to the neurosurgical unit was organised. The senior nurse sitting to one side started crying. I just said, thinking I would die soon, that all I wanted was to get my girls to adulthood and to my husband, 'you must marry again'.

## 10.2.4  Breaking the News

In shock my husband and I came up with some kind of plan to deal with the next 24 h. He had to go home and concoct a story about mum staying in hospital overnight: something about eyesight. Telling my family happened without any effort really. My twin sister happened to ring the house. My husband said I was in hospital and gave her the phone number. She phoned me on the ward. How do I tell my twin? I just blurted it out. 'I've got a brain tumour'—silence and disbelief. I tried really hard not to lose it and said my concern was for the girls. The family grapevine worked well. Telling my twin was a forerunner to telling the girls and for my twin telling our 80-year-old mother. Telling the girls was one of the most awful things I've had to do in my life. My childhood had been straightforward in terms of people not being ill and dying. What was this going to do to the girls? One of my sisters had been diagnosed with a melanoma when her children were teenagers. Her advice was to be honest. As I told them on my return from hospital, my 16-year-old daughter in a typically pragmatic way said 'we guessed mum'. My 14-year-old was devastated. The youngest has always said she took the news too well. Our lives changed in a moment of seconds.

In retrospect this was the right approach to take. My three daughters each with their own personalities took it in different ways. I don't think the shock could be lessened in any way. The anxiety of keeping a diagnosis under wraps could only increase the stress.

## 10.2.5  I Don't Want to Join This Club

"Hope" is the thing with feathers -
That perches in the soul -
And sings the tune without the words -
And never stops - at all -
And sweetest - in the Gale - is heard -
And sore must be the storm -
That could abash the little Bird
That kept so many warm

*Emily Dickinson* [3]

### 10.2.5.1  The Misunderstood View of Brain Tumours

The public view of brain tumours is that it is a death sentence, which of course it is, in varying degrees. There is no cure. The common belief is that there is only one type of brain tumour, which many people die swiftly from. Certainly, famous politicians such as Edward Kennedy and Mo Mowlam were reported to die quickly from their brain tumours. This misunderstanding of *all* brain tumours is perpetuated by TV drama and a general misunderstanding of brain tumours told as stories in the press. The notion that all brain tumours are the same does have ramifications at diagnosis. So, being admitted to a neurosurgical unit was, to say the least, very frightening. Over 48 h I learnt that I had a low-grade glioma, to which the blood supply was limited, and that this was a good feature. I could not comprehend at that time whether or not I could 'live' with a low-grade glioma—I thought I would die soon. This uncertainty is something which I continue to live with, and for me it underpins everything.

## 10.2.6  A Silver Lining: Hope but Not False Hope

On admission, two well-meaning patients told me that the bed I was allocated had been vacated by a lady expecting to die in 5 weeks and she was going to make the most of the time she had left. Their intention wasn't to scare me but to indicate the resilience of people who have brain tumours. There have been many poignant moments like this over time. I have hung on to them in order to back up my sense of hope and pragmatism.

Sleep didn't come but the duty night nurse did. I guess it's difficult to come up with the 'right' words to say to someone with a newly diagnosed brain tumour. But his silver lining was that I was lucky because brain tumours don't metastasise. Yes, I could be sitting here with a breast cancer, or cervical cancer, but this cancer won't spread.

Hope comes in many guises. The neurosurgeon says it will be all right, neurosurgery has been transformed by technology, advanced life-support systems have made neurosurgery so much safer, that there is just a 'fragment' of tumour remaining and that it was low grade but with the caveat that it would progress (transform) into a high grade at some stage. The decision he and I took not to touch on statistics, because they bear no relation to the individual and their unique brain tumour. New treatments are coming along all the time. He is a wonderful communicator with empathy in buckets. I didn't fear seeing him or feel dissatisfied. I trusted him, literally with my life.

I think trust is intertwined with hope. I know people who have approached a devastating diagnosis with scepticism and mistrust of their clinicians. Despite how my journey started, I consciously aimed to trust the clinicians. Although my past nursing experience helped inform me of this, I also concluded early on that I did not have the energy, or expertise, *not* to trust. Nonetheless, I have met people with brain tumours who have found a lot to be unhappy with about their whole experience. Sometimes I have thought that I've been too passive in accepting treatment and supportive care. When I hear people complaining about the same clinicians who also look after me, it is confusing. It doesn't bear relation to my experience.

## 10.2.7  The End of Deference: Trust and Its Contradictions

The truth that makes men free is for
the most part the truth which men[sic]
prefer not to hear.

                                                                                          (Agar 1965) [4]

When I started nursing in 1980, paternalism was in full swing. It was still the era of 'doctor knows best'. When the general surgeon came to do his weekly ward round, the nurse in charge would insist all students and auxiliary nurses were to be out of view. We were shuffled off to the sluice. The surgeon would come to the ward on a Christmas day to carve the turkey for the patients' Christmas dinner.

The end of paternalism did not just happen. The 1980s brought with it a radical shift in how the layperson experienced all kinds of expertise, including health care. In terms of health care, prior to this the experts' advice was heeded. David Held suggests that 'the decade and a half following the Second World War was characterized by many as an age of consent, faith in authority and legitimacy' [5]. Neoliberalism brought with it an enhancement of the client/patient. This reversal in authority brought with it a demand by the citizens over authority [6]. For the NHS the patient has become the consumer of health care who can challenge decisions and make informed choices.

This change in mentality and practice was not a bad thing. I had experienced the ward rounds when the doctor, standing as far away from the patient as possible, would tell the patient what to think and do and the doctor moving on to the next bed and the patient calling me back afterwards to explain what he had just said. This does not mean to say that it is perfect now, but there is an acknowledgement that doctors should not behave in a maverick way, and patients have the right to ask questions and make choices. The risk-benefit calculation that underpins all medicine is imperative. For some patients, there is a choice, an easy choice. For the person with a brain tumour, choice is not obvious—when there is no cure, choice is limited.

Choice is also contradictory. The chance to choose brings with it a certain freedom. The other side of that is the complexity of deciding and making the *right* decision. In the context of treatment for a brain tumour, the right decision is on a knife-edge. The multidisciplinary meetings for me have acted as a second opinion. No single doctor makes his or her own decision. I have trusted the clinicians to make the safest and best decision on my behalf. Trusting the neurosurgeons, anaesthetists, oncologists, nurses, radiologists, pathologists and all the other medical staff involved in my care (not mentioned here), for me, has been crucial to living with this tumour.

I think hope is an extension of trust. It can be a holistic, existential idea. It encompasses love, help and kindness and being kind to oneself, looking for the best in everything, even brain tumours. Not having hope, for me, is knowing this is a disease which, at this moment in time, has no cure. It resides in the brain where any insult impacts on the body and mind, bringing disability with it, and death. With that come sadness, anger and not emotionally existing. Having training in the philosophy of science and an understanding of the antagonism between positivism and emotion, I put that impenetrable dilemma to one side.

Hope and trust were and remain important to living each day with this thing in my brain. They underpin the enormity of this condition.

## 10.2.8 The Beginning of the Unknown: Treatment

### 10.2.8.1 Clearing My Diary

Being discharged home 48 h after being diagnosed with a very large brain tumour was surprising. There was nothing for me to do other than to keep taking the high-dose steroids. Surgery was planned for as soon as possible, so I was left in a state of limbo, waiting for a date.

I don't remember much about the month between diagnosis and surgery, but the things that were uppermost in my mind were to spend as much time with my husband and daughters and extended family. There was my youngest daughter's 12th birthday to celebrate. This took on much more poignancy, as did everything else.

The undergraduate marking that I was in the middle of a diagnosis had to be dropped. Looking for a job had to stop as did getting on with my PhD. My diary was becoming empty, as I had to say no to things. This was done with sadness and marked the beginning of a journey I had no idea I was to embark upon.

### 10.2.8.2 The Postoperative Period

After a 10-h surgery, I woke up in intensive care having expected to be taken back to the ward. (My consultant later told me he had scraped the tumour off my brainstem, hence intensive care.) I wasn't scared at all; in fact it was rather lovely. I was awake. I was alive. I remember coughing as the endotracheal (ET) tube was removed. So that's what it's like?

I woke with the anaesthetist at the end of my bed reassuring me. To his side were my husband and my twin sister with their arms around the girls. I delightedly told my sister I could move my left arm and leg. Twenty-four hours later, I was back on the neurosurgical ward and 4 days later discharged home. With intense pain from a dislocated jaw (temporal lobe tumour, they cut your mastoid muscles for one!) and gross swelling, I thought I'd be ok at home. From then on, my husband and our three daughters and I did our best to cope with someone (me) who was in shock, found doing anything with the pain difficult, such as eating or talking. I slept a lot. My family found this particularly distressing as I wasn't the same person I was when I left home that morning prior to surgery.

### 10.2.8.3 Identity: Am I Still Me?

My neurosurgeon refers to understanding of how the brain works, as 'the final frontier'. But in all of its biological complexity and so much that is not known, I think the brain comes down to being a mind and encompasses who we are as individuals.

This has been the enduring concern for me, from the beginning until now. Was I the person I was before the diagnosis? Things had certainly changed. Who was I with a brain tumour before diagnosis? Who am I now that people with good intentions have been inside my brain? Am I concerned about my mind or my brain? Where is the essence of who we are located in the brain? Do I have a soul and, if so, might it be in my brain? This tautology is exhausting and ultimately esoteric. Plato and philosophers thereafter have battled (and continue to battle) to understand and lay down what consciousness and the mind are, with no concrete answers. My youngest daughter, who has an old head on young shoulders, said to me a few years ago, 'Mum, none of us stay the same'.

Initially these questions consumed me. Ultimately, I was concerned with my characteristics and personality. I asked my family and close friends, constantly: Did I seem to be the person I was before the surgery? Was I rational? Did I make sense? Did I look the same? Was I still a mother who cared? Unless you have had neurosurgery, I don't think it is possible to 'imagine' what it might do to your sense of self. I certainly annoyed my family with this concern, and I suppose I began to reinforce it by this constant questioning. It became an acute problem for me when I interviewed for a job and was subsequently appointed. In a way I could start off being 'me' somewhere where nobody knew me. This should have been a positive thing; however, my new employers knew my diagnosis, and to them I was a brain tumour patient, rather than a person. I had been given a new identity, but its name was 'prove yourself'. Disease or injury to the brain brings with it connotations a person who is perceived to be unable to be independent, to think, to make sense and to be irrational. So, I had to continually prove myself. It was a tough job, and when my contract ended, it was with a sense of relief. In retrospect, I now know all of this was made harder by fatigue (see below).

## 10.3   Getting on with Life and on My Way to Acceptance

I don't remember with any great clarity the first 6 months after surgery. I slept a lot. My husband went back to work as his employer did not allow carers leave, and the girls went to school. My oldest daughter who was 16 at that time helped to organise the younger two. I have no idea who did the laundry and who cleaned the house or cooked our meals. The running of the house became a mystery. What I slowly became aware of, however, were changes in my physical as well as visual abilities.

The worst of these were the visual problems. I first noticed a worsening in my field of vision when I walked into rooms. Looking down as I entered a room, I missed people. A few seconds later, I would lift my head and see whoever was there. My husband and children would look at me with a puzzled look as I realised I had missed them. This was a shock, and I knew it hadn't been this bad before the surgery. I convinced myself I was going blind. The subtle double vision which I didn't realise I was experiencing at that time confused me even more. I have no doubt this experience lowered my mood and shattered my confidence. I didn't tell anybody about my fear of going blind. I felt my family had been through enough and we were just coping from day-to-day.

My 6th month surgical follow-up with my consultant revealed a slight worsening in my visual field, but he said it wouldn't worsen beyond that. Along with this came a warning, delivered gently, that getting my driving licence back could be difficult. However, he said I would drive again. The good news was that the 'double vision' could be corrected with prisms and to see my optician to organise this. My husband and I literally ran out of the hospital and went straight to the optician. The kindness that was shown when they picked up the tumour continued. A very empathic optician reassured me that the diplopia was easy to correct. I collected the glasses the next day. They changed my life. Seeing became sharp and everyday life became easier.

### 10.3.1 Fatigue

Fatigue is a vague and difficult condition to describe. Fatigue is not tiredness, and it is difficult to explain this to people. Fatigue is so much worse than that. The first time I was introduced to this term in the context of illness was by my GP. I am quite sure I experienced this before my diagnosis. Fatigue is now a huge part of my life. Some days are better than others. My experience of it is the feeling of having absolutely no power left in my limbs, 'jelly legs' as I call them, and having nothing else to give in terms of energy, emotional and cognitive input. Occasionally I have the thought that this is what it must feel like going towards death, when the body is closing down, but not giving up. The closest thing I could describe it to would be the first 12 weeks of pregnancy. The word fatigue is overused, as it seems everyone is fatigued—after exercise, a day at work, or too much to do. This is not to say people don't experience fatigue, but when it occurs on an almost daily basis, it drains momentum, resulting in some days being overwhelming.

Over the last 9 years, I have been offered advice from many people, professionals and lay people. Some of the advice has been contradictory, for example, exercise when you're feeling fatigued. Exercising when you feel depleted is so difficult. I have taken bits of the advice and used it to try and find what suits me and what I can fit into a 24-h period. When I was working, I didn't measure the fatigue; I just did what I had to, not what I wanted, for example, going to bed at 8 pm in order to be able to get up the next day at 7 am to prepare for work. This resulted in life being a cycle of work and sleep. Knowing it is inevitable that you will leave this life too soon—making the most of relationships, enjoying leisure and enjoying life—takes on more importance. So rather than just doing what you have to, doing what you want to becomes important. With the recurrence of the tumour and the onset of epilepsy, taking anticonvulsants and effects of recent radiotherapy, fatigue has changed and become more intense. The gaps between 'bad' days are getting shorter. Importantly, I have reached an emotional acceptance that it is a disability, and sometimes it will win on any particular day. I am now at the point that I measure my ability to do things very carefully. If I want to go shopping, for example, I will plan my route from the bus stop to each shop (no more than three!), with the last one close to the bus stop. It has taken a long time to accept that a taxi might be needed to get home, instead of taking a bus. If I want to swim, I will take the day before and after very easy. This is a tricky one. Exercise is supposed to help fatigue, but for me there is a price to pay, namely, more fatigue.

The most difficult element of fatigue is its invisibility. You're disabled but you look well. Is it real or is it imagined? People without a brain tumour likening their fatigue to yours—it's difficult to say, but it really is not the same. It matters ultimately, because understanding the limitations it places on the lives of people with brain tumours helps the sufferer. So, when I decline an evening out or have to renege on plans, it's accepted as authentic, especially as I quite often overestimate what I can manage in a day.

### 10.3.2 Employment

As stated, I was completing my PhD at the time I was diagnosed. The intention had been to finish the PhD and find work outside of nursing that would be fulfilling. Perhaps something that would still involve health care in some way. I had been to two interviews in the weeks before diagnosis, but unsuccessful. Hence, at diagnosis, I was unemployed and without a salary that would help pay the mortgage and household bills. I had asked my consultant at the first postoperative appointment when I could work, and he answered immediately there was nothing to stop me from working. I was surprised but delighted. I could start applying for jobs. However rather than improving my self-worth, it depleted it. I failed at three interviews, feeling useless. At the 1-year anniversary of my diagnosis, I secured my first job as a researcher. This was a bittersweet job. I gained a sense of achievement, but as previously alluded to, I was seen as 'a brain tumour'.

### 10.3.3 Understanding Disability

I hadn't understood that I was disabled or the impact the fatigue and my sight impairment would have on my ability to finish a week of part-time hours. I was helped to the acceptance of being disabled by a wise woman who had been disabled all of her life. She reiterated that we are disabled by society. This is the social model of disability [7]: societal norms 'disable' us, not our impairments (the semantics of disability versus impairment is complex and contested). People who have impairments are not inadequate; in fact people who are disabled persevere every day of their life and are resilient. The social model of disability [7], whilst not fully embraced by all of medicine, is part of disability legislation. The Disability Discrimination Act 2010 [8] sets out clearly that long-term illness which affects how we live on a daily basis is a disability. This really was news to me. Disability is still identified as the signage of the wheelchair on disabled toilet doors. I wish I had had this information at the point of looking for work and going back to work. It would have helped me avoid a huge amount of distress and the collapse of my self-esteem and self-worth.

At the point the epilepsy started, it coincided with the end of the academic year. The sedative effect of the anticonvulsants, the continuing fatigue and responsibility of the job helped me to make the decision to stop: I was not giving up, and I had reached an acceptance.

### 10.3.4 Not Driving

The Driver and Vehicle Licensing Agency (DVLA) [9] rules and regulations are complex. I was able to tick a box against craniotomy, having an unstable brain tumour, epilepsy, sight impairment and fatigue. Rationally I knew I was not safe to drive, but the emotional part for me was mourning the loss of independence. I have always told my daughters that passing my driving test was the best exam I have ever passed. It is one of those things; until you've lost it, you do not understand the value of it. My family did not understand my sadness at not being allowed to drive. I was alive—How could I place the inability to drive ahead of living? Not driving brought with it 'embarrassing' moments and frustration, explaining to people I wasn't driving because I had a brain tumour, not because I was a drunk driver. How does one say that in a rational and unemotional way? I missed not being able to help my children, getting them from A to B. Not being able to reciprocate lifts with other parents left me apologising profusely. Thank goodness for the Internet and online shopping! After a year of not driving, my consultant agreed that I should start reapplying for my licence. This is such a long story; it would need a book in itself to tell it all. Nonetheless, there are some key moments, which closely follow the Kubler-Ross' cycle of grief and loss [10] and the rollercoaster of my experience:

• Being told by a DVLA-appointed optician that my sight impairment meant I would never drive again and then being handed a small piece of paper with the number of the local Royal National Institute of Blind People (RNIB) branch! Devastation.
• Dealing with the DVLA as an organisation that does not deal with 'cases' but numbers, endless hours spent on the phone and subsequently being turned down three times in as many years.
• My consultant suggesting that I contact an undervalued organisation called Driveability [11]. They ended up being my advocate and gave me confidence to challenge the DVLA and to show I had 'adapted' to my sight impairment.
• Passing a driving test in a car I had never driven, on roads I had never driven on, after 3 long years of not driving, and I could only have one shot at this. I passed! Then finding out the DVLA was only renewing my licence for a year. Having my licence renewed twice, still going through rigorous tests to prove adaptation to my sight loss.
• A week after getting my licence *back*, one of my daughters was admitted to the hospital with a serious illness. Driving meant I could visit her every day for a long period of time.
• My first tonic-clonic seizure (leading to a subsequent diagnosis of epilepsy), occurring after a long journey to pick up one of my daughters from a university I had broken the journey up staying overnight with my sister. I thought I was rested enough to manage the next leg of the journey. My daughter and I left her university at 4 pm and got home 6 h later having made no breaks in driving despite my daughters' requests to have a break. We got home and I was tired and went straight to bed. My husband found me having the tonic-clonic seizure at

around 10.30 pm. My daughters too saw this happening. I had been so close to a car accident. It was a big wake-up call in recognising the seriousness of this disease. Giving up my licence was not difficult.

Since the start of epilepsy, I have not fought with myself about driving and have not asked the doctors their opinion on the possibility of getting my licence back. I think perhaps in reaching acceptance of not driving again, I have reached acceptance of having this tumour.

### 10.3.5  The Long View: Watch and Wait

I didn't search the Internet in terms of information and research on brain tumours. This was done very consciously. I did not want to frighten myself. My research training had also armed me with the knowledge of peer review and the ceaseless, erroneous information on the Internet. My consultant had also, in my opinion, delivered the plan for follow-up and results of MRIs in a way that didn't frighten me. Although I was put onto the protocol of 'watch and wait', he didn't give it that name. My passive approach and stable condition meant talk of the future was optimistic and to carry on with annual scans. I was happy to go along with this plan. Instead of thinking about the tumour immediately on waking up, looking forward to the day ahead took its place, just as my consultant had said it would. I was optimistic and continued to know I was lucky that my optician had picked up the tumour when she did, lucky to have a consultant who was prepared to go for a subtotal resection of the tumour (where others would have simply offered a diagnostic biopsy), lucky to have a loving family and friends and lucky to be alive. I had a stable low-grade glioma.

### 10.3.6  Recurrence: The End of Contempt for My Brain Tumour

Regarding this tumour as a 'stable, low-grade glioma' came to a traumatic end, with the onset of epilepsy. I was slightly bewildered but mostly not surprised. At that point, I was 6 years on from my diagnosis and resection. I had been close to my annual appointment with my consultant for results of the most recent MRI scan. I realised I was at a different stage of this disease but quickly burying it.

For my family, this phase matched the trauma of the postoperative period. At my annual review, I was told the tumour had started growing again and that the seizures were a result of this. I had a consultation with a doctor I had never met before, not 'my' surgeon. This new doctor reassured me that the plan was to continue with 6 monthly MRIs. Reassured? Not really, in fact, feeling the most nervous I'd felt since the postoperative period. This was not the best way to deliver this news: hearing it from a doctor I had never met and did not know; it should have been 'my' surgeon.

I went home and started to experience some strange episodes. Excessive gulping preceded by a warm feeling that travelled down to my stomach, what I imagined to be a panic attack. After my youngest daughter observed an episode of my jumbled speech over a 2-min period (expressive dysphasia), I secured an appointment with 'my' consultant. As ever he didn't frighten me with talk of where exactly the tumour was heading for. We discussed the next steps. He advised me that further surgery was too risky, with a high chance of inducing a stroke. He offered to do the surgery if I wanted it, but I needed no persuasion. At that appointment, I had what I have come to know as a complex partial seizure. Referral to a neurologist quickly followed, for medical management of my seizures. By the time I was seen, a lot of my day was peppered with complex seizures preceded by anxiety attacks.

The neurologist approached the diagnosis from a different perspective and was the first doctor to talk about timelines. I was looking at a survival of 10 years. It was a surprise to hear a doctor mention those numbers for the first time, although I had read enough at this point to have an idea of survival times. However, all the reading I had done could not buffer this news. It made all of my reading real, the power of face-to-face communication. From there I was referred to a neuro-oncologist who is now my main consultant. At my first appointment with her, the first thing she said was that I was unlucky. I think that says it well. There is no point going over what might have caused it. It gets you nowhere. It is a rare condition, and I am glad it's I and not one of my children.

A year ago, I completed a 6-week course of radical radiotherapy, my lifetime dose. The multidisciplinary team (MDT) had advised that the time had come to take action in the form of the aforementioned radiotherapy. I did not argue with this decision, my trust kicking in as ever. My tumour responded well to the radiotherapy— some of the swelling subsided—and the seizures have pretty much ceased. This has made a huge difference to my quality of life. The side effects of the treatment, however, have been an increase in my fatigue levels.

My ability to manage numbers is very poor now. My short-term memory is not great. At the time of writing this, I am not ready to accept the cognitive changes. The anticonvulsants were increased at the beginning of the radiotherapy, and this dose has not changed. My neurologist has told me that I am on a fairly high dose of anticonvulsants that probably contributes to my increased fatigue.

I have had a few episodes which, when I described them to my neurologist, we agreed were out of body experiences. I was glad he used that term first as it sounds like a story line from a movie. They have been frightening episodes, feeling myself slipping away and desperately trying to 'get back'. These episodes have felt real to me but I think also act as a metaphor for how brain tumours disrupt brain activity and play tricks on the 'mind'. Now is the time to acknowledge this tumour will kill me.

## 10.3.7 Carpe Diem: Seize the Day

There *are only two days in the year*
     *that nothing can be done.*
*One is called yesterday and the other*
     *is called tomorrow*
*So today is the right day to love, believe, do and*
     *mostly live.*

                                                                    ***The Dalai Lama*** [12]

A lot has happened in the last 9 years, and it has challenged (and to some extent changed) my family and me in profound ways. It has not been easy, and it has not just been about my journey either. Since my diagnosis, my mother has died, and my husband and one of my daughters have both been seriously ill. I have lost four dear friends to cancer over the last 5 years. The uncertainty of this filthy disease has at times pushed my family, and me, to our limits. This brain tumour has brought sadness and also a big shove into the world of reality with the loss of some dreams and aspirations.

But there have been good times too. We welcomed the sweetest cocker spaniel dog into our family. I have seen my three daughters reach adulthood, as hoped. I shared my 50th birthday with my twin. I have got back in contact with some very old friends and known the kindness of strangers. Most of all I am still here. This is not to gloss over having a brain tumour. It has been so hard at times. The saddest thing is the effect it has had on my daughters. How I wish this had not happened but with one caveat—I know the value of this life as I live it.

All the clichés come to mind, but there is so much to learn from taking a day at a time, living in the moment and really knowing that life is short.

## References

1. Michelangelo: creation of Adam. http://www.metmuseum.org/toah/hd/leon/hd_leon.htm.
2. Page RM. Altruism and the British Welfare State. Aldershot: Avebury; 1996.
3. Dickinson E. https://www.poetryfoundation.org/poems/42889/hope-is-the-thing-with-feathers -314.
4. Agar H. The perils of democracy. London: Bodley Head; 1965.
5. Held D. Power and legitimacy. In: McLennan G, Held D, Hall S, editors. State and society in contemporary britain: a critical introduction. Cambridge: Polity Press; 1984.
6. Rose N. Government, authority and expertise in advanced liberalism. Econ Soc. 1993;22(3):283.
7. Oliver M. The politics of disablement. London: Macmillan; 1990.
8. Gov.uk. https://www.gov.uk/definition-of-disability-under-equality-act-2010.
9. Driver and Vehicle Licencing Agency (DVLA). https://www.gov.uk/government/organisations/driver-and-vehicle-licensing-agency. Accessed 13 Dec 2017.
10. Kubler-Ross E. On death and dying. New York, NY: Scribner; 1969.
11. Driveability. http://www.eastangliandriveability.org.uk/. Accessed on 13 Dec 2017.
12. The Dalai Lama. https://simplereminders.com/20140711011601.html. Accessed on 12 Dec 2017.

# Holistic Needs Assessment and Care Planning

# 11

Karin Piil and Lena Rosenlund

**Abstract**

The complexity of symptoms, needs and concerns experienced by brain tumour patients and their informal caregivers requires a timely and coordinated response from healthcare services and providers. The holistic needs assessment is a systematic way of conducting an overall assessment together with the patient and caregiver, which involves an approach that covers all domains of care.

It is imperative that clinical specialists are familiar with the needs, preferences and interests of patients and their caregivers in order to provide the best possible care. Advance care planning involves (together with the patient and their caregivers) thinking about, talking about and planning for the future, including end-of-life decisions. Determining the appropriate timing for these discussions is, however, problematic and is discussed in this chapter.

This chapter presents key areas of interest when conducting a holistic needs assessment and emphasises the need to determine the future direction of advance care planning research within neuro-oncology in order to establish evidence-based, best clinical practice.

**Keywords**

Holistic needs assessment · Relatives · Symptom management · Concerns · Advance care planning · Tools · Measurements

K. Piil (✉)
Department of Oncology 5074, Copenhagen University Hospital, Rigshospitalet, Copenhagen Ø, Denmark
e-mail: karin.piil@regionh.dk

L. Rosenlund
Regionalt Cancercentrum Stockholm – Gotland, Stockholm, Sweden
e-mail: Lena.Rosenlund@sll.se

© Springer Nature Switzerland AG 2019
I. Oberg (ed.), *Management of Adult Glioma in Nursing Practice*,
https://doi.org/10.1007/978-3-319-76747-5_11

161

## Abbreviations

| | |
|---|---|
| ACP | Advance care planning |
| DT | Distress thermometer |
| EOL | End of life |
| EORTC | European Organization for Research and Treatment of Cancer |
| FACT-Br | Functional assessment of cancer therapy-brain |
| HADS | Hospital Anxiety and Depression Scale |
| HNA | Holistic needs assessment |
| HRQOL | Health-related quality of life |
| MBT | Malignant brain tumour |
| MDASI-BT | MD Anderson Symptom Inventory for Brain Tumour |
| MUIS-BT | Mishel uncertainty in illness scale-brain tumour |
| NFBrSI-24 | National Comprehensive Cancer Network/Functional Assessment of Cancer Therapy-Brain Symptom Index |
| PCI | Patient concerns inventory |
| PI | Prognostic information |
| PREM | Patient-reported experience measures |
| PRO | Patient-reported outcome |
| QOL | Quality of life |
| SNAS | Sherbrooke Neuro-Oncology Assessment Scale |
| SPARC | Sheffield Profile for Assessment and Referral for Care |

### Learning Outcomes
- To be able to identify and document complex needs and concerns from both patient and carers' perspectives, by utilising available assessment tools specific to brain tumours/glioma patients.
- To gain deeper insight into the clinical implications of assessing patients' complex needs and how to address these more readily in any clinical settings.
- To be able to provide resources such as specific patient information and tailored education and by providing early supportive care to enable them to deal with these complex issues more readily.

## 11.1 Introduction

Patients diagnosed with malignant brain tumour (MBT) experience a complex symptom burden and face a high mortality rate. The disease, surgical procedure and oncology treatments cause a variety of cerebral symptoms, and complications often occur. These include global cerebral symptoms (fatigue, nausea, headache and confusion), focal symptoms (hemiparesis, seizures and speech difficulties), neurocognitive deficits (impaired attention, concentration difficulties, reduced short-term memory and personality changes) and emotional symptoms (depression, anxiety and stress) [1]. This diagnosis, which is often frightening for the patient, involves both life-threatening cancer and a brain disease with neurological symptoms that can impact cognition, personality and overall quality of life [2]. The disease affects the entire family. As the tumour progresses, relationships, roles and responsibilities change, and the closest relatives often become the MBT patient's informal caregivers [2, 3]. The uncertain prognosis and severity of symptoms call for continued assessment and interventions based on the individual patient's situation. The complexity in needs experienced by brain tumour patients and their informal caregivers requires a coordinated response from healthcare services and providers. Neuro-oncology units consist of multidisciplinary teams including clinical nurse specialists or cancer care coordinator. The key to valuable nursing for patients with brain tumours is to provide proactive support, including the provision of information to both patients and caregivers, delivered at appropriate time points (which can be different for both the patient and the caregiver) throughout the disease period. Further, helping the patient and their caregivers to identify and manage symptoms and side effects increases their ability to cope with the disease and thereby improves quality of life [2] which is crucial.

## 11.2 Identifying Complex Needs and Concerns

One way of identifying the complex needs of cancer patients is through holistic needs assessment (HNA). The word "holism" derives from the Greek for whole, all or entire. Within the health sciences, holism is a philosophy that views human beings as having physical, social, psychological and spiritual properties, all of which are closely interconnected. The HNA is a systematic way of making an overall assessment together with the patient, which involves all domains of care. HNA is an important aspect of patient-centred care and involves specialists listening and responding to what matters for the patient. Clinical nurse specialists often take a leading role in implementing HNA, and it is common practice to co-operate with different healthcare specialists during the assessment. The HNA process helps patients to find the words to describe their complex situation, allowing greater facilitation of communication and therefore helps with the coping process. Starting HNA at the time of diagnosis is recommended, as is continuing it at certain key points or upon the patients' request. Key points during the trajectory are, for example, after being diagnosed, prior to the oncological treatment, at tumour progression, at the point of recognition of incurability and in the end-of-life (EOL) phase, as well as for caregivers upon bereavement.

## 11.3 Assessment Tools

An assessment tool used in combination with HNA can help ensure that all domains of care are covered, in addition to promoting conversation between patients, caregivers and the professional staff. A useful assessment tool can be a questionnaire or a checklist that allows patients to reflect on their situation prior to professional HNA. Another possible application is to use an assessment tool as a memory aid, comprised of questions for healthcare professionals to ask the patient. Possible tools that can support HNA are, for example, the National Comprehensive Cancer Network Distress Thermometer, Sheffield Profile for Assessment and Referral for Care and PEPSI COLA Aide Memoire (Table 11.1).

It is important to remember that patients with a brain tumour may experience not only general symptoms related to cancer but also brain cancer-specific symptoms. Generic tools run the risk of failing to address significant symptoms specific to patients with brain tumours. Incorporating assessment tools designed or modified for the population of adult brain tumour patients in the HNA process is essential. Rooney et al. [4] made a brain tumour-specific tool for HNA to be used prior to consultations in neuro-oncology outpatient clinics. This brain tumour Patient Concerns Inventory (PCI) captures problems absent from general cancer checklists and was used as part of HNA to focus on patient agenda [4]. Using patient-reported outcomes as a screening instrument can be a way to detect needs in malignant brain tumour patients. For example, there are validated measurement instruments (usually questionnaires) for patient with malignant brain tumours to self-report their health outcomes (PROs). To obtain quantifiable, actionable data, several studies are defining the efficacy and benefits of implementing PROs into the standard of care, including improved survival rates compared to standard care and the importance of early intervention of symptoms [5]. In this way, PROs can be used individually as part of an HNA and support interaction between the patient and the healthcare professionals and even for research and quality improvement. Table 11.2 lists examples of brain tumour-specific assessment tools, specifically developed or modified for brain tumour patients.

The HNA process serves as a communication and screening process detecting symptoms and concerns. During the HNA process for brain tumour patients, closest family members or caregivers should be involved. Caregivers can see important symptoms or concerns that are hidden to the patient because of cognitive impairment or to the healthcare professional who only sees the patient when visiting the clinic. This, and knowing that the closest family members eventually will become the patient's caregivers and have their own need for support, means that involving the family early is important. Therefore, assessing the family or caregiver also, using the HNA process, will support both the brain tumour patient and their family [13].

## 11.4 Care and Support Plan

HNA should always result in a care and support plan. The care and support plan is the patient's document and can be either a paper copy or electronic document or both. The care and support plan should contain a description of the patient's key concerns or needs, agreed actions to help address the needs, information to help the patient know who to contact for more help if a problem should arise and a record of

**Table 11.1**  Examples of tools to assist holistic needs assessment

| Assessment tool | Measure | Short description | Number of items | Developed by |
|---|---|---|---|---|
| National Comprehensive Cancer Network Distress Thermometer (DT) and Problem List for Patients (PL) | Holistic needs assessment (HNA) Suitable for self-report | DT is a screening tool for assessing psychological distress and for identifying rehabilitation needs in people affected by cancer. It contains a 45-item checklist regarding practical issues, family matters, emotional topics, spiritual or religious concerns and physical symptoms. It is also a scale from 0 to 10, where the patient estimates the level of distress experienced last week | 45 items and a self-reported level of distress scale and an area for free text/typing own questions | The National Comprehensive Cancer Network (USA) |
| Sheffield Profile for Assessment and Referral for Care (SPARC) | HNA Suitable for self-report | SPARC is a multidimensional screening tool for clinical assessment of supportive and palliative care needs, regardless of diagnosis or stage of disease. The self-reported questionnaire is divided in 9 dimensions: communication and information issues, physical symptoms, psychological issues, religious and spiritual issues, independency and activity, family and social issues, treatment issues and personal issues | 45 items and an area for free text/typing own questions | The Network Supportive and Palliative Care Group |
| PEPSI COLA Aide Memoire | HNA Aide memoire for the healthcare professional | An aide memoire **P** Physical **E** Emotional **P** Personal **S** Social support **I** Information and communication **C** Control and autonomy **O** Out of hours **L** Living with your illness **A** Aftercare | 9 domains of HNA | The Gold Standards Framework to support best practice for EOL care |

*DT* distress thermometer, *EOL* end of life, *HNA* holistic needs assessment, *SPARC* Sheffield Profile for Assessment and Referral for Care

**Table 11.2** Examples of brain tumour-specific assessment tools

| Assessment tool | Measure | Short description | Number of items | Reference |
|---|---|---|---|---|
| Brain tumour-specific Patient Concerns Inventory (PCI) | Holistic needs assessment (HNA) Suitable for self-reporting | PCI is a brain tumour-specific tool for HNA to be used prior to consultations in neuro-oncology outpatient clinics. The PCI is divided into three sections: <br> 1. A checklist of 48 items that allows patients to identify recent concerns involving practical, family, emotional, spiritual and physical issues <br> 2. Questions to patients regarding any need for a referral to a specialist, such as a dietician, palliative care services, a physiotherapist or social worker <br> 3. Allows the patient to prepare questions for the specialists | 48 items and an area for free text/ typing own questions | [4] |
| MD Anderson Symptom Inventory for Brain Tumour (MDASI-BT) | To assess the severity of symptoms and the impact of these symptoms on daily functioning Suitable for self-reporting | The MD Anderson Symptom Inventory (MDASI) is a tool to assess the severity of symptoms experienced by patients with cancer and the interference with daily living caused by these symptoms MDASI-BT is a diagnose-specific module for patients with brain tumour which has nine brain tumour-specific items added to the core questionnaire | 13 Core items, six interference items and nine brain tumour-specific items | [6, 7] |
| Mishel uncertainty in illness scale-brain tumour (MUIS-BT) | Uncertainties in illness Suitable for self-reporting | MUIS is applied to cancer patients during diagnostic and treatment phases to measure uncertainty. Six out of 33 items in the original MUIS were modified to better describe brain tumour patients' uncertainty. MUIS-BT is used to evaluate patients' cognitive state of uncertainty and its impact on mood, symptom severity and symptom interference | 33 items | [8] |

**Table 11.2** (continued)

| Assessment tool | Measure | Short description | Number of items | Reference |
|---|---|---|---|---|
| National Comprehensive Cancer Network/ Functional Assessment of Cancer Therapy-Brain Symptom Index (NFBrSI-24) | Identifies symptoms and level of severity Suitable for self-reporting | NFBrSI-24 is used for patients with malignant brain tumours during treatment and covers disease and treatment-related symptoms and function/well-being | 24 items | [9] |
| The European Organization for Research and Treatment of Cancer (EORTC) QLQ-BN20 is a quality-of-life assessment tool specific to brain tumours | Health-related quality of life Suitable for self-reporting | The European Organization for Research and Treatment of Cancer (EORTC) EORTC QLQ-C30 is an assessment tool for HRQOL for adult cancer patients. The brain tumour module, BN20, consists of 20 items specific to patients with brain tumours | 30 items and 20 items specific to brain tumour | [10] |
| The Functional Assessment of Cancer Therapy-Brain FACT-Br | Health-related quality of life Suitable for self-reporting | Functional Assessment of Cancer Therapy-General (FACT-G) consists of 27 items covering four domains: physical, social/ family, emotional and functional well-being. In addition, the brain tumour module consists of 23 items specific to brain tumour patients | 27 core items and 23 items specific to brain tumour | [11] |
| Sherbrooke Neuro-Oncology Assessment Scale, SNAS | Health-related quality of life Suitable for self-reporting | The questionnaire consists of seven multi-item scales, tapping into distinct dimensions of QOL: functional well-being, symptom severity/fear of death, social support/ acceptance of disease, autonomy in personal care, digestive symptomatology, neurocognitive function and pain | 30 items | [12] |

*EORTC* European Organization for Research and Treatment of Cancer, *FACT-Br* functional assessment of cancer therapy-brain, *HRQOL* health-related quality of life, *HNA* holistic needs assessment, *MDASI-BT* MD Anderson Symptom Inventory for Brain Tumour, *MUIS-BT* Mishel uncertainty in illness scale-brain tumour, *NFBrSI-24* National Comprehensive Cancer Network/ Functional Assessment of Cancer Therapy-Brain Symptom Index, *PCI* patient concerns inventory, *PRO* patient-reported outcome, *QOL* quality of life, *SNAS* Sherbrooke Neuro-Oncology Assessment Scale whether the patient has agreed to this information being shared with family and/or other health- and social care professionals in the team [14]. Patients with malignant brain tumours have complex symptoms and needs, and the care and support plan should cover all dimensions of care. Early in the diagnostic process, emotional support and information about the disease and treatment options are essential [2] and should be part of the care and support plan. During and after treatment, both patient and caregivers need to know how to manage medications and look for side effects or other complications depending on the patient's treatment and function [2].

The care and support plan should also include a focus on rehabilitation on how to improve functioning or compensating for possible permanent deficits. Cognitive testing can be helpful; identifying a cognitive deficit allows the patient, family and the healthcare team to include interventions to compensate for the deficits.

Fatigue is a common symptom of all patients with malignant brain tumour, known to have a negative impact on the patient's health-related quality of life (HRQOL), and can occur at any time during the disease course. Therefore, monitoring fatigue is recommended to always be part of the care and support plan, and the HNA can be used to follow up strategies and self-care [15].

Disease progression, physical disabilities, personality and behaviour changes and fatigue hinder many patients to be able to return to work, and their financial status may be compromised. Referral to social workers may help address financial concerns.

Safety concerns often need to be included in the care and support plan. Alterations to the home can be necessary to improve safety and reduce risk of injury for patients with physical or cognitive deficits. At home, family members need to know how to react and maximise safety during an episode of seizure activity. Patients who are forgetful and at risk for wandering may require door alarms, and child-proofing items may be useful. Both cognitive and motor deficits can impair a patient's ability to self-administer medication and take care of economics. Also, for safety reasons, many patients with a brain tumour are restricted from driving [16].

## 11.5   The Specific Needs, Concerns and Preferences of Patients and Informal Caregivers

Research has explored how patient and caregivers experience the disease and treatment trajectory, as well as the related needs. A recent study specifically examining patients diagnosed with high-grade glioma and their caregivers for 1 year [3, 17] shows that the needs of this group can be divided into three categories: information/education, rehabilitation and supportive care. Some needs are unique for either the patients or the caregivers, while other needs are shared.

## 11.6   Information, Education and Supportive Care

To manage the disease process, patients need supportive care tailored to their individual needs and preferences, as well as to their psychosocial abilities. The goal of the information is to increase the patient's ability to cope with the disease, motivate and facilitate rehabilitation and prepare and improve adherence to treatment. Several studies have described the importance of information provision; informed patients are more satisfied with care, have a higher sense of control and experience lower levels of affective distress and better HRQOL. Today, patient and relatives obtain patient information from different sources: in the meeting with healthcare professionals, written patient information, websites, patient associations, telephone counselling and contact with other patients and relatives, often via informal internet groups. Nonetheless, several studies show that patients and relatives often experience lack of information. Providing information that is congruent with patients' needs is challenging and requires communication skills and knowledge about how the disease affects HRQOL. The information needs of cancer patients vary by socio-demographic factors such cultural background, educational level, age, gender and clinical factors such cancer type, stage of disease and coping style. Newly diagnosed patients express feelings of distress and worry due to the unpredictability of their future. In this phase some patients seek to exchange experiences with other patients, while others try to avoid hearing patients' stories. Many countries have patient organisations and support groups for patients with brain tumours and their families that offer a variety of events, online services and support. Patients often also need practical help and support from family and friends.

Upon learning of the MBT diagnosis, patients and caregivers may respond and approach prognostic information (PI) differently, with some pursuing additional information and others limiting it. At times, the patient and the caregiver can have opposing strategies. People who want more information look for everything available online about, e.g. survival rates, the disease and symptoms. Others find the initial prognosis so emotionally devastating that they feel the need to control and limit the level of PI they receive. In general, information related to their prognosis needs to be offered at a pace in accordance with the rate at which they can assimilate and tolerate it.

During the MBT trajectory, patients may experience periods where the disease is stable and there is a lack of or few symptoms and/or complications. Eventually, however, symptoms increase in number and severity, resulting in neurological deterioration. At different points along the disease and treatment trajectory, patients describe how their awareness of the early symptoms of dementia gradually surfaces, accompanied by fear and distress. Symptoms of depression also appear in the symptom cluster that includes fatigue, disrupted sleep and cognitive impairment [18]. The literature recommends that future intervention studies include individually tailored communication and specialist support [19] to relieve emotional distress in patients with gliomas and stress among caregivers. After initially learning about the life-threatening MBT diagnosis, patients and caregivers often embrace a healthier lifestyle, e.g. increase physical activities, which they would like to discuss with a healthcare professional.

## 11.7  Multidisciplinary Rehabilitation

Evidence shows that patients need ongoing rehabilitation conducted by a multidisciplinary team of specialists. The goal of rehabilitation is for patients to improve symptom management and be as independent as possible for as long as possible. Examples of rehabilitation include cognitive training, physical exercise and speech therapy. Note that scant attention has been paid in literature to non-pharmacological rehabilitative and supportive care interventions targeting patients with MBT and/or their caregivers [20]. Preliminary evidence, however, shows that cognitive group therapy improves memory skills in patients with high-grade gliomas, while early physical training improves functional outcome and massage therapy reduces stress. As new interventions are designed and tested for feasibility, the depth and breadth of evidence will grow. Due to the complexity of symptoms, multidisciplinary rehabilitation programmes must target the limitations of patients and caregivers, as well as the identified needs. Patients feel that their ability to participate in ordinary physical rehabilitation programmes becomes limited because they have trouble understanding and following instructions, difficulty coordinating their movements and/or experience unpleasant symptoms when physically active. As a result multidisciplinary rehabilitation programmes must be tailored to the cognitive ability of the patients to allow active participation and to provide meaningful activities for the patient. The HNA can result in referral to rehabilitation services and referral to a cognitive assessment, e.g. the Montreal Cognitive Assessment [21] conducted by a neuropsychologist or an occupational therapist. Patients often prefer to attend local training programmes due to transportation issues, such as being barred from driving due to epilepsy and seizures. Moreover, due to the social aspect of exercise, some patients prefer to spend time with friends and family during training sessions.

Throughout the disease and treatment trajectory, symptoms gradually become more severe, altering the patient's lifestyle. Fatigue and cognitive and physical impairment restrict activities, not only socially but also with regard to work, daily activities and level of physical exercise. Through an ongoing process of, becoming aware of and adapting to their loss of functioning, patients can learn to adjust to the neurological disorders they face [3].

## 11.8 Specific for the Caregivers

When close family members take on the responsibility of administering care, their role shifts from being a close family member to becoming the primary and informal caregiver. Informal caregivers are at risk of neglecting their own physical and emotional needs and may have divergent preferences regarding the kind and level of information given by health professionals [3]. Taking on this role may often involve experiencing a sense of crisis and grief because the caregiver lives in a constant state of anxiety, fearing that the patient will die. Caregivers may feel a sense of powerlessness due to their inability to influence the situation. While the patient undergoes treatment, caregivers may experience fatigue, distress, economic worries, a lack of energy and physical ailments such as weight loss and disrupted sleep, causing their commitment to waiver. Caregivers can become frustrated when the patient's cognitive function declines to the point of memory loss that precludes meaningful conversation and sharing concerns. If the patient's dementia progresses and their level of awareness decreases, it places a constant and even greater responsibility on the caregiver. Because they often need to be readily available to assist the patient, caregivers can experience limitations in daily life. They are committed to their role as caregiver, but the immense burden they face nonetheless gradually tests their commitment as time passes. Guidelines that take these needs into consideration and that are implemented in clinical practice have the potential to improve patients' HRQOL and to support caregivers by involving them more actively in care and management.

The disease affects not only the patient but also the individual family members. Studies have shown that family members are the people who most closely witness the patients' actual condition. They support and assist the patient with a variety of needs, for instance, by accompanying them to treatments, by participating in medical consultations and by becoming the patient's primary caregiver as time passes. Caregivers are given immense responsibility and continually seek to manage this new life-threatening situation and the sheer burden that represents. Consequently, caregivers would benefit from supportive care interventions individually tailored to their psychosocial needs to ease their burden, for example, by receiving help and information from healthcare professionals to manage the new responsibilities they have taken on, e.g. financially, socially and with regard to care. They need information about how to manage problems and symptoms related to brain cancer and can benefit from an introduction to navigating the healthcare system. In general, caregivers experience a sense of encouragement when healthcare professionals acknowledge and support them as a vital resource [3].

If children are affected, it is recommended to include qualified specialists that focus on the children's needs so that they receive the appropriate support. Parents can also benefit from being advised on how to communicate with their children about the disease, etc.

## 11.9    Advance Care Planning

It is imperative that clinical specialists and researchers are familiar with the needs, preferences and interests of these patients and their caregivers in order to provide the best possible care. Presently, more evidence is being accumulated on how to provide the best advance care planning (ACP). Timely and appropriate ACP is essential for supporting caregivers and thus patients, during the final phases of the MBT trajectory. ACP includes, for instance, ongoing symptom management, monitoring and referral to palliative care teams to avoid inappropriate and expensive hospitalisations.

The European Association of Neuro-Oncology (EANO) guidelines (for the diagnosis and treatment of anaplastic gliomas and glioblastoma) cover palliative care including speaking with patients and caregivers at an appropriate stage [22, 23]. ACP involves thinking about, talking about and planning for the future, including EOL decisions such as a living will. The issues of greatest importance are the ones that affect the caregiver's situation at a later stage and also at bereavement. Determining the appropriate timing for discussing EOL issues, however, is problematic when it involves patients and caregivers. If initiated at an early stage of the disease, patients and caregivers might see them as irrelevant, inappropriate or as destroying their sense of hope [3]. If postponed until late in the disease trajectory, there is the risk that the patient will be unable to contribute actively due to progressive neurological symptoms, e.g. cognitive dysfunction, speech difficulties and dysphasia. One study found that, after being diagnosed with malignant glioma, more than 50% of patients have an impaired capacity to make treatment decisions [24], which supports the importance of discussing EOL issues early. Moreover, Diamond et al. [25] stress that patients with primary MBTs may not derive the optimal benefit from multidisciplinary hospice care due to being referred too late in their treatment trajectory, which the other research also indicates [26]. Preferences for PI have been identified as individual. Opposing preferences between the patient and the caregiver make the timing for introducing EOL issues even more complex. The present study, however, shows that bereaved caregivers preferred referral to palliative care at an early stage and would have appreciated being encouraged to speak openly about difficult issues during the disease trajectory. Fritz et al. [27] conclude that future feasibility studies are necessary to decide the best timing and content of ACP. Walbert and Pace [28] advocate for a future definition of the best timing and appropriate interventions to better prepare people for the EOL stage, including improved neuro-oncology education for care providers. Spiritual support is an essential component in ACP, and interventions designed to manage uncertainty have been shown to improve mood and symptoms.

## 11.10  The Expression and Meaning of Hope

Hope is essential for patients' HRQOL, which is why they require help to obtain, maintain or redefine hope and to discuss hope with professionals. Hope is expressed in various ways, e.g. quantity of life or QOL. Many say that they hope that they can live a normal everyday life for as long as possible by participating in everyday activities.

Research confirms the need for hope to be sustained, showing that a balance must be struck between fostering realistic hope and unethically creating unrealistic expectations of survival [29, 30]. Many clinicians find it difficult to combine hope with honesty; some are more willing to inspire patients with hope than others [31]. Hope is a source of strength that helps individuals to keep going [32, 33], brings purpose and meaning to life, encourages a positive attitude and improves psychological well-being [34].

## 11.11  Prognostic Information and Preparing for Bereavement

Patients and their caregivers need prognostic information (PI) in accordance with their individual preferences, which means taking into consideration how much information can be tolerated and the pace at which it can be assimilated. Research shows that there is a significant correlation between accurate PI and reduced psychological distress in patients with advanced cancer [35, 36], which is in accordance with other findings indicating that PI preferences can act as a catalyst to ease the individual's adjustment to receiving the MBT diagnosis [3]. PI may facilitate EOL planning [37], but there is a risk of causing increased distress instead. PI needs to be based on a strategy that accounts for individual preferences and approaches to managing a life crisis [19]. The literature refers to this strategy as prognostic awareness, which is defined as a patient's capacity to understand the prognosis and the likely illness trajectory [38]. Individuals with a low level of prognostic awareness are too emotionally burdened and postpone dealing with their mortality until a future point. Gradually, a higher prognostic awareness can be developed through interactions with skilled clinicians [38]. In addition, the impaired cognitive capacity of patients with MBT interferes with the ability to prioritise and understand information and communication that can have either a negative or positive influence on the experience of cancer.

## 11.12  Perspectives on Bereavement

Given that the MBT trajectory is burdensome and impacts caregivers negatively, it is important to support bereaved caregivers to aid their reintegration into their social network activities and working life. Reflecting on their experience with giving care, bereaved caregivers mention that early referral to palliative care is preferable in order be better prepared for the rapid decline phase of the disease trajectory. These results indicate the need for an increased focus on empowering caregivers in the future, for instance, by educating and supporting caregivers to embrace their caregiver role. In addition, bereavement interventions designed to help former caregivers to reintegrate into their social and working life are also called for.

## 11.13  Clinical Implications

There is a need for interventions that improve symptom management due to the various cancer-related difficulties that patients report. It is possible that a higher level of HRQOL can be achieved and maintained among MBT patients through an early palliative approach with the aim to improve life planning [39]. Whether a prolonged survival time or improvement of HRQOL should be prioritised depends on individual preferences and needs. As a result actively involving patients in treatment decisions regarding depression is crucial considering the various therapeutic options that are available [40]. Patient involvement has the potential to contribute to a better adaption process to having MBT [41]. Eventually, this may lead to a positive effect on HRQOL among terminally ill MBT patients.

Providing bereavement consultations with recognised healthcare professionals is one way of supplying the opportunity to discuss the care provided and decisions that took place, in addition to answering any questions related to the disease and treatment trajectory. Considering the enormous caregiver burden (during the time of care), we suggest that general practitioners or clinical nurse specialists offer follow-up health-care consultations to ensure a healthy and normal grieving process. Finally, a stratifi-cation of those who are able to cope with understandable sadness versus those facing a complicated grieving process would indicate who has the greatest need of support from healthcare providers. This chapter points out key areas of interest from that per-spective, emphasising the need to determine the future direction of ACP research within neuro-oncology in order to establish evidence-based, best clinical practice.

## 11.14 Conclusions

Patients with MBT differ from patients with other cancer diagnoses due to the pro-gressive neurological deterioration resulting in changing and complex symptoms along the disease and treatment trajectory. A multidisciplinary approach has the potential to meet the variety of needs that emerge as a result of this life-threatening situation. The needs and preferences of patients and caregivers include rehabilita-tive and supportive interventions designed to maintain or achieve the highest func-tional level possible, a redefinition of hope during the disease trajectory, implementation of health-promoting activities, provision of psychological care, application of symptom management strategies and carrying out life planning. As evidence begins to emerge, there is a need for well-designed longitudinal and ran-domised controlled trials of non-pharmacological interventions in MBT patients and their caregivers in order to develop clinical guidelines for supportive and reha-bilitative approaches in this unique population.

## References

1. Molassiotis A, Wilson B, Brunton L, Chaudhary H, Gattamaneni R, McBain C. Symptom experience in patients with primary brain tumours: a longitudinal exploratory study. Eur J Oncol Nurs. 2010;14(5):410–6.
2. Cahill JE, Armstrong TS. Caring for an adult with a malignant primary brain tumor. Nursing. 2011;41(6):28–33. quiz-4
3. Piil K, Juhler M, Jakobsen J, Jarden M. Daily life experiences of patients with a high-grade glioma and their caregivers: a longitudinal exploration of rehabilitation and supportive care needs. J Neurosci Nurs. 2015;47(5):271–84.
4. Rooney AG, Netten A, McNamara S, Erridge S, Peoples S, Whittle I, et al. Assessment of a brain-tumour-specific Patient Concerns Inventory in the neuro-oncology clinic. Support Care Cancer. 2014;22(4):1059–69.
5. Basch E, Deal AM, Kris MG, Scher HI, Hudis CA, Sabbatini P, et al. Symptom monitoring with patient-reported outcomes during routine cancer treatment: a randomized controlled trial. J Clin Oncol. 2016;34(6):557–65.
6. Armstrong TS, Mendoza T, Gning I, Coco C, Cohen MZ, Eriksen L, et al. Validation of the M.D. Anderson Symptom Inventory Brain Tumor Module (MDASI-BT). J Neuro-Oncol. 2006;80(1):27–35.
7. Armstrong TS, Cohen MZ, Eriksen L, Cleeland C. Content validity of self-report measure-ment instruments: an illustration from the development of the Brain Tumor Module of the M.D. Anderson Symptom Inventory. Oncol Nurs Forum. 2005;32(3):669–76.

8. Lin L, Acquaye AA, Vera-Bolanos E, Cahill JE, Gilbert MR, Armstrong TS. Validation of the Mishel's uncertainty in illness scale-brain tumor form (MUIS-BT). J Neuro-Oncol. 2012;110(2):293–300.

9. Lai JS, Jensen SE, Beaumont JL, Abernethy AP, Jacobsen PB, Syrjala K, et al. Development of a symptom index for patients with primary brain tumors. Value Health. 2014;17(1):62–9.

10. Aaronson NK, Ahmedzai S, Bergman B, Bullinger M, Cull A, Duez NJ, et al. The European Organization for Research and Treatment of Cancer QLQ-C30: a quality-of-life instrument for use in international clinical trials in oncology. J Natl Cancer Inst. 1993;85(5):365–76.

11. Weitzner MA, Meyers CA, Gelke CK, Byrne KS, Cella DF, Levin VA. The Functional Assessment of Cancer Therapy (FACT) scale. Development of a brain subscale and revalidation of the general version (FACT-G) in patients with primary brain tumors. Cancer. 1995;75(5):1151–61.

12. Goffaux P, Boudrias M, Mathieu D, Charpentier C, Veilleux N, Fortin D. Development of a concise QOL questionnaire for brain tumor patients. Can J Neurol Sci. 2009;36(3):340–8.

13. Northouse L, Williams AL, Given B, McCorkle R. Psychosocial care for family caregivers of patients with cancer. J Clin Oncol. 2012;30(11):1227–34.

14. The National Health Service N. Holistic needs assessment for people with cancer. London: NHS; 2011. p. 2011.

15. Asher A, Fu JB, Bailey C, Hughes JK. Fatigue among patients with brain tumors. CNS Oncol. 2016;5(2):91–100.

16. Doherty L, LaFrankie DC. Patient safety concerns for cognitively impaired patients with brain tumors. Clin J Oncol Nurs. 2010;14(1):101–2.

17. Piil K, Jakobsen J, Christensen KB, Juhler M, Jarden M. Health-related quality of life in patients with high-grade gliomas: a quantitative longitudinal study. J Neuro-Oncol. 2015;124(2):185–95.

18. Fox SW, Lyon D, Farace E. Symptom clusters in patients with high-grade glioma. J Nurs Scholarsh. 2007;39(1):61–7.

19. Lobb EA, Halkett GK, Nowak AK. Patient and caregiver perceptions of communication of prognosis in high grade glioma. J Neuro-Oncol. 2011;104(1):315–22.

20. Piil K, Juhler M, Jakobsen J, Jarden M. Controlled rehabilitative and supportive care intervention trials in patients with high-grade gliomas and their caregivers: a systematic review. BMJ Support Palliat Care. 2016;6(1):27–34.

21. Nasreddine ZS, Phillips NA, Bedirian V, Charbonneau S, Whitehead V, Collin I, et al. The Montreal Cognitive Assessment, MoCA: a brief screening tool for mild cognitive impairment. J Am Geriatr Soc. 2005;53(4):695–9.

22. Weller M, van den Bent M, Hopkins K, Tonn JC, Stupp R, Falini A, et al. EANO guideline for the diagnosis and treatment of anaplastic gliomas and glioblastoma. Lancet Oncol. 2014;15(9):e395–403.

23. Pace A, Dirven L, Koekkoek JAF, Golla H, Fleming J, Ruda R, et al. European Association for Neuro-Oncology (EANO) guidelines for palliative care in adults with glioma. Lancet Oncol. 2017;18(6):e330–e40.

24. Triebel KL, Martin RC, Nabors LB, Marson DC. Medical decision-making capacity in patients with malignant glioma. Neurology. 2009;73(24):2086–92.

25. Diamond EL, Russell D, Kryza-Lacombe M, Bowles KH, Applebaum AJ, Dennis J, et al. Rates and risks for late referral to hospice in patients with primary malignant brain tumors. Neuro-Oncology. 2016;18(1):78–86.

26. Song K, Amatya B, Voutier C, Khan F. Advance care planning in patients with primary malignant brain tumors: a systematic review. Front Oncol. 2016;6:223.

27. Fritz L, Dirven L, Reijneveld JC, Koekkoek JA, Stiggelbout AM, Pasman HR, et al. Advance care planning in glioblastoma patients. Cancers (Basel). 2016;8(11):E102.

28. Walbert T, Pace A. End-of-life care in patients with primary malignant brain tumors: early is better. Neuro-Oncology. 2016;18(1):7–8.

29. Hagerty RG, Butow PN, Ellis PM, Lobb EA, Pendlebury SC, Leighl N, et al. Communicating with realism and hope: incurable cancer patients' views on the disclosure of prognosis. J Clin Oncol. 2005;23(6):1278–88.

30. Clayton JM, Hancock K, Parker S, Butow PN, Walder S, Carrick S, et al. Sustaining hope when communicating with terminally ill patients and their families: a systematic review. Psycho-Oncology. 2008;17(7):641–59.
31. Rosenblum ML, Kalkanis S, Goldberg W, Rock J, Mikkelsen T, Remer S, et al. Odyssey of hope: a physician's guide to communicating with brain tumor patients across the continuum of care. J Neuro-Oncol. 2009;92(3):241–51.
32. Coolbrandt A, Sterckx W, Clement P, Borgenon S, Decruyenaere M, de Vleeschouwer S, et al. Family caregivers of patients with a high-grade glioma: a qualitative study of their lived experience and needs related to professional care. Cancer Nurs. 2015;38(5):406–13.
33. Sterckx W, Coolbrandt A, Clement P, Borgenon S, Decruyenaere M, De Vleeschouwer S, et al. Living with a high-grade glioma: a qualitative study of patients' experiences and care needs. Eur J Oncol Nurs. 2015;19(4):383–90.
34. Sutton K. The impact on quality of life for people with brain tumours of entering a research trial involving new anti-cancer agents. Eur J Oncol Nurs. 2013;17(4):396–401.
35. Innes S, Payne S. Advanced cancer patients' prognostic information preferences: a review. Palliat Med. 2009;23(1):29–39.
36. Thompson GN, Chochinov HM, Wilson KG, McPherson CJ, Chary S, O'Shea FM, et al. Prognostic acceptance and the well-being of patients receiving palliative care for cancer. J Clin Oncol. 2009;27(34):5757–62.
37. Applebaum AJ, Kolva EA, Kulikowski JR, Jacobs JD, DeRosa A, Lichtenthal WG, et al. Conceptualizing prognostic awareness in advanced cancer: a systematic review. J Health Psychol. 2014;19(9):1103–19.
38. Jackson VA, Jacobsen J, Greer JA, Pirl WF, Temel JS, Back AL. The cultivation of prognostic awareness through the provision of early palliative care in the ambulatory setting: a communication guide. J Palliat Med. 2013;16(8):894–900.
39. Temel JS, Greer JA, Muzikansky A, Gallagher ER, Admane S, Jackson VA, et al. Early palliative care for patients with metastatic non-small-cell lung cancer. N Engl J Med. 2010;363(8):733–42.
40. Boele FW, Verdonck-de Leeuw IM, Cuijpers P, Reijneveld JC, Heimans JJ, Klein M. Internet-based guided self-help for glioma patients with depressive symptoms: design of a randomized controlled trial. BMC Neurol. 2014;14:81.
41. Hubbard G, Kidd L, Donaghy E. Preferences for involvement in treatment decision making of patients with cancer: a review of the literature. Eur J Oncol Nurs. 2008;12(4):299–318.

# Communication Skills: The Patient as Co-pilot

Helen Bulbeck

**Abstract**

Daily interactions with patients and caregivers who are living with a brain tumour reveal that self-management practices, whilst being provided routinely in some places, tend to be on an ad hoc basis, reactive and unplanned. Patients do not know what support is available to them, where to seek help or what questions they should be asking. A shift to being empowered begins at the point of diagnosis, with a collaborative and interactive relationship between patients and healthcare professionals, which empowers patients to take on responsibility for their condition with the appropriate clinical support. This chapter explores why shared engagement is a prerequisite for optimised clinical care, what this looks like and how to achieve it so that it becomes the cornerstone of every communication between people living with a brain tumour and their clinical team.

**Keywords**

Communication · Glioma · Coaching · Shared engagement

**Learning Outcomes**
- Gain insight and deeper understanding of the core aspects of good communication.
- Learn about basic communication skills and how to put these skills into daily practice.
- Understand the vital importance of open, honest communication and why shared engagement is a prerequisite for optimised clinical care.

---

H. Bulbeck (✉)
Brainstrust – The Brain Cancer People, Cowes, Isle of Wight, UK
e-mail: helen@brainstrust.org.uk

© Springer Nature Switzerland AG 2019
I. Oberg (ed.), *Management of Adult Glioma in Nursing Practice*,
https://doi.org/10.1007/978-3-319-76747-5_12

- Understand how neuro-psychosocial support can improve outcomes for glioma patients and what steps are required to ensure you offer your patients this level of support.

A move from "what's the matter?" to "what matters to you?' [1].

Communication is central to human interaction. Without it, people cannot relate to those around them, make their needs and concerns known or make sense of what is happening to them. A survey [2] has highlighted gaps for the brain cancer community. It has very simple asks about communication. It wants:

- Clear signposting of care in the community
- The right information at the right time
- Public understanding
- Clear expectations
- A more equal relationship with my doctor
- More honest discussions sooner
- To know how to get what I want out of a discussion
- To not be alone
- To feel in control
- To know how to deal with death and dying

Currently, patients and their caregivers do not know what support is available to them, where to seek help or what questions they should be asking. They are unable to move from the position of seeing the healthcare professional just as an expert giving advice to an enabler who supports the person they are caring for to achieve their goals and the challenge of patients seeing themselves as passive recipients of care, to becoming activated and taking responsibility for their own contribution to improving their health and well-being outcomes and being empowered to do so. Knowledge alone is not power: knowledge + skills + beliefs = power.

Clinicians know what the issues are around effective communication with their patients and families. These do not need to be revisited. This chapter will explore how everyone (clinicians, patients and caregivers) can use communication so that we can all:

- Be an enabler for others
- Be secure with uncertainty
- Be open with not knowing and taking risks
- Ensure that inner dialogue is constructive
- Be nondefensive by having nothing to prove and no agenda

It will investigate **why** effective communication is key for developing a proactive relationship between all parties; **what** the communication strategies are that can help to achieve a better quality of life, prolonging overall survival; and **how** these can become part of everyone's toolkit when they are living with a brain tumour. It focuses on achieving specific, immediate goals, which relate to precise challenges, for example, weighing up the pros and cons of having a particular treatment, overcoming a problem with caring or coming to terms with entering the next stage of treatment. All of these are effective forms of self-management, and all rely on effective communication, which should be routinely embedded into daily clinical practice.

## 12.1 Why

Brain cancer is unique. Brain tumours are infiltrative, affecting our complex, integrated information-processing and control systems. The burden of these tumours is considerable for the individuals, their families and the healthcare system. Poor survival for many tumour types results in a disproportionate number of years of life lost compared to other cancers [3]. High attrition is the norm as many patients become disabled or die as a result of progressive disease. Therefore a greater burden of epilepsy, neurological deficit, cognitive impairment and, often, mortality is observed in a person living with a brain tumour than in systemic cancer. Losses of health, independence, identity and hopes that can accompany a diagnosis of a brain tumour are also relevant. Emotional states of change include feeling low, diagnosed depression, anxiety, loneliness, uncertainty, decreased self-esteem and fears about recurrence and relationship problems.

Support for brain tumour patients and their caregivers is crucial and needs to be founded in shared experiences. For example, in the UK in 2016 [4], only 26% of patients diagnosed with a brain tumour were given a care plan. This means that 74% patients never received a care plan. Only 42% of patients felt their clinical team worked together all of the time to give them the best possible care, and 38% came away from their consultation without fully understanding the diagnosis. At this point, feeling lost and scared, they desperately need someone to talk to—someone who truly understands [2]. There is little available through the usual channels of clinicians for this support—only 43% of neuro-oncology multidisciplinary teams have access to neuropsychiatry services [5].

The National Institute for Health and Care Excellence (NICE) guidelines for brain and CNS tumours (2004) recommend that "patients, their relatives and carers should have the opportunity to be involved in the decision making process about management and care", and the Brain Tumour Patients' Charter of Rights also states that patients should "be included in the decision making process for their care". Further to this, the National Health Service (NHS) has a vision for patients to be more actively involved in treatment decisions—shared decision-making—and it has the principle of "no decision about me without me" at its heart [6]. This means that if the patient wishes, they can be an active participant in discussions and decisions about their care with their clinicians. A clearer understanding of their diagnosis and what it means for them will encourage patients to participate in this shared decision-making. Whilst not everyone wants to play an active role in their care, most surveys suggest that a majority do [7]. There is strong evidence that patients and caregivers value—and benefit from—receiving accurate and relevant information [8].

The diagnosis of a brain tumour is devastating. As a rare cancer, patients and families find themselves suddenly in a situation that is complex and bewildering. They feel very isolated, not knowing anyone else in the community with whom to share their anxieties. At times they find it difficult to make decisions about their care due to the uncertainty surrounding their prognosis (which is bleak if the diagnosis is a glioblastoma—only 14% are alive after 5 years) and their perceived lack of treatment alternatives. Patients therefore require support to achieve their desired level of involvement in decision-making. A qualitative longitudinal study of 26 patients with diagnosed high-grade glioma between the years 2006 and 2007 tells us that [9–11]:

- The period surrounding diagnosis is one of immense distress and uncertainty:

  *You have this churning in your stomach and this horrible feeling that your life's never going to be the same again.* (63-year-old man, GBM)

- Participants felt ill informed during this crisis period, a source of anxiety and distress for them:

  *Sometimes you feel like you're dragging teeth to get, to get some kind of information out of them.* (46-year-old male, GBM)

- Participants sought clear, direct yet sensitive information about what was happening and what to expect to help alleviate anxiety borne from uncertainty:

  *I think that I should have been told at that stage, more about erm, the nature of the beast, erm, and the seriousness of it. And I still haven't been told anything of that nature by the hospital, I've had to find that out myself on the internet.* (58-year-old male, GBM)

  *Well for me, no matter how bad it is I think I'd rather know what it was than have it camouflaged in some way.* (65-year-old male, GBM)

- However, participants acknowledged they were not always ready to hear difficult information or retain it during the early weeks surrounding diagnosis:

  *Part of you is frightened to ask too much 'cos you don't really want to know.* (66-year-old female, suspected glioma)

  *Anybody who was talking to me, it was 'blah, blah, blah'. I wasn't taking anything in, you know. I was operating on automatic pilot.* (Wife of a 46-year-old male, GBM)

Following diagnosis and treatment for a brain tumour, patients will have differing trajectories, which may be predicted ranging from recovery, stable situation or progression. Research shows that neuro-rehabilitation and neuro-psychosocial support improves outcomes for patients diagnosed with a brain tumour [12]. For improved survivorship, close collaboration is required between clinicians involved with neuro-rehabilitation, supportive care, quality of life and psychological and palliative care to plan transition points in care. This requires coordination of different specialties and expertise from symptom management to end of life care. We know that patients and caregivers who are coached and engaged with shared decision-making are better able to manage the complexity of their journey and have more resilience and a better quality of life. They are significantly more likely to attend screenings and regular check-ups and adhere with treatments and actions and significantly more likely to engage in healthy behaviours like eating a healthy diet [13, 14] or taking regular exercise [15–18]. Conversely, less engaged patients are significantly less likely to have prepared questions for a visit to the doctor, to know about treatment guidelines for their condition or to be persistent in asking if they don't understand what their doctor has told them [19]. They are also two to three times more likely to have unmet medical needs and to delay medical care compared with more highly engaged patients, regardless of income, education and access to care [16].

Having greater control over our health and care is a good thing: autonomy, or the ability to exercise control over the forces that affect our lives, is an essential part of a good life. In healthcare self-directed support is only now starting to break through into mainstream services, but there are strong grounds for extending it. Healthcare services should support people to lead independent lives, rather than forcing them to fit their lives around the services on offer.

So, there is a straightforward moral case for empowering people in health and care—but there is an instrumental case as well. Empowerment produces better health outcomes, more satisfied patients and caregivers and much-needed financial savings. Research has shown that patient "activation [having the knowledge, skills and confidence to manage one's own health] is strongly related to a broad range of health-related outcomes, which suggests improving activation has great potential" [13]. This is because patients with chronic conditions like brain cancer live with their condition 24/7 and only spend a fraction of their time visiting clinical experts: the rest of the time, they have to manage their condition themselves.

### 12.1.1  Patient Satisfaction

Research has shown that patients who are engaged in their health and healthcare—through health literacy, shared clinical decision-making and self-management—are more likely to say that their healthcare is of high quality and are less likely to report experience of medical errors [20].

### 12.1.2  Saving Money

Giving people the support and information they need to avoid getting ill, or when they have a chronic condition to self-manage it effectively, should save the National Health Service (NHS) money by reducing demand on acute care. If people are not equipped and supported to self-manage, they are effectively left on their own and can end up with complications, health crises, preventable trips to the general practitioner (GP) or accident and emergency (A&E), avoidable suffering and even premature death. Around 20% of emergency admissions to hospital are thought to be potentially preventable, and many of these involve chronic conditions [21].

The most robust evaluations of empowerment programmes focused on peer support and redesigned consultations have been estimated to reduce acute care costs by 7%. Nesta (an innovation charitable foundation) estimates that this, which it describes as a conservative estimate, would save the NHS £4.4 billion a year across England [22].

## 12.2 What

Communication is key and never more so when there are so many complex things at play. But it is human nature to feel unsure about how to talk with someone who is distressed or in difficulty. It can also be hard to know how to talk when you are in crisis. Questions about the illness, its symptoms, its meaning or its impact can be hard to ask. And there are others too involved who might struggle to have a voice, such as the caregiver.

But patients and caregivers do have the capacity to take control of their situation to secure the best possible outcomes for their situation. Empowering people through coaching brings autonomy, a better quality of life, and more patient satisfaction, and with these comes a strong health economic argument—it saves the NHS money.

Empowerment models such as choice and entitlements have focused on responding to a person's needs rather than developing their capabilities. This is common across the NHS, where services have been established with a "deficit" mindset: hospitals exist to provide patients with medical treatment at times of acute need, and doctors exist to diagnose illnesses and provide medications. High-impact coaching takes a different starting point: it rejects the view of the patient as principally a "service user" with needs that the NHS must meet. This approach tends to infantilise and disempower people, creating dependency cultures, in which people's best hope for improving their lot is to wait for a paid professional to step in. Instead, there are capabilities in everyone, and these can be mobilised by discussing a person's needs and aspirations and then exploring what resources are available to help meet these. Coaching does this.

There is clear evidence to show that coaching works. High-impact coaching helps brain tumour patients and caregivers to feel anchored, focused and strong in their approach to managing their brain cancer and the interventions offered. Navigation to support decision-making and improve understanding and information has been shown to be associated with better knowledge, a better understanding of diagnosis and treatment, better ability to cope and improved distress levels [9]. Coached patients felt by preparing through coaching for consultations, a discussion of personalised key issues, broader than the prime focus of the consultation, resulted. Patients felt more informed and utilised coaching materials to aid memory and information gathering and understanding. Clinical feedback revealed that coaching led to more effective consultations and facilitated communication within consultations by giving insight into information gaps. Telephone follow-up was effective for information and support, and psychoeducation increased feelings of mastery [23].

Evidence therefore suggests that when we are no longer able to change a situation, we are challenged to change ourselves. You are the person who is ultimately going to have the greatest impact on your life. A coaching relationship enables people who are living with a brain tumour to face their challenges, so that they learn how to develop resilience and utilise resources, and those of others, to their full potential.

The coaching relationship is built on collaboration; it is not essential that the coach has more experience of the coachee's situation than the coachee and will use questions to facilitate the coachee's thinking. At *brainstrust*, for example, we listen, listen some more and then ask questions. We focus on achieving specific immediate goals which relate to specific areas, for example, weighing up the pros and cons of having a particular treatment or overcoming a problem with caring. We also know that, through coaching, clients can also experience a sense of healing, as they make courageous decisions about their lives and work. Coaching focuses on the future and the development of a workable solution. It's about developing strategies and clarity to achieve a better quality of life. Our approach further enables patients and caregivers to engage in their care and gain a deeper understanding of what they're facing in terms of treatment and prognosis (if they wish to know).

Qualitative studies [9, 10, 24] show that patients and caregivers want to be fully involved in:

- Understanding their illness
- Exploring their options for treatment and for living with the illness
- Sourcing information, knowledge, help and advice

After a coaching conversation with a *brainstrust* coach, patients and caregivers feel resourced, in control and clear, and they have positive actions to take forwards, as a small selection of testimonials attests to:

> *Wow, for the first time I feel like someone has heard my pleas and actually listened....I feel quite overwhelmed at your kind response and how your thoughtful suggestions actually make sense ... Thank you once again, just knowing you are there has brightened my day*
>     Patient, Lincolnshire

> *Thank you so, so much for your help and advice the other day, I think the best thing is I feel more in control now as I have a plan of action as such, whilst before I was floundering, and I don't have any support network to help me with things*
>     Patient, Belfast

> *I have re-read your reply several times and know you understand how I feel. You brought up some very valid points for me, and I could not see the wood from the trees and my perspectives became obscured because of the panic ... I have made a list from the points you make and I am using this as my plan of action, so I can keep focussed on the solutions to this instead of the worry all the time ... You made me think about things differently in your reply and I am very grateful that you took the time and effort to help me and what I am going through at this time*
>     Patient, London

## 12.3 How

How can this be achieved when there is that fine line between telling the truth and nourishing hope? No matter what your role (in any conversation about a life-limiting illness), you are having to respond to emotion; involve people in decision-making, when their decisions might be different; deal with stress caused by meeting expectations; and give hope when the situation is bleak. The complexity of the interaction can create serious miscommunication, which in turn thwarts understanding expectations of treatment or involving others in treatment planning.

Firstly there is the need to develop a supportive community. Social support is an important contributor to the general well-being of patients and particularly caregivers, and it acts as a buffer. A supportive healthcare community that transcends on- and offline boundaries can drive a measurable improvement in brain tumour patients' and caregivers' understanding of their condition, their treatment and their care.

People affected by a brain tumour need a community because being a rare disease, patients and caregivers are unlikely to know someone in their local community or friendship group who also has a brain tumour. Furthermore, brain cancer cannot be compared to other cancers as it brings with it progressive neurological disease, and therefore support from someone with another kind of cancer would not be as valued. Online support is necessary to enable them to find others in the same boat. Online support is not bound by geographical boundaries and does not prevent those geographically isolated or those unable to get out due to disabilities from accessing support. It is also important that these online interactions can be carried across from the virtual to the real world wherever and whenever possible.

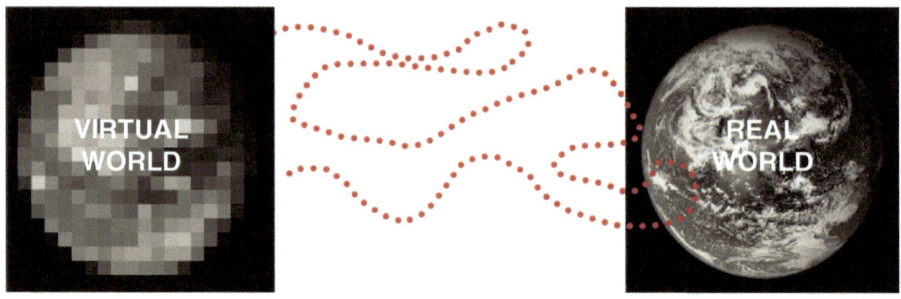

There are many situations where health communities (on- and offline) aid patients. These benefits include improved quality of life, better decision-making and patients who feel less alone and more empowered. Indeed, the availability of online health communities is especially appreciated by individuals with impaired mobility, potentially difficult medical conditions or caregiver responsibilities that may prohibit them from receiving adequate face-to-face medical and emotional support.

A community has a life of its own that goes beyond the lives of the residents in it, something that is beyond its very components. It is on-going—people join and people leave. There are communities within communities. A community is not a harmonious unity (it is comprised of individuals with differences, i.e. gender; age; education; different roles (patient/caregiver); different tumour types, grades and prognosis; different treatments), but what underpins a community is the shared narrative; peer support programmes prove that support from others who have been through a similar experience can help to reduce the negative impacts of living with a brain tumour [25, 26]. Such sharing of experiences and the sense of belonging impact significantly and positively on well-being, bringing improved satisfaction with medical care, improved mood, positive psychological states and healthier behaviour.

However, the success of communities depends on the quality of the interaction. Effective communication has to extend beyond just transferring knowledge. Being able to create the moment where the conversation can take place can be a real gift, and being able to work at abstraction level, where the conversation data is used to characterise the patient's values, wishes and stories, can deliver outcomes that could never have been imagined. But having created this moment, then what do you do to achieve this? What follows are some effective and successful tools which have been transformative for patients, caregivers and their clinicians and are easily absorbed into practice.

## 12.4 How to Hold Difficult Conversations

There are always critical times in the treatment of brain cancer when there are difficult conversations that need to take place. There are key tools that can be used that ensure we can have better, more focused conversations, one of which is simply planning the conversation. Eighty-two percentage of people say it is important to communicate their wishes when ill, but only 23% actually do this [27]. Great conversations work better if they are planned and rehearsed even if this just stays in the mind of the person who is planning to have the conversation.

### 12.4.1 Being Ready

Explore in your own mind:

- Why do you want to have the conversation? What is important to you in doing this?
- Why now?
- What do you need to say?
- What do you believe the other person needs to hear?
- What do you need to be ready to have the conversation?
- How can you resource yourself?
- Where should you have the conversation? What is important about the environment?

### 12.4.2 Doing It Well

There are four stages of awareness that shift the scope of a conversation from individual reflection to shared insight:

1. Concrete information—the facts
2. The emotive responses—the feelings
3. Their interpretation—where the deep grappling is done to find the meaning
4. The decision—where implications and decisions are discussed [28]

### 12.4.3 Concrete Information: The Facts

| Focus of the questions | The facts about the brain tumour—the medical and situational external reality |
|---|---|
| What it does for you both | Ensures that everyone deals with the same body of data and all of the aspects |
| Questions are in relation to: | The senses: what is seen, heard and touched |
| Key questions | What do you see? What words or phrases stand out? What happened? |

### 12.4.4 The Emotive Responses: The Feelings

| Focus of the questions | Internal relationship to the brain tumour |
|---|---|
| What it does for you both | Reveals internal responses |
| Questions are in relation to: | Feelings, moods, emotional tones, memories or associations |
| Key questions | What do you spend time thinking about? How does it make you feel? Where have you struggled? |

### 12.4.5 Their Interpretation: Where the Deep Grappling Is Done to Find the Meaning

The interpretative responses build on the facts, plus associations or feelings from the reflective level.

| Focus of the questions | The meaning of it all |
|---|---|
| What it does for you both | Draws out the significance from the facts for you both |
| Questions are in relation to: | Layers of meaning, purpose, significance, implications and values. Considering alternatives, options and the plan |
| Key questions | What is happening here? What is this all about? What does it mean for us? How does this affect us? What are our insights from this? |

### 12.4.6 The Decision: Where Implications and Decisions Are Discussed

Here some kind of resolve brings the conversation to a close. The questions allow for conscious choices to be made.

| Focus of the questions | Resolution, implications and new directions |
| --- | --- |
| What it does for you both | Makes the conversation relevant for what you both want in the future |
| Questions are in relation to: | Clarity, planning and action |
| Key questions | What therefore do we want? What decision is called for? What are the next steps? |

A more detailed overview of how to plan and prepare for a difficult conversation can be found at http://www.brainstrust.org.uk/advice-resources.php#Difficult Conversations.

## 12.5 The GROW Model and the Problem Outcome Framework

Other resources which can create shift in our interactions, whether you are a patient, a caregiver or a healthcare practitioner, are the GROW model and the problem outcome framework. Both of these tools follow a structure and, through simple and effective questioning, bring clarity and move people from feeling out of control to owning their situation. They create a more meaningful dialogue at every touch point. Caregivers are able to use support resources more effectively; they feel more resilient and are better able to deal with the challenges they face.

GROW [29] stands for:

- **G**oal
- **R**eality as it is now
- **O**ptions—what are they?
- **W**ill—what is your will or way forward?

The model was originally developed in the 1980s by business coaches Graham Alexander, Alan Fine and Sir John Whitmore. It is linear in feel, like a journey, where the first step is to establish a goal and then explore what the current reality is, so that you have an end point and a start point. The options about how you might reach your goal are then determined, and as a way forward, or will, the one that is most realisable is defined and worked through. But what underpins all of this is the value of the questions that you ask at each stage of the process. The questions outlined here have been specifically designed for the brain tumour community.

## 12.6   How to Use GROW

1. Establish the goal. Don't skimp the time spent on this area. If you spend 70% of your time establishing the goal, you are doing well. There is no point in having the conversation if the goal is not meaningful and relevant. Reassure the patient or caregiver that barriers are irrelevant at this stage. Questions you can ask to ascertain the goal include:

- What do you want to discuss?
- What's your goal?
- What do you want?
- What would you like to achieve in this conversation?
- What would need to happen for you to walk away feeling this was time well spent?
- Is that realistic?
- What will be of real value to you?
- What would be different?
- What would you class as a successful outcome for this session?

2. Examine the current reality. This is important, as it is in this stage that often a solution will begin to emerge. Too often people try to solve a problem or reach a goal without considering their starting point so they will never reach their goal. Useful coaching questions include:

- What is happening at the moment?
- When does this happen? How often?
- What other factors are relevant?
- Who else is relevant?
- What is their perception of the situation?
- What else?
- What have you tried so far?
- What are the implications?
- What is your starting point?
- What do you know?
- What are the clinical facts?
- What do you understand about your condition?
- How much do you want to know?
- What have you found out for yourself?
- What have you heard others say?
- What are the words/phrases that keep playing over in your mind?
- What are you frightened of?
- Describe your cancer. What's the metaphor you use?
- How much do you want to be involved?
- Describe how you feel when you are with your:
  1. Clinicians
  2. Intimate family
  3. Friends and helpers
- When do you feel powerful?
- When have you felt powerful?
- How did you think/believe when you felt powerful?

- What was your sense of self?
- Where do you feel safe?
- Right now, here in this conversation today – how are you?
- Who's in your team?
- What do you need from each person in the team?
- What do you need to do to make sure you get that?
- What conversations do you need to have with:
  1. Your clinicians
  2. Your intimate family
  3. Your caregivers
  4. Your children
  5. Your friends
  6. Your colleagues
- What's your relationship to the cancer?
- What's your life motto?
- How do you see yourself now?
- What can you see?
- What now stands out?
- What's on the horizon?
- What has swamped you?
- Who has rescued you?
- Where's your sanctuary?
- Where's your anchor?
- What helps you most?
- Who helps you most?
- Coach—what I sense is…

3. Exploring the options. Once the current reality has been defined, it's time to move forward to explore options. What will help reach the goal? Put everything on the table. These questions will elicit the options.

- What could you do?
- What else?
- What alternatives are there and which might work?
- What have you seen or used before in similar circumstances?
- Who can help you?
- Would you like suggestions from me?
- What are the benefits or pitfalls of doing that?
- Of these, which interests you?
- Would you like to choose one to act on?
- Which one would you like to discuss?

4. Establish the will or way forward. The time has come to commit specific actions so that the person can move forwards towards their goal. This will help them to think about their motivation, commitment and desire to move forward.

- What are the next steps?
- Precisely when will you do them?
- What might get in the way?
- What support do you need?
- How and when will you enlist that support?
- How committed are you to this solution?
- What might stop you and how can you deal with that?
- How will you measure success?
- What is already in place?
- What are you missing?
- What are the sources of information that will help you to fill in the gaps?
- Who are the people who can help?

Powerful questions can be used at any stage of the person's illness. These questions encourage insight when you are living with a life-limiting illness and relate to specific scenarios.

Dealing with a close person who is terminally ill:

- What has made you a strong partnership?
- Where are you both strong for each other?
- What do you bring to each other?
- What do you admire in each other?
- What strength do you gain from each other?
- What does the other person do that is getting in the way?
- What do you need from each other at this time?
- What is going to be hard to talk about?
- How have you managed disagreements in the past?
- What's important to get right?
- What's going to get you through tough decisions?
- What role do you want the other person to play?
- What milestones would you like to achieve?
- Are there any circumstances worse than death that you need to talk about?

Coming to terms with a specific prognosis:

- What do you not want to regret?
- Who do you want to be in the time left?
- How do you want to think about these next few months?
- What will help you be prepared?
- What questions do you need to ask or get answers to?
- What do you need to get in order to talk about with your loved ones?
- What do you (and your loved ones) want to remember about the next few weeks/months/years?

Finally try to plan a review meeting to discuss progress. Things can go off course when living with a critical illness, so there may be a need to be agile about the approach if things don't work quite as planned. The problem outcome framework can help here.

## 12.7    The Problem Outcome Framework

The *problem outcome framework* is really useful as it enables people to stop being stuck. It gets them to think about how they are approaching the problem. We are always able to say what it is we don't want, but rarely can we say what it is we do want, often just because we don't have the space to think, let alone articulate this. We are too bound up in life's intercession of chance and react to things, never more so when we are caring for someone. This frame enables people to think about what it is they want and how they might move forward. It's useful as a starting point. The problem questions focus on the problem. The outcome questions are solution oriented, so focused on goals, which is where energy should be placed. Decisions then become aligned, as people know what their focus is. These questions are not focused on why the problem exists but what is wanted and how to achieve it.

### 12.7.1  How to Use It

Ask the first set of questions to elicit the problem, without sharing the second set (which will elicit the outcome or the solution). Allow about 20–30 min for this. Many will have a need to tell their story. When these questions have been exhausted, move them to the second set. If anything these are more important.

When they have finished exploring the questions, take some feedback. Start with a generic question about the difference between the two conversations. Ask them if the conversations felt different? What was it that made them feel different?

**What about me?** Feedback tends to be focused on the person as a caregiver or patient. People rarely talk about themselves as a person. Raise this. You may get some emotion at this point.

Is it realistic for you to do anything for yourself? Where and when do we discount our own needs in service of others? How could this look different? Be different?

Talk about the need for a sanctuary. What does their sanctuary look like? What are the enablers for them using this? Give them permission to take time out from being a caregiver/patient/healthcare practitioner.

| Problem | Outcome |
| --- | --- |
| What type of tumour are you living with? | What do you want to achieve in the next few months? |
| How long have you known about it? | What will help you to progress? |
| What has been hard? | Who can help you? |
| Who or what is at fault here? | What skills or experience can you call upon from other parts of your life that will be useful to you here and now? |
| What is not going as you would wish? | What would be a good first step? |

## 12.8   Conclusion

This chapter has defined why there is a need to have better conversations about what it means to be living with a brain tumour. It has explored the role that coaching can play in creating the space to have these conversations and shared tools that will enable everyone to embrace the change that is needed.

There is a critical need for patients, caregivers and their families to be able to self-manage so that they can make informed choices about their treatment pathway. Even if individuals spend as much as 6 h a year in a clinic or health professional's office, that leaves them 8760 h when they are "on their own" to manage their diet, physical activity, medications, stress and other factors. In discussion with healthcare professionals including neurosurgeons, neuropathologists, neuro-oncologists and neuro-oncology nurses and patients and families, a picture has emerged as to what is needed to help people at the point of diagnosis and throughout their treatment in order to empower them to take control of their situation.

Caregivers and patients don't understand how an emphasis can be placed on restoring or maximising independence with activities of daily living, mobility, cognition and communication. Although goals change as the stage of illness advances, being proactive can maintain independence in patients who undergo treatment and who have potential loss of function. If patients and caregivers were more informed about the progression of the disease, they could be better prepared and intervene earlier. They could be more specific and more proactive in their asks of the support services, outlining specifically what the problem is so that additional help can be targeted effectively. It is difficult to ask for support if you don't know what is available. This could so easily be addressed. A key question which should be asked regularly is "what are you struggling with the most?" Once this is articulated, it is easy to define what is needed. This chapter should enable everyone to engage more meaningfully in the conversations that are being held about the needs of people who are living with a brain tumour, so that the challenges are better faced, resilience is built and everyone feels resourced.

## References

1. Barry M, Edgman-Levitan S. Shared decision making – the pinnacle of patient-centered care. N Engl J Med. 2012;366(9):780–1.
2. brainstrust. Quality of life: what the brain cancer community needs [Internet]. Cowes: brainstrust; 2015. Updated 2 Apr 2015. https://issuu.com/brainstrust/docs/150309_what_the_community_needs_fin. Accessed 26 Aug 2017
3. Burnet N, Jefferies S, Benson R, Hunt D, Treasure F. Years of life lost (YLL) from cancer is an important measure of population burden – and should be considered when allocating research funds. Br J Cancer. 2005;92(2):241–5.
4. Quality Health. National cancer patient experience survey 2016: national results summary [Internet]. Chesterfield: Quality Health; 2016. [updated 2016]. http://www.ncpes.co.uk/index.php/reports/2016-reports/national-reports-1/3572-cpes-2016-national-report/file. Accessed 26 Aug 2017
5. Rooney A. Challenges and opportunities in psychological neuro-oncology. Oncol News. 2011;2011(4):133–5.
6. Department of Health. Equality and excellence: liberating the NHS, vol. 57. London: Department of Health; 2010.
7. Flynn K, Smith M, Vanness D. A typology of preferences for participation in healthcare decision making. Soc Sci Med. 2006;63(5):1158–69.
8. National Institute for Clinical Excellence. Improving supportive and palliative care for adults with cancer: The manual [Internet]. London: National Institute for Clinical Excellence; 2004. p. 70. [Updated 24 Mar 2004]. https://www.nice.org.uk/guidance/csg4/resources/improving-supportive-and-palliative-care-for-adults-with-cancer-pdf-773375005. Accessed 26 Aug 2017
9. Shepherd SC, Cavers D, Wallace LM, Hacking B, Scott SE, Bowyer DJ. Navigation' to support decision making for patients with a high grade brain tumour. A qualitative evaluation. Neuro Oncol. 2012;14(2):4.
10. Cavers D, Hacking B, Erridge S, Kendall M, Morris P, Murray S. Social, psychological and existential well-being in patients with glioma and their caregivers: a qualitative study. Can Med Assoc J. 2012;184(7):E373–82.
11. Cavers D, Hacking B, Erridge S, Morris P, Kendall M, Murray S. Adjustment and support needs of glioma patients and their relatives: serial interviews. Psycho-Oncology. 2012;22(6):1299–305.
12. Bartolo M, Zucchella C, Pace A, Lanzetta G, Vecchione C, Bartolo M, et al. Early rehabilitation after surgery improves functional outcome in inpatients with brain tumours. J Neuro-Oncol. 2011;107(3):537–44.
13. Greene J, Hibbard J. Why does patient activation matter? An examination of the relationships between patient activation and health-related outcomes. J Gen Intern Med. 2012;27(5):520–6.
14. Hibbard J, Stockard J, Mahoney E, Tusler M. Development of the patient activation measure (PAM): conceptualizing and measuring activation in patients and consumers. Health Serv Res. 2004;39(4p1):1005–26.
15. Becker E, Roblin D. Translating primary care practice climate into patient activation. Med Care. 2008;46(8):795–805.
16. Hibbard JH, Cunningham PJ. How engaged are consumers in their health and health care, and why does it matter? Health Syst Change Res Briefs. 2008;8:1–9.
17. Hibbard J, Mahoney E, Stock R, Tusler M. Do increases in patient activation result in improved self-management behaviors? Health Serv Res. 2007;42(4):1443–63.

18. Mosen DM, Schmittdiel J, Hibbard J, Sobel D, Remmers C, Bellows J. Is patient activation associated with outcomes of care for adults with chronic conditions? J Ambulat Care Manag. 2007;30(1):21–9.
19. Fowles J, Terry P, Xi M, Hibbard J, Bloom C, Harvey L. Measuring self-management of patients' and employees' health: further validation of the Patient Activation Measure (PAM) based on its relation to employee characteristics. Patient Educ Couns. 2009;77(1):116–22.
20. Edgman-Levitan S, Brady C, Howitt P. Partnering with patients, families, and communities for health: a global imperative – report of the family engagement working group 2013 [Internet]. Ar-Rayyan: World Innovation Summit for Health; 2013. [Updated 2013]. http://dpnfts5n-brdps.cloudfront.net/app/media/387. Accessed 26 Aug 2017.
21. Blunt I. Focus on preventable admissions: trends in emergency admissions for ambulatory care sensitive conditions, 2001 to 2013 [Internet]. London: The Health Foundation and the Nuffield Trust; 2013. http://www.qualitywatch.org.uk/sites/files/qualitywatch/field/field_doc-ument/131010_QualityWatch_Focus_Preventable_Admissions.pdf
22. Nesta. The business case for people powered health [Internet]. London: Nesta; 2013. [Updated 8 Apr 2013]. https://www.nesta.org.uk/sites/default/files/the_business_case_for_people_pow-ered_health.pdf. Accessed 26 Aug 2017
23. Piil K, Juhler M, Jakobsen J, Jarden M. Controlled rehabilitative and supportive care interven-tion trials in patients with high-grade gliomas and their caregivers: a systematic review. BMJ Support Palliat Care. 2014;6(1):27–34.
24. brainstrust. Share aware pinboard [Internet]. Cowes: brainstrust; 2013. http://www.brainstrust.org.uk/pinboard/. Accessed 26 Aug 2017
25. Campbell H, Phaneuf M, Deane K. Cancer peer support programs—do they work? Patient Educ Couns. 2004;55(1):3–15.
26. Hoey LM, Leropoli SC, White VM, Jefford M. Systematic review of peer-support programs for people with cancer. Patient Educ Couns. 2008;70(3):315–37.
27. California Healthcare Foundation. Final chapter: CAL' attitudes and experiences with death and dying [Internet]. Oakland, CA: California Healthcare Foundation; 2012. [Updated Feb 2012]. http://www.chcf.org/~/media/MEDIA%20LIBRARY%20Files/PDF/PDF%20F/PDF%20FinalChapterDeathDying.pdf. Accessed 26 Aug 2017
28. Stanfield RB, editor. The art of focused conversation: 100 ways to access group wisdom in the workplace. Montreal, QC: The Canadian Institute of Cultural Affairs; 1997.
29. Alexander G. [2006]. Behavioural coaching—the GROW model. In: Passmore J, editor. Excellence in coaching: the industry guide. 2nd ed. London/Philadelphia: Kogan Page; 2010. p. 83–93. ISBN 9780749456672. OCLC 521754202.

# The Mental Capacity Act/Deprivation of Liberty Safeguards and Their Relationship to Adult Safeguarding

Heather Ayles

**Abstract**

This chapter describes the Mental Capacity Act and its relevance when applied to people receiving healthcare within England and Wales. It explains the circumstances in which additional safeguards are triggered, in the form of the Deprivation of Liberty Safeguards (2009). In our roles as the providers of care and treatment to patients, we have a responsibility to both follow the Act and be able to demonstrate that its use is embedded in our practice. We are required to use the Act to promote our patients' involvement in decisions related to their care and treatment. Only when we have evidence that this expectation cannot be met are we legally permitted to follow the guidance in the Act in order to make decisions on another adult's behalf.

In this context, the Act has implications for all of us—clinicians and patients—by stipulating measures that must be taken before decisions are made on any individual's behalf. By providing the tools to empower people for whom decision-making may be problematic, the Act also offers protection for those involved in caring for people who are unable to advocate fully for themselves. It covers the whole range of decisions to be made, from everyday issues to healthcare and financial matters.

**Keywords**

Mental capacity · Healthcare · Safeguarding · Consent · Advocacy · Decision-making · Autonomy · Interventions · Legal framework · Best interests · Least restrictive option

H. Ayles (✉)
Addenbrooke's Hospital, Cambridge University Hospital NHS Foundation Trust, Cambridge, UK
e-mail: Heather.ayles@addenbrookes.nhs.uk

© Springer Nature Switzerland AG 2019
I. Oberg (ed.), *Management of Adult Glioma in Nursing Practice*,
https://doi.org/10.1007/978-3-319-76747-5_13

**Learning Outcomes**
- To gain an oversight of the Mental Capacity Act and its processes in the UK—a case illustration will provide you with a more concrete example of how the process works.
- To understand the differences between varying processes such as the Mental Capacity Act, best interest decisions, deprivation of liberties and the varying legal services surrounding the Mental Capacity Act in the UK.
- To gain insight and knowledge into the legal decision-making processes involved in emergency situations whereby the rights of the patient are safeguarded, along with safeguarding the clinician from potential liability.
- To know how/where to find support and information and how to escalate issues if you are worried about your patient's mental capacity to make safe decisions surrounding their care and treatment.

## 13.1    Introduction

The Mental Capacity Act 2005 provides a legal framework to promote the decision-making autonomy of all adults over the age of 16 who usually reside or are present in England or Wales. In Scotland, the Adults with Incapacity (Scotland) Act 2000 provides a similar framework. This legislation safeguards people's right to independence by bringing together core elements of pre-existing legislation relating to the equality of individuals (Equality Act 2010) and their basic human rights (Human Rights Act 1998). In this context, the Act has implications for everyone—clinicians and patients—by stipulating measures that must be taken before decisions are made on any individual's behalf. By providing the tools to empower people for whom decision-making may be problematic, the Act also offers protection for those involved in caring for people who are unable to advocate fully for themselves. It covers the whole range of decisions to be made, from everyday issues to healthcare and financial matters.

This chapter describes the Mental Capacity Act and its relevance when applied to people receiving healthcare within England and Wales. It explains the circumstances in which additional safeguards are triggered, in the form of the Deprivation of Liberty Safeguards (a 2009 amendment to the Mental Capacity Act 2005). In nurses' roles as the providers of care and treatment to patients, they have a responsibility to both follow the Act and be able to demonstrate that its use is embedded in practice. Nurses are required to use the Act to promote their patients' involvement in decisions related to their care and treatment. Only when there is evidence that this expectation cannot be met are health professionals legally permitted to follow the guidance in the Act in order to make decisions on another adult's behalf.

## 13.2    Background

For most people, admission to hospital for acute medical care is an unwelcome yet bearable experience. If, as a result of expert assessment of their clinical needs, a patient were to be faced with this recommendation, he/she would instinctively place his/her trust in those who have been trained to deliver medical care and treatment. And whilst they'd hope for the experience not to be too unpleasant, and that there would be a positive outcome, their understanding and engagement in the detail of the process might essentially be quite passive—after all, the specialists know best.

Public confidence in the healthcare system has historically been based upon trust. Healthcare professionals attain high levels of expertise; their roles are perceived as vocational, and their intentions are construed as honourable and selfless. The underlying premise is that as experts in a complex arena, to challenge clinical opinion would be inappropriate and to request the evidence behind decision-making would be unnecessary. A traditional paternalism embedded in the culture of medical services has encouraged this; those with expertise must convince others of their competence and reassure them with their command of the situation.

However, this approach to building confidence can be at the cost of patient participation in making genuine choices about care and thus may not fulfil all the obligations of valid consent. Furthermore, a certain tension can arise between traditional clinical confidence and legal responsibilities. The foundation for a practitioner's legal position is the need to represent the individual's point of view. As a result, practitioners may become polarised by their differing frames of reference—the urge to do what is best for the individual based upon scientific expertise versus the intention of representing a person's view and promoting the right for that view to be upheld, wise or unwise though it may be in the opinion of others.

Recent developments in social care have signalled a shift towards more person-centred assessments and care provision (The Care Act 2014). This intention to promote autonomy also makes healthcare professionals more accountable to the wishes of the individual and has boosted a strategy that is being driven forward across the health and social care economy on several fronts. Public enquiries into systemic failings within our healthcare system have been partly responsible. The national UK scandals of Mid-Staffordshire Heath Authority and Winterbourne View care home exposed failings in the delivery of care and treatment by paid professionals working in healthcare settings. The subsequent enquiries shone a light on the darkest extremes of brutality and ignorance within services that were primarily set up to care for and protect vulnerable people with limited ability to advocate for themselves but became dysfunctional, neglectful and abusive. The Francis Report, amongst its core recommendations, drew attention to the importance of involving patients in decision-making around their healthcare—i.e., no decision about me without me [1].

> Good communication involves better listening and shared decision-making—no decision about me without me.

The need to challenge dogmatic authoritarianism and to promote transparency within the provision of healthcare services was recognised and has become a focus of legal effort, and a core element of the Nursing and Midwifery Council Code of Practice in the UK since 2013.

It is everyone's right to receive the information and explanation required to understand and participate in decision-making associated with their medical care and treatment. For many that simply involves a conversation and perhaps the signing of a consent form. For some individuals there will be barriers to the process of providing straightforward consent. Disability or sensory impairment may impact on an individual's ability to process information. Methods of communication may not be straightforward, requiring specialist equipment or the support of other services to interpret or represent them. By definition, consent must be accompanied by an understanding of both the benefits and the disadvantages of an intervention and must be obtained in a timely manner and without coercion. Ensuring that these conditions are truly met can present challenges for both practitioner and patient. These issues lie at the heart of the Mental Capacity Act 2005 and are also embedded in the protective strategy we know as 'Adult Safeguarding' (Care Act 2014 s. 42).

## 13.3    An Overview of the Mental Capacity Act (2005)

### 13.3.1  What Is Mental Capacity?

Mental capacity is the ability to make a decision. This is not an overarching condition—people often lack capacity to make some decisions but not others, and their ability to do so can fluctuate, especially when they are ill. Decision-making relates both to consent and refusal of interventions—for good reasons, bad reasons or simply no reason at all. The ability of an individual to take part in this process should be fully explored and recorded. If a clinician ignores this requirement, they risk committing assault. This in itself is a direct challenge to paternalistic attitudes and previously held assumptions that the trained professional must automatically know what is best for the patient.

Clearly, circumstances exist in which obtaining valid consent is not possible, perhaps because of the urgent nature of the need for intervention or because of the patient's inability to participate. The Mental Capacity Act provides health professionals with the legal framework for use in the care and treatment of patients in emergency situations such as these. It protects the rights of the patient and also safeguards the clinician from liability.

### 13.3.2  Principles of the Mental Capacity Act (2005)

There are five basic principles underpinning the Mental Capacity Act. Embedded as standards in the Code of Practice, they provide the basis of all capacity assessments:

1. A person must be assumed to have capacity unless it is established that they lack capacity.

Every adult has the right to make their own decisions if they are able to do so. Capacity is assumed in an individual unless it is established otherwise. One is never required to prove that someone *has* capacity—one assesses in order to establish if capacity is *lacking*.

2.  A person is not to be treated as unable to make a decision unless all practicable steps to help them do so have been taken without success.

Capacity is decision-specific. One cannot tell whether or not someone is able to make a specific decision unless they have tried to help them make it. In healthcare this may mean addressing one or several obstacles—perhaps relating to language or communication. Support from specialist services such as linguistic interpreters or speech and language therapists may need to be sought. Easy-read literature, sign language and use of electronic communication devices would all feature here too.

3.  A person is not to be treated as unable to make a decision merely because he/she makes an unwise decision.

People have the right to do lawful things that others don't agree with or to take risks that others don't approve of. Eccentric decisions that may be regarded as unwise by professionals should not be taken as an indication that the person lacks capacity.

4.  An act done, or decision made under this Act, for or on behalf of a person who lacks capacity must be done or made in his/her best interests.

'Best interests' decision-making is a process and not a simple assertion. Guidance on best interest decision-making is laid out in full in the Mental Capacity Act Code of Practice [2].

5.  Before the act is done, or the decision is made, consideration must be given to whether the purpose for which it is needed can be as effectively achieved in a way that is less restrictive of the person's rights and freedom of action.

All care and treatment of an individual, including interventions and future planning, should be constructed in a form that follows these five principles. When decisions are made on behalf of someone, their lives are being stepped into by that person, and they should seek to intrude as little as possible.

There may be several options to choose from, and priority should be given to the options which will be less restrictive of the patient, for example, administering medication in oral form rather than injection or regularly toileting someone rather than catheterising them. Sometimes clinicians, with the benefit of their foresight and experience, struggle to allow what they see as unwise decisions. On occasions where the patient is demonstrating that a decision has been made with full adherence to the stages of the assessment, they need to allow the patient to follow their own path regardless of clinicians 'better judgement'.

### 13.3.3  How to Assess Mental Capacity: A Functional Test

Every individual must be assumed to have capacity unless there is good reason to think otherwise. If a practitioner has concerns about someone's ability to make a particular decision, further assessment should take place. Ideally, the assessment should be undertaken by the 'decision-maker', that is, the person who will undertake or authorise the intervention. Following this principle, a nurse will assess a patient to whom she intends to administer a pain-killing injection or provide personal care; a physiotherapist assesses the patient's agreement to engage with therapy; and a social worker may assess someone's ability to consent to a care package.

Obtaining consent in this way is usually a routine and instinctive part of the professional's practice, something they do many times a day in the course of their work. What may be less familiar is the need to break the assessment down into its component parts and work methodically through each stage. Recording the detail of the steps taken illustrates the efforts made to engage the person in decisions about their care and treatment and ensures that the extent of their ability to give consent competently is evidenced.

In order to meet the criteria for assessment of mental capacity, the person must fulfil the two-stage criteria:

- There is an impairment or disturbance of the person's mind or brain, either temporary or permanent.
- The impairment or disturbance is sufficient that the person may lack capacity to make that particular decision at that particular time.

Once these criteria are met, formal assessment using the guidance from the MCA should follow. The suggested format places emphasis on *how the decision is reached*, rather than *what the decision is*. As already defined (in the five principles above), a decision judged by others as 'unwise' does not necessarily indicate a lack of capacity. The four stages of a capacity assessment are closely mapped to the principles. They require a person faced with a specific decision to be able to:

- *Understand* the information relating to that particular decision.
- *Retain* the information—with support in any form required, for long enough to make the decision.
- *Weigh up* the information—use the information to consider the risks and benefits involved.
- *Communicate* their decision, by whatever means possible—again, with the use of any of the support mechanisms required.

Failure to complete any of the four stages indicates a lack of capacity to make that particular decision at that particular time. However, there are several potential pitfalls for the assessor in this situation. To disagree with the person in the light of superior clinical knowledge does not mean that they lack capacity. To 'want to act in their best interests' does not mean that they lack capacity and can be overruled. Details of the conversation for each step taken should be recorded—reducing the assessment to a tick-box exercise is indefensible and does not constitute valid consent.

### 13.3.4  When to Formally Assess Mental Capacity

Reflecting on the scope of the two-stage test helps identify the kind of patient to whom the Act applies. Some individuals will have identified impairments, such as learning disabilities or long-term brain injuries. Other people may be living with dementia or degenerative diseases that progressively rob them of their cognitive ability. A wide variety of circumstances also have the potential for impact on decision-making. Medications, infections, pain and anxiety may all alter an individual's ability to understand, retain, weigh up and communicate decisions.

Where possible, professionals should defer decision-making to a later point when the patient is able to take part, but in hospital this is not always practical or advisable. It has been established that the delivery of urgent or life-threatening treatment is authorised within the Act; in all other circumstances, the care and treatment of patients should be accompanied by their consent or authorised by the mental capacity safeguards.

Decisions should be specific—it is rare that someone totally lacks capacity. Care should be taken to promote the highest level of autonomy possible for the patient—for example, they should be able to choose meals or when to sit in the bedside chair and whether or not to listen to music or watch TV. If an approach to the delivery of care that actively promotes patient involvement is established, there will be a clearer picture the patient's ability to be involved. It may become apparent that more complex decisions are not possible, and formal assessments will then be triggered.

Fluctuating capacity may affect many people with conditions that occasionally worsen or in situations that increase the demands on the person to a point where decision-making is affected. Occasionally this may be predictable, e.g. someone who always develops a period of confusion after anaesthetic or someone with dementia who is more confused at the end of the day. Medication, infection or even a severe shock can temporarily affect a person's ability to make certain decisions.

Ongoing and progressive illnesses may steadily rob a patient of cognitive ability, or the person may experience periods of fluctuating capacity that lessen temporarily but leave behind an overall deterioration. It is important to judge when to have conversations and enable decisions to be made in a timely manner, taking advantage of moments when the person is able to engage competently. These considerations may include making advanced decisions to refuse further treatment or appointing a 'power of attorney'.

### 13.3.5 Setting the Scene for Assessment

Identifying the decision to be made and ensuring that it is communicated to the patient clearly and concisely are key. Choosing when and where to do this will be based upon the individual's circumstances. The time of day, the number of people present and the environment itself should all be considered, justified and documented. The length of time taken is also crucial, and the practitioner should be willing to repeat the exercise if necessary—the patient only needs to be able to hold the information for long enough to make the decision, but if short-term memory is impaired, revisiting the issue would be a good practice to ensure that the outcome of assessment is consistent.

The practitioner must be able to demonstrate that they understand the risks and benefits involved in the patient's decision, relating to any and all options available. This may require research or sharing documentation. Information must be delivered in a way that the person understands—using an interpreter or visual aids as necessary—and it is important to ensure that both patient and practitioner have every resource to hand that is needed. Glasses, working hearing aids and a peaceful environment are amongst the essentials that may aid in the preparation for assessment. In some cases, a patient may wish for family members to be present. If this is the case, the assessor must not allow family to speak for the patient or exert undue pressure as a result of their own opinions. In cases where family members are known to have strong opinions, it may be necessary to reinforce this fact before the assessment by explaining the importance of avoiding any coercion.

The assessor must assure themselves that the information has been understood by the patient, e.g. by asking the patient to paraphrase the discussion after a short while. Evidence that the person has been able to 'weigh up' the information is also required and can be a challenge to represent. One solution might be to ask, 'How did you come to that conclusion?' or to prompt the patient for feedback regarding the risks and benefits of the options associated within the decision being made. One way to make this more meaningful is to introduce the subject from the perspective of others—'What concerns does your daughter have? Why do you think she feels that way? What thoughts do you have around this?', etc.

Communicating the outcome of the decision may itself require support if the person has disabilities that prohibit the usual methods of communication. Speech may be inhibited in someone who has had a glioma, or it may be normal for the person to be non-verbal. The use of aids such as a whiteboard or more sophisticated assistive technology may be required or support enlisted from speech and language therapy, a sign-language practitioner or family member or carer who knows the patient well and can interpret for them. However, if the barriers to communication are relatively new—for example, as a result of stroke or acquired brain injury—it should be borne in mind that human nature invests us with a deep sense of positivity for our loved ones. This may introduce an element of interpretation about the cognitive ability of the patient that is based more on optimism and personal conviction than evidenced ability.

Inability to demonstrate any step in the assessment indicates that the patient lacks capacity to make that particular decision. The assessment should be clearly documented, and the patient should not be made to feel that they have 'failed' or caused disappointment in any way. A view must be taken about the prospect of the patient's capacity improving and whether or not the decision could be postponed until a point when the patient might be better able to participate. If neither is the case, a best interest decision should be made.

## 13.4 The Best Interests Process

The Mental Capacity Act Code of Practice outlines the steps required to ensure that a decision made on behalf of another person follows the recommended process and is in keeping with the spirit of the Act. It involves obtaining information from all of those with a connection to the patient who may be able to offer a perspective on the decision being made. Where the patient has no family or friends (or there is a strong belief that those people are not acting in the best interests of the patient), and the only people eligible to take part are paid professionals, the appointment of an IMCA (Independent Mental Capacity Advocate) should be considered within those UK countries where the Mental Capacity Act is relevant. This is essential for issues relating to serious medical treatment or a change of residence for the patient.

Attendees at a best interest meeting will address the specific decision to be made. After listening in turn to the information from each member present, an overall picture of the risks and benefits within the situation can be built. Individual opinions on the decision should not be gathered until the end of the meeting, after everyone has had their chance to comment. Rules of etiquette are emphasised—everyone must feel able to speak their mind freely, without fear of reprisal or ridicule, and confidentiality is key. The intention is that by 'walking in the person's shoes', a decision will be made that, if capacity were present, the patient would have made for themselves. If possible, the patient should be included in proceedings. A record is kept of all that has been discussed, and a checklist is available from the Code of Practice which should ideally be completed to provide evidence that all points were covered and due process followed.

## 13.5 Deprivation of Liberty Safeguards (DoLS 2009)

### 13.5.1 The Background

In some situations, providing safe care may involve submitting the patient to a level of restriction or restraint. Where the patient 'lacks capacity to consent to care and treatment, is under continuous supervision and control and is not free to leave', this is known as the 'acid test', and additional safeguards, known as the Deprivation of Liberty Safeguards (DoLS), are triggered. Importantly, the safeguards are related to the patient's location and only authorise the necessary detention of the patient in that place. They do not authorise the care and treatment interventions directly; these should be undertaken in line with the broader guidance of the MCA, with assessments and best interest decisions for all serious decisions that need to be made at that time.

DoLS were not introduced into the Act until 2009. Their inclusion was prompted by the outcome of a specific court case (R. v Bournewood Community and Mental Health NHS Trust [1997] EWCA Civ 2879). This had implications in terms of human rights and autonomy of decision-making. Although the broad framework of the safeguards continues to apply, the legal landscape is evolving and has been shaped by the outcome of further legal challenges heard by the supreme court (most specifically Cheshire West and Chester Council v P [2011] EWCA Civ 1257). There has also been acknowledgement by government that the DoLS process represents an unwieldy burden on services in terms of time and resources [3]. A bill proposed by the Law Commission [4] to reform and streamline the current safeguards is currently under consideration.

The DoLS process provides for an overview of individuals in care settings who are unable to provide informed consent to be there. Although in receipt of care and treatment deemed necessary by professionals, the application of the safeguards triggers objective scrutiny of their circumstances, in order to ensure that they are not subject to unwarranted and thus unlawful restrictions of their liberty. Local authority-sponsored assessors ('Best Interests Assessors') review the patient and ensure that the measures being taken are necessary and proportionate and that the Mental Capacity Act provides the correct legal framework for the care setting to use for the patient at that time.

DoLS applies in all circumstances where an individual is said to be in receipt of 'putative care', i.e. care delivered by the state. Primarily this applies to care homes and hospitals, but more recent case law has extended the sphere of application to include those at home in receipt of large state-funded care packages. Originally only applicable to those aged 18 and above in England and Wales, the age range has also extended, and there are now an increasing number of cases where the legislation has been used for 16- and 17-year-olds.

## 13.5.2 When to Apply DoLS

The safeguards do not apply in life-saving situations. In hospital, professionals are no longer required to make applications for patients in critical care areas when intervention is vital and could not be delivered using alternative measures. In such situations the conditions of treatment would be applicable to anyone, regardless of their premorbid ability to consent, as adjudicated in R (Ferreira) v HM Senior Coroner for Inner South London [2017] EWCA Civ 31.

For other patients, the safeguards are triggered by care plans introducing a certain level of restriction or restraint. Where this level of supervision and control is deemed necessary over a period of time (described in law as 'non-negligible'), consideration should be given to a DoLS application. Organisations are asked to interpret this time frame locally, and in acute care a suggested time frame of 7 days has been deemed as the appropriate 'non-negligible' period.

Patients who are not free to leave and who are being restricted in terms of confinement to the ward or bed area should be considered for DoLS if they are unable to give informed consent for these measures, particularly if there are additional restrictions in place.

Examples of additional restrictions range from 'falls mats' to 'posey mitts' or splints that may be in use to prevent the patient from pulling out invasive equipment required for their care. Arterial lines, intravenous lines and tracheostomy tubes are all examples of vital equipment that may be dislodged by an agitated and confused patient, and measures are sometimes required to prevent this from happening. In keeping with the spirit of the Mental Capacity Act, such measures should represent the lesser restriction, and the care plan should be regularly reviewed in an attempt to reduce their intensity as soon as possible. Clear differentiation should be made between those restrictions that are essential and those that relate to potential risk.

The use of force within a plan of patient care, either physical or with the use of sedation, significantly increases the likelihood of a patient's suitability for DoLS application. Covert administration of medication (when drugs are administered without the patient's awareness or consent) and instances where the patient is being physically returned to the ward or bedside are all suggestive of deprivation.

Other factors with an impact on liberty relate to the access to the patient by family or friends. Circumstances where visiting is restricted or banned, or where a patient is not allowed to leave for a period of time with visitors or reasons of safety, should indicate to staff that there may be a need for DoLS application.

An intense level of patient observation such as 1:1 care or the use of a locked ward or tag alarm indicates a high level of control over a patient's movements and care. It is important to note that the patient's physical ability to leave is irrelevant; someone who is bedbound with total dependence on staff for all care, although unable to physically make that move, is nevertheless subject to the safeguards.

Case law has provided much of the guidance for the DoLS process, and currently it is in circumstances where the 'acid test' is met that an application should be made. Since a hospital is not a long-term living arrangement, the use of the combined urgent and standard form is recommended. In the first instance, the acute trust is able to authorise 7 days of restriction, based upon the measures laid out in the care plan. The acute trust then asks the relevant local authority to endorse those measures and extend the time frame for a suitable period during which professionals are authorised to continue delivering care. If capacity is regained or the restrictions no longer apply, the local authority is notified, and the process is discontinued.

Restriction and restraint of a patient are not necessarily a bad thing, and where there is good evidence to support their use, DoLS application provides legal endorsement and does not indicate fault on the part of the care provider. However it is important to note that the local authority assessors will seek to assure themselves that measures in place are both necessary and representative of the least restrictive option possible. On no account must restrictions be in place for punitive reasons or for staff or organisational convenience—they must be demonstrably in the patient's best interests. Neither should the safeguards be used nor extended as a result of delays in transfers of care or other discharge planning issues.

In addition to the six assessments undertaken before an authorisation is granted, the local authority will also appoint a 'relevant person's representative (RPR)' for the patient'. In most cases this will be a family member or friend who can be depended upon to advocate for the patient. Other safeguards imposed under the DoLS process are the right to challenge the deprivation and access to support from an independent mental capacity advocate (IMCA).

An IMCA referral should be made for people who may lack capacity to make some important decisions autonomously and who do not have the support of a family member or friend. The IMCA ensures that the standards of the MCA are adhered to and that the best interests' process is followed when decisions are being made on behalf of the patient. The details of the IMCA role are fully laid out within the terms of the Act, which also authorises the IMCA to examine confidential information relating to the patient such as medical notes and social care records. In acute care settings, an IMCA should be requested for any patient who is unable to participate in decision-making around serious medical treatments. An IMCA may also be involved in cases where a patient is likely to have a change of address upon discharge, such as a care home. If family is not felt to be acting in a patient's best interests, an IMCA referral may be made, but this should be clearly the case— IMCA will not become involved just because the family does not concur with medical opinion. However, in adult protection cases, an IMCA may be instructed even where family members or others are available to be consulted.

## 13.6    Case Study

Please note that the following case study is fictitious and intended as a guide only. It illustrates the considerations outlined above and explains measures that could be taken to address such circumstances. It is not a prescribed template and does not represent any known case.

### 13.6.1 Background

P is a 46-year-old gentleman who has previously been treated for glioma and who has re-presented with seizures and expressive dysphasia. Fully able to engage with discussions relating to treatment, he is able to consent to admission to hospital for a course of high-dose steroids and anticonvulsant therapy. This leads to improvements in both his seizure activity and his dysphasia, and he subsequently has surgery to partially resect residual glioma tissue.

## 13.6.2 Relevance of MCA

At P's presentation, formal assessment of his ability to consent to care and treatment in hospital is indicated as it's known that he has an 'impairment of the mind or brain' that could potentially impact upon that ability, thus meeting criteria for the two-stage test detailed in the MCA Code of Practice. His ability to give valid consent for admission is recorded, as is his consent for treatment and for surgery.

Unfortunately, P then suffers a postsurgical ischaemic stroke, leaving him with significant cognitive impairment and no longer able to participate in decision-making around the details of his clinical management.

## 13.6.3 Advocacy

P's progress under the care of the inpatient neurological rehabilitation services is slow but, in the opinion of the team, steady. Discussions at the multidisciplinary meetings indicate that the therapists feel continued inpatient rehabilitation should be offered to the patient in an attempt to regain some of his neurological function via neurogenesis (retraining of the brain pathways) in order to maximise his quality of life. P's wife does not concur with this approach. She is unconvinced that there is any sustained functional improvement in her husband's condition and is exhausted by the lengthy travelling necessary to visit him in hospital. She feels that 'enough is enough' and wants him to be discharged as soon as possible to a nursing home near to her and the family. However, such a move would bring an end to active therapy. P's wife does not have power of attorney.

## 13.6.4 MCA Considerations Within Care Planning

P's stroke alters his circumstances considerably. His increased dysphasia makes communication with him more difficult, and expert help from speech and language therapists is required, thus fulfilling the second MCA principle by ensuring that everything possible is done to facilitate communication and enable decision-making by the patient whenever possible.

Mental capacity assessments are conducted by therapists engaged in his care and by all members of the treating team at the initiation of interventions. Outcomes are recorded and demonstrated that at times P has awareness and a connection with his surroundings and is able to participate in care willingly. This assent is taken as an indication that in times when he is less alert, routine care can take place in his best interests.

In fact P retains a knowledge of where he is, and why, for some of the time. He is able to nod his agreement for basic care and treatment and shows no sign of agitation or resistance to intervention. Deprivation of Liberty Safeguards is considered and deemed not to be of issue. His wife and family visit regularly, are actively involved in discussions related to his management and clearly demonstrate that they care deeply about his welfare. He therefore does not require an IMCA.

### 13.6.5 Tackling Differences of Opinion When a Patient Lacks Capacity

P's wife disagrees with the team on the subject of his ongoing treatment plan, feeling that further intervention is not justified and that P should now be 'left in peace'. Her view is respected by the team, who initially ensure that she has an opportunity to observe P's interaction with therapy and is fully aware of his function and his level of participation. P's wife does not always have an opportunity to see him in therapy—his sessions often take place before she arrives, and result in his fatigue during her visits, giving a distorted view of his function and engagement. P's ability to decide for himself with regard to rehabilitation is also assessed by the lead consultant, who concludes that he lacks capacity to make this decision.

### 13.6.6 Best Interests

The best interests process draws together those with a part to play in P's care and future planning. The purpose is to objectively consider the identified decision to be made—rehabilitation—and to come to a conclusion that all present all those with a part to play in his current care and treatment, and his family, feel able to support. The patient's lack of capacity to engage with this decision is formally confirmed at the outset of the meeting. The attendees on this occasion include the consultant, the physiotherapist, the speech and language therapist, the occupational therapist, a nursing sister and P's wife and son.

P indicates that he does not wish to attend, but the consultant, in the company of P's family, speaks to him before and after the meeting to explain the process and outcome.

Consideration is given in the meeting to P's previous beliefs and wishes and those of his family, alongside the clinical recommendations and the risks and benefits they potentially hold. In order to develop a plan that meets P's healthcare needs, promote his autonomy and safeguard his liberty and dignity, due regard is also given to the least restrictive way forward. This could be interpreted as going home rather than being subjected to further institutional care. After hearing how the therapists view her husband's prognosis, and when the risks and benefits of further treatment and rehabilitation are considered, P's wife and family are able to agree with the team that these measures represent overall benefit to the patient and are justifiable and proportionate. The outcome of the meeting is that it is in P's best interests to continue with active inpatient therapy in a dedicated rehabilitation setting. Additional contingencies such as the facilitation of weekend leave and open visiting are planned as added measures to restrict deprivation and connect P with family life as speedily as possible.

### 13.6.7 Conclusion

This case study shows how the Mental Capacity Act framework can be used to provide structure and momentum in the care planning of a patient who lacks capacity to engage fully in that process. Aspects of the legislation will require differing emphasis according to the case under consideration, but the underpinning principles of promoting autonomy and avoiding undue restriction are implicit throughout all of the mechanisms it contains. The best interests process ensures that the views of all those with relevant connection to the patient are heard but still keeps that individual at the centre of proceedings. Solutions can be found and stalemate avoided if the principles are effectively applied.

The remainder of this chapter details the legal services provided within the Act that underpin and support the framework.

## 13.7  Legal Services and the MCA

### 13.7.1 The Office of the Public Guardian

Legal powers can be given by an individual (donor) to a person or people of their choice (donee/s) to enable decisions to be made on their behalf in the event of capacity being lost. Known as a 'lasting power of attorney' (LPA) under the terms of the Mental Capacity Act, this formal authorisation must be initiated whilst the person still has capacity to engage in the process. LPAs replace the previous 'enduring power of attorney' system in use prior to the introduction of the Act, but do not invalidate them. An individual may choose to give all powers to one person or to ask a number of people to share the responsibility.

LPAs cover a range of decisions including those relating to property and financial affairs and health and welfare. Whereas financial decisions may be made with the permission of the donor before capacity is lost, health and welfare decisions may not. The detail of the authorisation is specific to the individual and constructed according to their wishes.

In order for an LPA to be legally binding, it must be completed on a regulatory template issued by the Office of the Public Guardian and then registered with that body. The donee must be aged 18 or above and be willing and capable of fulfilling the terms of the LPA. Signatures of donor and donee must be in place, along with an independent certificate confirming that the donor understands the document and has not been subject to any undue pressure or coercion in its making. The person who signs this document is known as a 'certificate provider'. The certificate provider can be someone the donor has known for at least 2 years or someone with relevant professional skills to assess their capacity such as a financial adviser, doctor, nurse, will writer or solicitor.

Within the detail of an LPA, the donor can stipulate areas where they do not wish the LPA to act. There are also restrictions related to life-sustaining treatment. A donee with power of attorney for health and welfare may only make decisions related to life-sustaining treatment if authorised by the specific terms within the LPA. Even so, they are not empowered to make any decisions that might bring about the patient's death. If there are doubts about the integrity of a donee, or concerns that they may not be acting in the donor's best interests, application should be made to the Court of Protection for support with decision-making.

### 13.7.2 The Court of Protection

Known as a 'superior court of record', the Court of Protection (CoP) advocates on behalf of individuals who may lack capacity to make decisions about their affairs at the point when they need to be made. Capacity must be assessed according to the principles of the MCA, including confirmation of the initial criteria, in accordance with the two-stage test and following the principles for assessment. Covering both health and welfare, the CoP may make declarations and decisions specifically around the capacity issue itself or may order certain actions related to the individual's circumstances.

The CoP may also rule on the validity of an LPA or an EPA (Enduring Power of Attorney) and may appoint deputies to act for a person with no advocacy already in place. Equally, where there are concerns about the effectiveness or integrity of an existing deputy, the CoP can remove those individuals from their position of authority and replace them with others of its choosing.

Application to the CoP is usually only required in health and welfare cases of extreme complexity or where discord and disagreement run so deep that it cannot be resolved in any other way. This is rare, as the principals of the MCA, if applied efficiently, will be effective in bringing resolution to most circumstances.

In contrast, financial matters or those related to property and affairs are likely to need referral for a court order if someone lacks capacity to make necessary decisions and does not have an appointed LPA or EPA.

It is usual to ask for prior permission from the CoP before making an application. Permission is likely to be granted in cases where an individual is challenging a decision that they lack capacity or where professionals are in dispute about that fact. Also likely to be heard are cases related to care and treatment where the patient lacks capacity and there are differing opinions related to providing life-sustaining treatment or where serious medical intervention is not felt to be in the patient's best interests. Whilst a court decision is awaited, healthcare professionals would be expected to continue delivering treatment necessary to ensure the patient's stability.

## 13.8   Conclusion: The Impact of Safeguarding

In the context of the 2014 Care Act, 'safeguarding duties' apply to an adult who has 'needs for care and support' and as a result of those needs is unable to protect themselves from 'either the risk of or the experience of abuse or neglect'. Further enquiry into such circumstances is led by the local authority relevant to the patient, who may in turn request support from health or police colleagues.

Whilst these circumstances occur all too frequently in every aspect of modern life, use of a broader definition of safeguarding also proves useful in the clinical setting. The experience of illness, diagnosis, treatment and recovery can be lengthy and traumatic for the individual. Often described as a 'journey', each stage can involve uncertainty, pain and distress. Whilst the patient sits at the centre of events, everyone in their sphere is touched by the situation—like ripples spreading outwards. For those closest to the patient, there are likely adjustments to be made and added pressures to be absorbed. As the journey progresses, an emotional burden accumulates for all but the most distant observer.

This 'pebble in the pond' effect not only impacts on the patient's loved ones but also on medical professionals. Decisions about treatment options could just as easily be overlaid with preferences on the part of the skilled professional as subject to secondary concerns from the partner. After decisions about treatment, there may be decisions related to a future place of residence or a level of care in the community. Typically, family members are very invested in safety and support for their loved ones—indeed they may be even more concerned than the patient about avoiding future risks. These layers of complexity exist even before the effects of illness and treatment on the patient are considered. Periods of confusion or low mood may be prevalent, times when the patient cannot reliably speak for themselves and interventions are likely to be in their 'best interests'.

A vital common factor in all cases is that the patient's voice should remain at the heart of everything professionals undertake, and it should not be displaced or overly influenced by the opinions of others, however well meaning. To 'safeguard' the patient in this wider context, the Mental Capacity Act is a powerful tool. It imposes upon healthcare providers a statutory obligation to ensure that the patient's own views are sought and acted upon. It assures everyone that the patient's best interests have been acted on and provides evidence of individual efforts for use in any future challenge. By providing the legal framework and the toolkit for practical application, the MCA advocates powerfully for individual autonomy at every step of the patient journey. It should therefore be embraced and ensured it is at the heart of our practice.

## References

1. Francis R. Report of the Mid Staffordshire NHS foundation trust public inquiry (Report). House of Commons. 2013. https://assets.publishing.service.gov.uk/government/uploads/system/uploads/attachment_data/file/279124/0947.pdf.

 2. Department of Constitutional Affairs. Mental capacity act 2005 code of practice. 2007 Final ed. London: The Stationery Office; 2017.
 3. Doyle-Price J. Government Interim response to the Law Commission report on mental capacity and deprivation of liberty: written statement–HCWS202. House of Commons. 2018. https://www.parliament.uk/business/publications/written-questions-answers-statements/written-statement/Commons/2017-10-30/HCWS202/.
 4. Law Commission. Mental capacity and deprivation of liberty. Law Commission. 2017. https://s3-eu-west-2.amazonaws.com/lawcom-prod-storage-11jsxou24uy7q/uploads/2017/03/lc372_mental_capacity.pdf.

# Radiotherapy

**14**

Kate E. Burton

**Abstract**

The majority of adult patients diagnosed with a primary brain tumour will receive radiotherapy as part of their management plan. This chapter aims to explore what radiotherapy is and define the various forms of radiotherapy used in the treatment of gliomas. It will give an overview of the factors involved in patient selection for different tumour grades and describe the typical radiotherapy planning and treatment pathway.

The potential acute and long-term toxicity from radiotherapy to the brain will be addressed and appropriate management and support for patient undergoing treatment described.

**Keywords**

Radiotherapy · Glioma treatment · Brain tumour treatments · Concomitant RT · Adjuvant RT · Radiotherapy side effects

**Learning Outcomes**
- To gain a deeper understanding of what radiotherapy is.
- To understand the various forms of radiotherapy used in treatment of brain tumours, in particular when used to treat gliomas.
- To gain deeper insight into the radiotherapy planning and treatment pathways of a glioma patient.
- To gain insight and knowledge into some of the more common side effects of radiotherapy (early, as well as late), how to clinically recognise them, as well as adequately managing them.

K. E. Burton (✉)
Oncology Centre, Addenbrooke's Hospital, Cambridge University Hospitals NHS Foundation Trust, Cambridge, UK
e-mail: Katherine.burton@addenbrookes.nhs.uk

© Springer Nature Switzerland AG 2019
I. Oberg (ed.), *Management of Adult Glioma in Nursing Practice*,
https://doi.org/10.1007/978-3-319-76747-5_14

213

## 14.1   Introduction

Following a histological diagnosis of a primary glioma, many adult patients will be referred for consideration of post-operative external beam radiotherapy. Very occasionally radiotherapy may be offered without a histological diagnosis and based on radiological diagnosis alone. For many years radiotherapy alone has been the standard of care following surgery, but following the publication of a number of studies [1–3], it has become more common for the combination of chemotherapy either during the radiotherapy (concomitant) or as an adjuvant therapy to be recommended. This chapter will outline different forms of radiotherapy, patient selection, the radiotherapy planning and treatment pathway and support and care of the patient receiving radiotherapy to the brain.

## 14.2   What Is External Beam Radiotherapy?

External beam radiotherapy (EBRT) is the controlled use of high-energy radiation beams that are specifically targeted to damage the deoxyribonucleic acid (DNA) of tumour cells. A number of different forms of radiation may be used, and these include photon beam (high energy X-ray) or proton beam (positively charged particle therapy).

### 14.2.1 Photon Beam (High-Energy X-Ray)

This is the most common form of EBRT currently in clinical use. The majority of modern, clinical radiotherapy is delivered using machines called megavoltage (MV) linear accelerators (commonly abbreviated to Linacs); these produce a 4–20 MV X-ray beam. This is the form of radiotherapy that is most likely to be used for adult patients being treated for a primary brain tumour. There are a number of different forms of photon EBRT; these include the following:

#### 14.2.1.1   Stereotactic Radiosurgery (SRS) and Stereotactic Radiotherapy (SRT) Treatment

These are terms applied to a highly conformal form of radiotherapy that is used for treatment of small volume, well-defined intracranial tumours. SRS aims to ablate (cause necrosis) the tissue within the target volume and so is not suitable for larger tumours or tumours where the edge of the lesion cannot clearly be determined on imaging, e.g. gliomas. SRS is normally defined as a single treatment, and the term SRT is used where the radiotherapy is delivered in a small number of treatments (<5). A number of different manufacturers produce technology and software to deliver SRS, and systems currently available include Gamma Knife, CyberKnife and specialist Linac-based platforms. In the UK, current oncological indications for the use of SRS include cerebral metastases and small, benign tumours of the skull base. Due to the diffuse, infiltrating nature of gliomas and the large volume of brain tissue that needs to be included in the target volume, SRS or SRT is not recommended for patient receiving radiotherapy for these types of tumours.

### 14.2.1.2 Intensity-Modulated Radiotherapy (IMRT) Photon Therapy

This is a form of external beam radiotherapy that is highly conformal in three dimensions and shapes the beam to the target (tumour) volume. This allows reduction of dose to the normal brain tissue that is lying adjacent to the tumour and also provides the ability to create a concave (U-shaped) target volume. In brain tumours it allows reduction in dose to critical normal structures like the optic apparatus and brainstem.

## 14.2.2 Proton Beam Therapy (PBT)

This is a form of radiotherapy that uses positively charged, subatomic particles called protons. These particles are produced in a machine called a cyclotron or synchrotron, and the proton beam produced can be focussed to treat tumours. Unlike X-ray beams that cannot be stopped but are gradually attenuated as they travel through tissue and have an entrance and exit dose, protons deliver only a small dose of radiation during their journey to the target and then come to a halt, releasing a final sudden burst of energy. This is known as the Bragg peak, and beyond this point the beam completely stops, so there is no exit dose [4]. This may allow higher doses to be delivered to tumours that lie close to critical normal structures (e.g. brainstem and spinal cord).

Current indications for the use of PBT are mainly for the paediatric population where dose to normal, developing tissue should be avoided or minimised to reduce risk of long-term toxicity in survivors. In the adult population, the indications include skull base tumours that are radioresistant and require high dose to achieve cure but lie adjacent to critical, dose-limiting structures, e.g. chordoma. Currently no randomised, controlled studies exist that support the use of PBT in adult gliomas [5] although there is interest in whether they may have a role for younger patients with low-grade lesions where prognosis is better and long-term toxicity could potentially be reduced [6]. In 2018 the UK will open its first National Health Service (NHS)-funded proton facility, and an aim of the proposed national service is to record and assess long-term toxicity and identify conditions where this treatment offers the greatest benefits.

## 14.3  Dose and Fractionation

The aim of the radiotherapy is to try to deliver a high (tumouricidal) dose to the tumour cells but to minimise wherever possible the dose to the normal tissue that is surrounding the tumour. Delivering the radiotherapy in small doses per treatment will reduce the effect of radiation on the normal tissue and allow a higher total dose to be delivered to the tumour. In radiotherapy the term 'fraction' is normally applied to each treatment session, and fractionation is a combination of total dose (measured in gray (Gy) the derived unit of ionising radiation dose in International System of Units (SI), number of treatments and the overall length of treatment course (in days or weeks). There are a number of different RT fractionations in common usage for adult glioma in the brain. The choice of fractionation will depend on histology, treatment intent, performance status (PS) of the patient, use of concomitant therapy and patient choice. Common examples of radiotherapy fractionations used in the treatment of glioma are 60 Gy delivered in 30 treatments over 6 weeks or 40 Gy delivered in 15 treatments over 3 weeks or 30 Gy in six treatments in 2 weeks.

Radiotherapy is normally delivered in an outpatient setting and requires patients to travel to the hospital for each planning and treatment session. For patients who live some distance away from their radiotherapy centre, there is often on-site hostel accommodation.

## 14.4   Patient Selection

Until recently the recommendation for post-operative radiotherapy and selection dose/fractionation schedule has been based mainly on the 2000 World Health Organisation (WHO) classification of tumours of the nervous system that used a grading system based on histological diagnosis [7]. The increasing use and understanding of molecular markers in diagnosis is, however, leading to changes in standard of care and treatment recommendations; for more details on the classification and grading criteria, see Chap. 7.

Location and size of tumour may also influence radiotherapy recommendation particularly if there is evidence of disease spread through the corpus callosum or multifocal disease. Both of these features demonstrate an aggressive, infiltrative disease and lead to a worse prognosis, often measured in a few months. In situations such as these, it is important to measure the probable small survival benefit of a 6-week course of radiotherapy against the likely toxicity and impact on quality of life for the patient undergoing the radiotherapy.

Additionally, patient pre-existing co-morbidities must be taken into consideration; examples of this include a patient with significant memory impairment (dementia) where it may not be safe to leave them alone in a treatment room for the procedure or a patient who has severe breathing difficulties due to unrelated chest conditions that may not be able to lie flat for the length of time it takes to deliver the radiotherapy.

It is very important to discuss all radiotherapy treatment options with patients ensuring they have an understanding of the likely outcomes in terms of prognosis, likelihood of improvement of neurological function and potential treatment-related toxicity. Although radiotherapy and /or chemotherapy rarely provides a cure for any grade of glioma, the term 'radical' (implying curative intent) is still commonly used when referring to longer RT fractionations (>3 weeks).

## 14.4.1  WHO Grade IV Glioma (Glioblastoma or GBM)

### 14.4.1.1  Radical Radiotherapy Plus Concomitant Temozolomide

Following surgical resection or biopsy, patients who are newly diagnosed with a WHO grade IV glioma (GBM) and are WHO performance status (PS) 0–1 (see Table 14.1) are normally referred for consideration of 6 weeks of daily (Monday–Friday) radiotherapy with concomitant temozolomide chemotherapy (daily including weekends). Temozolomide is a form of cytotoxic chemotherapy used to treat gliomas; it is given in tablet form, and patients will be given this to take either on their journey in for radiotherapy or at home. For further information on chemotherapy treatments in adult gliomas, please see Chap. 15.

For patients aged 65 or older or patients with neurological deficits (e.g. hemiplegia or cognitive deficit), the 6-week chemo-radiation regime can be intensive, and many struggle to complete the course. Recently a study by Perry et al. [3] investigated the use of TMZ alongside a shorter 3-week (15 daily fractions) course of radiotherapy for patients with newly diagnosed GBM aged 65 or older. Published results from this study show an overall survival benefit when compared to 15 fraction radiotherapy alone for patients who have tumours that are DNA repair protein O6-methylguanine-DNA methyltransferase (MGMT) methylated (see Chap. 7 on molecular markers from more information on tumour biomarkers and how they influence response to treatment).

In newly diagnosed GBM patients with a WHO PS of 2 or 3, the option of a palliative, short course of radiotherapy is attractive. A common fractionation used in the UK is a course of six radiotherapy treatments delivered over a 2-week period. This means a reduction in the number of hospital visits is required and is generally well tolerated.

## 14.4.2  WHO Grade III Glioma (Anaplastic Glioma)

Traditionally for newly diagnosed grade III gliomas (also termed anaplastic glioma), the recommended management has been maximal, safe surgical resection plus a 6-week course of adjuvant radiotherapy alone. Increasing knowledge of the significance of a chromosomal 1p/19q co-deletion on improved prognosis and

**Table 14.1**  WHO performance status classification

| WHO performance status classification | |
| --- | --- |
| The WHO performance status classification categorises patients | |
| 0 | Able to carry out all normal activity without restriction |
| 1 | Restricted in strenuous activity but ambulatory and able to carry out light work |
| 2 | Ambulatory and capable of all self-care but unable to carry out any work activities; up and about more than 50% of waking hours |
| 3 | Symptomatic and in a chair or in bed for greater than 50% of the day but not bedridden |
| 4 | Completely disabled; cannot carry out any self-care; totally confined to bed or chair |

response to chemotherapy is leading to changes in practice. The evidence of a 1p/19q co-deletion is established from the tumour tissue taken at the time of diagnosis (debulk or biopsy) and cannot be made from blood tests. This molecular profile is also in keeping with an anaplastic oligodendroglioma rather than an astrocytoma.

For anaplastic oligodendrogliomas that demonstrate a chromosomal loss of 1p/19q, the planned management of surgical resection (or biopsy) plus 6 weeks of radiotherapy followed by adjuvant chemotherapy using a combination of procarbazine, lomustine (CCNU) and vincristine (PCV regime) has become the standard of care following publication of updated results from the EORTC 26951 [8] and RTOG 94-02 studies [9]· For more details on PCV and other chemotherapy regimens, please refer to Chap. 15.

Patients with grade III gliomas that are 1p/19q non-co-deleted are currently offered surgery plus radical radiotherapy alone. A recent randomised clinical trial (EORTC 26053-22,054, BR14 CATNON in the UK) was designed using a 4-arm randomisation model to investigate the role of TMZ chemotherapy both alongside the radiotherapy (as for GBM) and in the adjuvant setting. This trial is now in the data analysis phase, and results from the concomitant arm of the study are still awaited. Early, published results from the adjuvant arm [10] have suggested a survival benefit, and patients who are grade III 1p/19q non-co-deleted are now being offered 6 weeks of radiotherapy plus up to 12 cycles of adjuvant TMZ.

For grade III patients with a WHO poor performance of 2 or above, the option of short course radiotherapy may also be a consideration to minimise treatment-related toxicity and offer stabilisation or temporary improvement of symptoms.

### 14.4.3 WHO Grade II Glioma

The role of radiotherapy for low-grade gliomas remains controversial, and more clinical studies are required to ascertain timing of radiotherapy and combination with other oncological treatments. A randomised EORTC clinical trial [11] investigated the timing of radiotherapy, and results showed no overall survival benefit in early RT although it did demonstrate an improvement in disease-free survival (time until tumour progression).

In larger, inoperable lesions, the option of radiotherapy may be attractive to try to minimise progression of neurological symptoms. Unlike high-grade lesions, radiotherapy may improve neurological deficits and seizure activity [11] and may be a reason to opt for early treatment. In tumours that are operable and a maximal surgical resection is achieved, the decision to delay radiotherapy (and the potential toxicities) may appear attractive. However recent results from the RTOG 9802 trial [2] showed a median overall survival benefit (13 years versus 8 years) for good prognostic patients treated with RT plus adjuvant PCV when compared to RT alone and may mean increasing numbers of low-grade glioma patients are recommended for early treatment in the future.

For low-grade gliomas, the survival time following treatment is likely to be measured in years to decades, and the need to carefully optimise the radiotherapy treatment plan and minimise dose to normal tissue is imperative. The use of IMRT is generally utilised for these tumours, and there is also interest in the potential benefit of proton beam therapy for this patient group in order to achieve reduction of dose to normal tissue.

## 14.5 Radiotherapy Pathway

Prior to delivering a course of radiotherapy to the brain, a number of planning steps are required. These include patient immobilisation (production of an individualised mask), imaging to assist volume definition, delineation (outlining) of the target volume and production of a radiotherapy treatment plan. Depending on the intent of the treatment and complexity of the radiotherapy, these steps may take a few days or a few weeks.

### 14.5.1 Immobilisation (Mask Making)

Patients who are to receive radiotherapy to the brain will require some form of immobilisation (often termed a mask or beam direction shell) to ensure an accurate, reproducible and consistent set-up position. It is important that the head position established when the patient has their planning imaging can be reproduced on a day-to-day basis when they attend for their treatment and the immobilisation device should also assist the patient in not moving during their radiotherapy session. An additional benefit is that all the markings required to set up the radiotherapy can be placed on the mask and patients do not need pen marking or permanent skin markings.

The process of manufacturing the mask may vary depending on the system chosen by individual RT departments. Many centres now use a thermoplastic material that when placed in a hot water bath becomes flexible and mouldable and can be stretched over the patient's head to form a bust. This process takes approximately 20 min and has the benefit of not requiring multiple visits to produce the mask. Although the mask will be attached to the RT treatment couch, it is easily removable at any time during the treatment process, and the patient is able to breathe normally throughout. It is not uncommon for patients to experience feelings of claustrophobia or anxiety about the mask, and a number of techniques can be employed to support the patient including hypnotherapy, mindfulness and meditation. Occasionally patients will require a low dose of antianxiety medication in order to be able to proceed with RT (Fig. 14.1).

### 14.5.2 Radiotherapy Planning Imaging

Imaging is required at the time of RT planning to demonstrate the extent and position of either the tumour (in biopsy only cases) or the extent of resection and/or residual tumour following a surgical resection. Planning imaging will also provide the

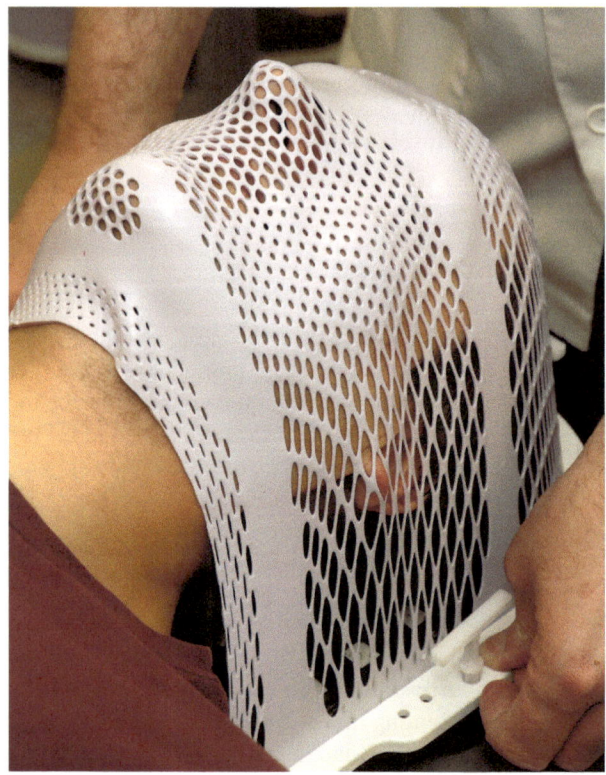

**Fig. 14.1** Radiotherapy mask preparation

location and size of organs at risk or structures to avoid in the RT planning process. All patients will have a computerised tomography (CT) scan; normally this is performed in the intended treatment position with the patient immobilised in their mask.

Additionally many patients will also have a further post-operative, contrast-enhanced, magnetic resonance scan (MRI) to assist in target volume delineation. Ideally the planning imaging should be done as close to the start of radiotherapy as possible, particularly for high-grade gliomas where tumours may increase in size in a very short period of time.

The planning CT and MRI scan will be electronically co-registered to allow for accurate delineation of the target volume and normal critical structures.

### 14.5.3 Target Volume Delineation and Plan Selection

The aim of radiotherapy is to deliver a high dose (tumouricidal) to the target volume (gross visible tumour on planning imaging plus a margin for suspected microscopic tumour spread) but to minimise or keep within tolerance the dose to the critical

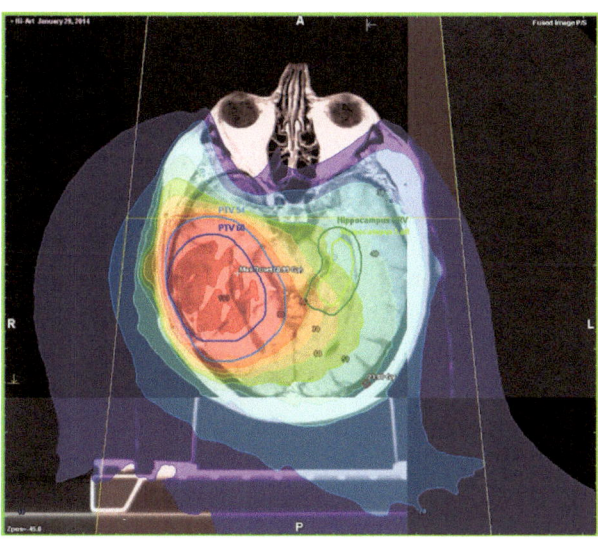

**Fig. 14.2** Radiotherapy dose plan for a right-sided GBM showing the high-dose target volume (red) and planning of dose away from the orbits

normal structures and normal surrounding brain tissue. In brain irradiation, there are a number of structures that have dose-limiting tolerances (often termed organs at risk or OARs), and these must be considered when producing RT plans. These include the eyes, optic nerves and optic apparatus, brainstem and spinal cord, pituitary gland and hypothalamus, lacrimal glands and potentially the hair follicles (to minimise risk of permanent alopecia). Acceptable doses to OARs will depend on a number of factors including intent of treatment, expected prognosis and patient co-morbidities.

The oncologist responsible for the patient's radiotherapy will electronically outline or delineate on the RT planning imaging a number of different volumes and structures; this process is called target volume delineation. The tumour target volume will comprise of the gross tumour volume (GTV) which is the visible abnormality on imaging plus a margin for microscopic tumour spread (clinical target volume or CTV). It is also necessary to outline the normal brain tissue and structures (OARs) that should be avoided or dose minimised as much as possible.

For each patient receiving RT to the brain, an individualised, computer-generated radiotherapy plan will be produced (see example in Fig. 14.2). For patients receiving long-course, radical radiotherapy, it is becoming the UK standard to use IMRT techniques, but for shorter course, palliative RT, the use of simpler RT plans, may be used to reduce the time to start radiotherapy.

## 14.5.4  Treatment Delivery

Once the treatment plan is produced and accepted for treatment, the patient will begin their radiotherapy. The patient will be positioned, in their mask on the treatment couch, and LASERs (light amplification by stimulated emission of radiation) are used to align the couch in the correct position. Often once the patient is in the treatment position, on-treatment imaging (cone beam CT) will be performed to verify the patient's position is correct prior to delivery of the treatment beams; this is termed image-guided radiotherapy or IGRT.

The complexity and number of beams utilised will depend on the intent of treatment, diagnosis and location of the lesion. Normally the patient will be in the treatment room for 10–20 min although 'beam-on' time is less than 5 min. Although the patient will need to be alone in the room during the treatment delivery, they will be monitored using closed-circuit television (CCTV), and an intercom will allow the radiographers to communicate with them if needed. The patient will not feel any sensation or pain during the radiotherapy and will not be radioactive following the treatment.

## 14.6 Side Effects and Patient Support Through Radiotherapy

As with any treatment, the side effects from radiotherapy will vary from patient to patient. For RT they are often related to volume of tissue irradiated, location within the brain of the target volume, dose and fractionation, radiotherapy plan selection and performance status of the patient prior to commencing treatment. Additionally the need to travel to the hospital on a daily basis can increase both the physical and psychosocial impact of radiotherapy.

This section looks at the toxicity associated with radiotherapy alone, but patients that are receiving chemo-radiation will also have the potential to experience chemotherapy-related side effects such as haematological toxicity and risk of immunosuppression. For more information on chemotherapy side effects, see Chap. 15.

Most radiotherapy centres offer patients a weekly on-treatment review either with their oncologist or a specialist therapeutic radiographer or clinical nurse specialist. This will provide opportunity to assess, record and manage any toxicity that occurs but also to give the patient time to discuss any questions or concerns relating to their diagnosis or treatment. The use of holistic needs assessment and quality of life tools in these clinics is increasing to identify the physical and psychosocial concerns of the patient and to signpost to appropriate support services.

### 14.6.1 Acute Toxicity

Acute toxicities are the side effects of the treatment that occur during the course of the treatment or in the immediate weeks following completion of radiotherapy. Common acute toxicities include:

#### 14.6.1.1 Fatigue/Lack of Motivation
The vast majority of patients receiving radiotherapy report fatigue although it is variable in severity and often there are multiple causes including the distance a

patient may need to travel to the RT department and steroid dosage. As fatigue is also one of the most common symptoms experienced by patients with a high-grade glioma [12], this side effect can be particularly difficult for patients to manage during their treatment. Like the majority of RT side effects, fatigue is cumulative and often at its worse in the weeks following completion of the treatment.

Traditionally, cancer patients undergoing radiotherapy were encouraged to rest during their treatment, but evidence has revealed that gentle, aerobic exercise appears to have some benefit in management of fatigue both during and posttreatment [13]. To minimise the fatigue, patients should be encouraged to stay as active as possible and to undertake daily physical activities (e.g. gentle walking). As many glioma patients may be on corticosteroid medication and experiencing muscle weakness (myopathy) as a result, the importance of keeping as active as possible should be discussed with patients and if necessary referral made to exercise referral or physiotherapy for support. Some patients may also report a lack of motivation, so activity diaries and encouragement to plan small achievable tasks may be helpful.

A small number of adult patients may also experience somnolence syndrome in the weeks following radiotherapy. Somnolence syndrome is a collection of symptoms consisting of drowsiness, lethargy and fatigue; it generally occurs approximately 6–8 weeks after completion of radiotherapy. For many patients, it is self-limiting and settles after a couple of weeks, but if it is severe, patients may need to increase their steroid dose to be able to perform their activities [14].

### 14.6.1.2  Skin Toxicity and Alopecia (Hair Loss)

The extent of skin reaction is dependent on both intrinsic factors (e.g. ethnic origin, presence of infection, smoking and co-existing disease) and extrinsic factors (e.g. treatment dose and fractionation, site of target volume, beam energy and direction). It is rare for patients to report any visible reaction before at least 2 weeks of treatment, and in general most patients will only experience a grade 1 toxicity which is defined as faint or dull erythema and dry desquamation using the Common Terminology Criteria for Adverse Events or CTCAE [15]; see Table 14.2. Occasionally if the ear is included in the treatment field, the patient may develop a small area of moist desquamation (grade 2 toxicity) behind the treated pinna. The external ear canal may also be affected, and use of simple ear drops may minimise irritation.

Hair loss will only occur where the radiotherapy fields are directed and the dose is high enough to cause alopecia. This is normally at the beam entry portals, but occasionally the exit dose may also be high enough to cause patchy hair loss. Alopecia will not occur until 3 weeks from the start of radiotherapy and for patients receiving short course 2-week RT will occur after completion of the radiotherapy. With modern-day radiotherapy techniques and standard fractionations, hair loss is rarely permanent, but it will take some months before patients will see visible hair regrowth after completion of the treatment.

To minimise the skin reaction, the patient should be encouraged to gently wash their hair and scalp and to use a gentle shampoo and avoid using a hairdryer during their course of radiotherapy. Frequency of hair washing has no impact on extent of

**Table 14.2** Common Terminology Criteria for Adverse Events (CTCAE) [15] for radiation skin reactions

| Common Terminology Criteria for Adverse Events (CTCAE) Version 4.0 [15] | | | |
|---|---|---|---|
| Grade of event – radiation dermatitis: cutaneous inflammatory occurring as a result of exposure to biologically effective levels of ionising radiation | | | |
| 1 | 2 | 3 | 4 |
| Faint erythema or dry desquamation | Moderate to brisk erythema; patchy moist desquamation, mostly confined to skin folds and creases; moderate oedema | Moist desquamation in areas other than skin folds and creases; bleeding induced by minor trauma or abrasion | Life-threatening consequences; skin necrosis or ulceration of full thickness dermis; spontaneous bleeding from involved site; skin graft indicated |

hair loss or skin reaction [16]. To reduce scalp dryness and irritation, the patient should regularly apply a sodium lauryl sulphate-free moisturiser to the area [17]. They should also avoid sun exposure and once the radiotherapy is completed should be encouraged to apply a high-SPF sunblock to the irradiated skin. If moist desquamation is identified, the use of an antibacterial ointment such as silver sulfadiazine (Flamazine) may be helpful but should not be applied directly before RT and should be discontinued as soon as skin is intact. All patients treated within the UK National Health System are eligible for wig referral.

### 14.6.1.3 Increase of Neurological Symptoms

Radiotherapy may cause some inflammation and/or oedema in the area of the brain being irradiated. This may lead to worsening of the patient's neurological symptoms including seizure activity. This is rare in patients who have had a surgical resection as the post-operative cavity allows for swelling without the patient experiencing symptoms. Occasionally the effect of radiotherapy may cause symptoms of raised intracranial pressure including headache, nausea and vomiting.

If patients start to develop increased neurological symptoms, an increase in their steroid dose is normally required to resolve or return symptoms back to baseline. If seizure frequency or severity increases, a review of the patient's antiepilepsy medication as well as consideration of increase in steroid dose should be undertaken. If seizure control proves problematic and patients require more than a single antiepileptic medication, referral to the neurology team is recommended. A sudden, acute deterioration may indicate an intracranial haemorrhage (ICH), and CT imaging should be requested to exclude this. If ICH is confirmed on imaging urgent, referral to the neurosurgical team should be made.

### 14.6.1.4 Nausea and Taste Changes

It is rare for patients receiving radiotherapy to the brain to experience nausea or vomiting, but some patients do experience a loss or change of taste that leads to them reporting a loss of appetite. If this occurs, they should be encouraged to eat small amounts often and to try different foods including spicy or citrus flavours. If oral intake is significantly reduced, dietetic input should be sorted.

Taste changes or an unpleasant taste may also occur as a result of oral candidiasis (thrush). This is a common side effect for patients on dexamethasone (steroid), and on examination there is commonly evidence of white patches (plaques) in the mouth and on the tongue. The patient may also report a sore tongue or throat which will be unrelated to the radiotherapy. If oral candidiasis is present, the patient should be prescribed an appropriate antifungal medication.

## 14.6.2 Late Toxicity

Late toxicities are the side effects that may occur months to years following radiotherapy.

### 14.6.2.1 Cataract Formation and Optic Neuropathy

Tolerance of the lens to radiation is low, and dose of <6Gy can lead to an increased risk of cataract formation. Patients should be counselled to this risk, but with the availability and effectiveness of cataract removal surgery, the dose to the tumour should not be compromised to spare the lens dose.

With standard radiotherapy doses, the risk of long-term damage to the optic apparatus (visual impairment or blindness) is very low provided careful radiotherapy planning is used to minimise dose to below tolerance. In tumours that are located adjacent to the optic apparatus, the patient may need to be counselled to the risk of long-term damage versus the higher risk of tumour recurrence if dose to this area is reduced.

### 14.6.2.2 Lacrimal Gland

The lacrimal glands are located in the upper, lateral area of the eyelid, and if these are included in the high-dose RT region, the patient may experience a dry eye (reduction in tear production) as result of treatment. The frequent application of eye drops may be required to minimise irritation and dryness.

### 14.6.2.3 Pituitary Dysfunction

If the pituitary gland is included in the high-dose radiotherapy volume, the patient is likely to experience hormone failure in the years following radiotherapy. Routine pituitary function tests should form part of the follow-up protocol for longer-term survivors and referral to endocrinologists made if/when hormone levels become abnormal. All of the affected hormones can be replaced with appropriate hormone replacement therapy. Radiotherapy to the brain does not directly impact on fertility, but if the sex hormones are affected as a result of pituitary dysfunction following radiotherapy, the patient may require assisted conception techniques in order to become pregnant.

### 14.6.2.4 Cognitive Dysfunction

The risk of neurocognitive damage and decrease in intellect as a direct result of radiotherapy alone for adult gliomas patients is poorly documented. This is due to the complex nature of the disease and the many factors that may lead to decrease in cognitive function. These factors include the tumour itself (location and size), surgical interventions, concurrent medications, chemotherapy, tumour progression and psychosocial considerations. Klein et al. [18] looked at cognitive function in low-grade gliomas (LGG) comparing patients with patients who had haematological malignancies and healthy controls. This showed worsening cognitive function in the LGG group who received radiotherapy but also showed an association with use of antiepileptics.

In patients with an expected long-term survival, it is important to consider carefully the use of radiotherapy to the brain and to use techniques such as IMRT to minimise the risk of cognitive dysfunction. Baseline pre-RT neuropsychological testing is useful to allow objective follow-up, and increased use of these outcome tools will allow a better understanding of the effects of radiotherapy.

## References

1. Stupp R, Mason WP, van den Bent MJ, et al. Radiotherapy plus concomitant and adjuvant temozolomide for glioblastoma. N Engl J Med. 2005;352:987–96.
2. Buckner JC, Shaw EG, Pugh SL, et al. Radiation plus procarbazine, CCNU and vincristine in low-grade gliomas. N Engl J Med. 2016;374(14):1344–55.
3. Perry JR, Laperriere N, O'Callaghan CJ, et al. Short-course radiation plus temozolomide in elderly patients with glioblastoma. N Engl J Med. 2017;376(11):1027–37.
4. Ncri.org. Clinical and translational radiotherapy research working group (CTRad) Proton beam therapy – information for a lay audience [Internet]. 2016. http://ctrad.ncri.org.uk/wp-content/uploads/2014/01/CTRad-PBT-consumer-information-Jan-2016.pdf. Accessed 29 Oct 2017.
5. Combs SE. Does proton therapy have a future in CNS tumors? Curr Treat Options Neurol. 2017;19(3):12.
6. Harrabi SB, Bougatf N, Mohr A, et al. Dosimetric advantages of proton therapy over conventional radiotherapy with photons in young patients and adults with low-grade glioma. Strahlenther Onkol. 2016;192(11):759–69.
7. Kleihues P, Cavenee WK, editors. World Health Organisation classification of tumours, pathology and genetics of tumours of the nervous system. Lyon: IARC Press International Agency for Research on Cancer; 2000.
8. Van den Bent MJ, Brandes AA, Taphoorn MJ, et al. Adjuvant procarbazine, lomustine, and vincristine chemotherapy in newly diagnosed anaplastic oligodendroglioma: long-term follow-up of EORTC brain tumor group study 26951. J Clin Oncol. 2013;31(3):344–50.
9. Cairncross G, Wang M, Shaw E, et al. Phase III trial of chemoradiotherapy for anaplastic oligodendroglioma: long-term results of RTOG 9402. J Clin Oncol. 2013;31(3):337–43.
10. Van den Bent MJ, Baumert B, Erridge S, et al. Interim results from the CATNON trial (EORTC study 26053–22054) of treatment with concurrent and adjuvant temozolomide for 1p/19q non-co-deleted anaplastic glioma: a phase 3, randomised, open-label intergroup study. Lancet. 2017; https://doi.org/10.1016/S0140–6736(17)31442–3.
11. Karim AB, Afra D, Cornu P, et al. Randomized trial on the efficacy of radiotherapy for cerebral low-grade glioma in the adult: European Organization for Research and Treatment of Cancer

Study 22845 with the Medical Research Council study BRO4: an interim analysis. Int J Rad Oncol Biol Phys. 2002;52(2):316–24.

12. Fox SW, Lyon D, Farace E. Symptom clusters in patients with high-grade gliomas. J Nurs Scholarsh. 2007;39(1):61–7.

13. Cramp F, Byron-Daniel J. Exercise for the management of cancer-related fatigue in adults. Cochrane Database Syst Rev. 2012;2012(11):Art. No.: CD006145. https://doi.org/10.1002/14651858.CD006145.pub3.

14. Faithful S, Brada M. Somnolence syndrome in adults following cranial irradiation for primary brain tumours. Clin Oncol (R Coll Radiol). 1998;10(4):250–4.

15. Nih.gov. Common terminology criteria for adverse events (CTCAE) V4.03 [Internet]. 2010. https://evs.nci.nih.gov/ftp1/CTCAE/CTCAE_4.03_2010-06-14_QuickReference_5x7.pdf. Accessed 29 Oct 2017.

16. Westbury C, Hines F, Hawkes E, et al. Advice on hair and scalp care during cranial radiotherapy: a prospective randomized trial. Radiother Oncol. 2000;54:109–16.

17. Society and College of Radiographers. Skin care advice for patients undergoing radical external beam megavoltage radiotherapy. SCoR professional document [Internet]. 2015. https://www.sor.org/learning/document-library/skin-care-advice-patients-undergoing-radical-external-beam-megavoltage-radiotherapy-0. Accessed 25 Oct 2017.

18. Klein M, Heimans JJ, Aaronson NK, et al. Effect of radiotherapy and other treatment-related factors on mid-term to long-term cognitive sequelae in low-grade gliomas: a comparative study. Lancet. 2002;360(9343):1361–8. Erratum in: Lancet 2011;377(9778):1654).

# Chemotherapy for Gliomas

15

Hanneke Zwinkels

**Abstract**

Standard treatment approaches for adult gliomas consist of surgery, radiotherapy and chemotherapy, based on the histological diagnosis and molecular profile of the specific glioma. Patient performance status and other prognostic factors are also taken into consideration when deciding upon treatment options.

Temozolomide (TMZ), procarbazine, vincristine and lomustine (PCV) are all types of alkylating (e.g. damaging the DNA, affecting the ability of cancer cells to multiply) chemotherapy agents frequently used in the treatment of gliomas. They can be given as initial treatment (either in combination with or adjuvant to radiotherapy) or administered at recurrence. Oncology specialist nurses work closely together with patients receiving chemotherapy, as well as their caregivers. Effective education by the oncology nurse of the patient and his/her caregiver(s) promotes patient safety and well-being, helps maintain optimal dosing and ensures accurate assessment and evaluation of side effects and toxicities. Specialist nurses evaluate the process and initiate supportive therapies as required, such as fatigue management, nutritional advice, psychosocial support and physiotherapy.

Temozolomide, lomustine and procarbazine can cause myelosuppression (also known as bone marrow suppression) and require careful monitoring of full blood counts to prevent complications associated with neutropenia, thrombocytopenia and lymphopenia. Other side effects such as nausea and fatigue are manageable, neuropathy is a specific side effect of vincristine, but all can have significant impacts on quality of life. These side effects and their nursing implications and considerations will be explored in more detail in this chapter.

Interventions such as treatment delay may lead to recovery of the bone marrow function and blood counts. Dose adjustments—if deemed necessary—may allow

H. Zwinkels (✉)
Haaglanden Medisch Centrum, Antonius Hove, Leidschendam, The Netherlands
e-mail: h.zwinkelsvan.vliet@haaglandenmc.nl

© Springer Nature Switzerland AG 2019
I. Oberg (ed.), *Management of Adult Glioma in Nursing Practice*,
https://doi.org/10.1007/978-3-319-76747-5_15

the patient to continue chemotherapy treatment as long as there is no evidence of tumour progression during treatment. Should a patient's tumour progress whilst on active chemotherapy treatment, the treating physicians and specialist nurse will need to help manage the patient's expectations and adjust their goal settings.

**Keywords**
Glioma · Patient education · Temozolomide · Lomustine · Side effects · Management · Thrombocytopenia · Lymphopenia · Nausea · Fertility

**Learning Outcomes**
- To have better insight into the varying kinds of chemotherapy used in the treatment of adult gliomas and gain a deeper understanding of why this is used as an adjunct to radiotherapy and as a stand-alone treatment.
- To know the most common side effects associated with chemotherapy use for gliomas and how to monitor for and manage these effectively.
- Gain insight into first- and second-line chemotherapy options for adult glioma patients and when to commence and/or halt such treatments.
- To understand the importance of patient education as a whole, but especially around alerting the patient and carers to common and more serious side effects of chemotherapy treatments, along with those requiring immediate medical intervention.

## 15.1  Introduction

The use of chemotherapeutic agents in the treatment of primary brain tumours and malignant gliomas has been at the forefront of clinical trials for at least 30 years, in both the adjuvant (immediately following surgery and radiotherapy) and recurrent settings. It was a long-held belief in the brain tumour community that chemotherapy would not be effective for the treatment of gliomas as it did not sufficiently penetrate the blood-brain barrier, which has a protective mechanism and thereby is difficult to cross by certain agents [1, 2]. Agents such as procarbazine, lomustine, vincristine and temozolomide appear to be able to cross the blood-brain barrier, and in subsequent clinical trials, they have a proven prolonged survival in the adjuvant setting and at recurrence of a previously treated glioma [2, 3]. However, despite efforts in improving treatments of gliomas, their prognosis remains poor, albeit there is a prognostic difference for oligodendrogliomas (averaging 15- to 20-year survival) as compared to glioblastomas (averaging 9- to 16-month survival).

Current knowledge of histological and molecular diagnoses of gliomas brought new insights into the treatment options and expected survival of glioma patients. This resulted in new pathology guidelines being issued (see Chap. 7 on molecular classification), which included concomitant and adjuvant oncology treatment options based on tumour profiling [4].

## 15.2    Historical Overview

Gliomas are the most frequently occurring primary malignant brain tumours in adults, and their prognosis remains poor, particularly in patients diagnosed with the most aggressive type, a glioblastoma (GBM). In the past century, standard treatment approaches consisted mainly of surgery and radiotherapy, and the benefit of chemotherapy has long been debated. Treatments and outcomes varied greatly for the different types of glioma, and chemotherapy had shown minimal benefit in the treatment of high-grade gliomas at the beginning of the twentieth century. Several agents were studied in various clinical trials for different types of glioma, searching for a better outcome towards survival [1, 2]. Additional research undertaken in the past decade, however, has revealed new insight into why and how some subtypes of glioma respond better towards treatment than others.

The use of PCV has been extensively studied in glioma patients and showed some overall survival benefit with regard to anaplastic gliomas, whether it be an anaplastic oligodendroglioma or anaplastic astrocytoma. However, patients with a GBM did not seem to benefit. After a longer follow-up period, research data clearly highlighted that adjuvant PCV (after initial surgery and radiotherapy treatment) *specifically* showed a benefit in the treatment of anaplastic oligodendrogliomas (with a deletion of chromosome 1p/19q) [3, 5]. Meanwhile, TMZ had proven effective in *recurrent* anaplastic gliomas and later in newly diagnosed GBM.

The current standard treatment for a GBM is based on a landmark study by Stupp in 2005 [6]. The results of this study showed a prolongation of the median survival of GBM towards 16 months, which exceeded the expected median survival until then of 9–12 months. Treatment consists of radiotherapy combined with oral temozolomide chemotherapy (TMZ) and is known as the concomitant phase. Additional cycles of TMZ (after completion of the concomitant phase) is known as the adjuvant phase, sometimes also referred to as the maintenance dose.

Recently, researchers found that molecular characteristics of the tumour cells have a great impact on survival. It has been established that glioma patients with a codeletion (or combined deletion) of 1p and 19q chromosomes have a pure oligodendroglioma and, with that, a better long-term prognosis [4]. In tumour cells of patients with either low-grade gliomas, anaplastic gliomas or secondary GBMs (a low-grade glioma that has subsequently transformed into a GBM), discovery of a mutation in the two genes isocitrate dehydrogenase (IDH1 and IDH2) appeared to be related with a longer overall survival. In turn, survival seemed even better in patients with both an IDH-mutated (i.e. IDH-positive) oligodendroglioma. In addition, it appeared that a part of the original classified low-grade gliomas that do *not* have a mutation of IDH (i.e. they were IDH negative) had a worse prognosis, similar to that of a GBM. Currently, besides using the original histological subtypes of gliomas (e.g. whether it is an astrocytoma or an oligodendroglioma), mutations in IDH status and a combined loss of 1p/19q are used to identify low-grade gliomas which have a better prognosis [3, 5].

Recent studies into the importance of molecular data and profiling have resulted in a new histological and molecular classification of gliomas [4]. These are explored in

**Table 15.1** Karnofsky performance score

| 100 | Normal, no complaints, no evidence of disease |
|---|---|
| 90 | Able to carry on normal activity, minor signs or symptoms of disease |
| 80 | Normal activity with effort, some signs or symptoms of disease |
| 70 | Cares for self, unable to carry on normal activity or do active work |
| 60 | Requires occasional assistance but is able to care for most of his/her personal needs |
| 50 | Requires considerable assistance and frequent medical care |
| 40 | Disabled; requires special care and assistance |
| 30 | Severely disabled; hospital admission is indicated although death not imminent |
| 20 | Very sick, hospital admission necessary; active supportive treatment necessary |
| 10 | Moribund; fatal processes progressing rapidly |
| 0 | Dead |

more detail in Chap. 7. In turn, these new classifications have altered treatment options for gliomas based on the histological and molecular diagnosis of the specific glioma and dependent on patient prognostic factors such as age, tumour size, focal deficits, Karnofsky performance score (KPS; see Table 15.1) and cognitive function [7].

## 15.3 Glioblastoma

In the landmark study by Stupp et al., newly diagnosed GBM patients (aged between 18 and 70 years of age) were randomized to receive radiation therapy alone, versus radiotherapy with concurrent TMZ (known as ChemoRT), followed with up to six cycles of adjuvant TMZ [6].

The results showed statistically significant benefits with overall 2-year survival at 26% for patients undergoing ChemoRT and adjuvant cycles of TMZ. This was compared to overall survival of 10% over the same 2-year period for patients receiving radiotherapy alone. Toxicity of the combined (ChemoRT) treatment showed limited acute severe grade III and IV adverse events (according to the National Cancer Institute Common Terminology Criteria for Adverse Events, version 3.0) [8], consisting of neutropenia and thrombocytopenia at 4% and 3%, respectively, with thrombocytopenia increasing to 11% in the adjuvant TMZ phase [6]. Molecular analysis of the tumour samples showed that patients with a methylation of the methyl-guanine-DNA methyltransferase (MGMT) promotor (i.e. patients who were MGMT positive) had a greater benefit of TMZ with regard to survival (18.2 months versus 12.2 months).

Another trial, looking at elderly patients (>65 years of age) with a newly diagnosed GBM, was randomly assigned to receive either radiotherapy alone or ChemoRT and adjuvant TMZ. Findings showed that the addition of TMZ resulted in a longer survival, especially in patients with MGMT methylation (MGMT positive). Toxicity of TMZ was limited to grade III and IV events of lymphopenia (27%), thrombocytopenia (11%) and neutropenia (8%) [9].

Since 2005, the standard treatment for patients with a GBM (KPS > 70) consists of radiotherapy (see Chap. 14) and daily TMZ (75 mg/m$^2$/day) in the concomitant

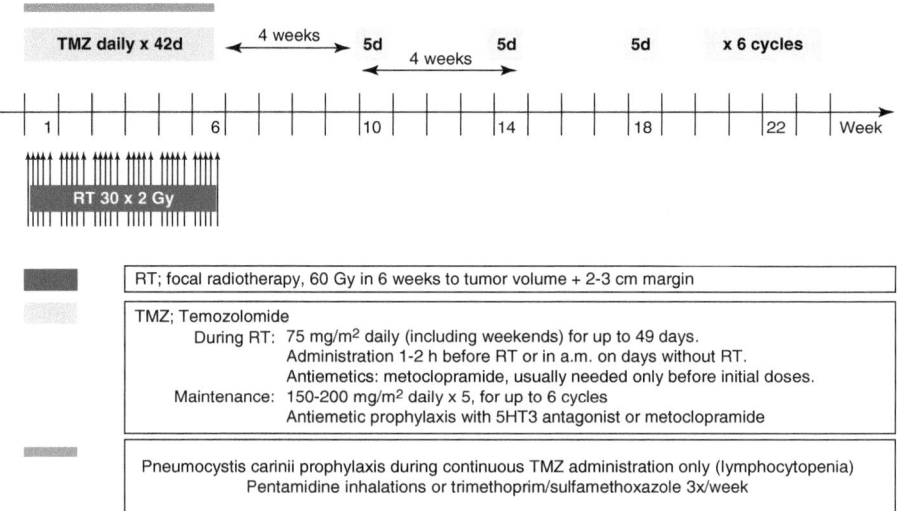

**Fig. 15.1** Stupp schedule

phase. After a 4-week rest period to allow for sufficient bone marrow recovery, the adjuvant phase is commenced, comprising of day 1–5 TMZ (150–200 mg/m²/day) every 4 weeks, for six cycles (Fig. 15.1). When patients are older than 65 years of age and have worsening neurology (KPS < 70), other prognostic factors such as tumour size, focal deficits, cognitive disturbances and methylation status will guide standard of care.

At the time of GBM recurrence, a multidisciplinary tumour board (MDT) will decide the best treatment options, dependent on factors such as the overall condition of the patient and the treatments received. Re-challenging with TMZ is an option and can be administered in a 5-day cycle every 4 weeks (150–200 mg/m²/day). However, when the tumour recurrence is shortly after (or during administration of) adjuvant cycles, it is commonly decided to switch from TMZ to lomustine monotherapy (90–110 mg/m², day 1, every 6 weeks) or lomustine in combination with procarbazine (60 mg/m²/day, day 8–21, every 6 weeks) and vincristine (1.4 mg/m² intravenously, day 8 and 29 every 6 weeks) (PCV).

Temozolomide, procarbazine, vincristine and lomustine are alkylating agents and are administered up to 6 (lomustine or PCV) or even 12 (TMZ) cycles, as long as there is no evidence of tumour progression during this interval and as long as the patient tolerates the treatment without grade III/IV adverse events.

## 15.4 Low-Grade and Anaplastic Gliomas

Low-grade gliomas have a lower prevalence than GBMs, and they are associated with a better prognosis as compared to anaplastic gliomas. Low-grade gliomas are rare slow growing but malignant tumours frequently occurring in young adults (20–40 years of age). After biopsy or resection, treatment decisions are dependent

A.

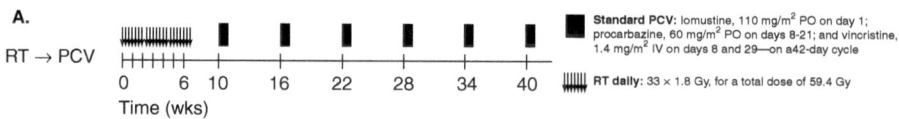

RT → PCV

0    6  10    16    22    28    34    40

Time (wks)

**Standard PCV:** lomustine, 110 mg/m² PO on day 1; procarbazine, 60 mg/m² PO on days 8-21; and vincristine, 1.4 mg/m² IV on days 8 and 29—on a42-day cycle

**RT daily:** 33 × 1.8 Gy, for a total dose of 59.4 Gy

**Fig. 15.2** Schedule for (anaplastic) oligodendroglioma

on the presence of unfavourable prognostic factors such as age (older than 40–45 years of age), tumour size (>5–6 cm), focal and cognitive deficits and uncontrollable seizures [7].

Treatment options for a patient with an oligodendroglioma and unfavourable prognostic factors consist of radiotherapy and adjuvant chemotherapy. Normally PCV is administered for up to six cycles [10] (see Fig. 15.2). For patients with an astrocytoma and an IDH mutation, TMZ will be the choice of treatment (up to 12 cycles), adjuvant to radiotherapy. Recently it became clear that patients without a 1p/19q deletion and without an IDH mutation (IDH wild type) have an even worse prognosis, similar to a GBM [11]. Therefore, these patients will be treated as if they had a GBM, with radiotherapy and concomitant TMZ followed by six adjuvant cycles of TMZ.

Anaplastic oligodendrogliomas are (for some reason) more sensitive to chemotherapy; hence researchers are trying to define the reason why. Typical genetic alterations appeared to be responsible for this sensitivity, and further research led to the discovery of MGMT and IDH mutations. Both studies of van den Bent and Cairncross showed an improved outcome after adjuvant PCV chemotherapy for anaplastic oligodendroglioma. Thus, treatment of all 1p/19q codeleted oligodendrogliomas should consist of resection, followed by radiotherapy and adjuvant PCV chemotherapy (see Fig. 15.2) [3, 5].

The interim analysis of the EORTC CATNON trial [12], randomizing patients with non-codeleted 1p/19q anaplastic gliomas into four arms, showed a survival benefit for patients receiving radiotherapy alone, followed by 12 cycles of adjuvant TMZ. Another similar study [13] showed no difference in survival between adjuvant PCV and TMZ following completion of radiotherapy. The higher toxicity rates of PCV (mainly cumulative bone marrow suppression) often lead to discontinuation of treatment. Besides, TMZ is better tolerated by patients; hence it is often the treatment of choice in these scenarios.

Once a glioma has recurred or transformed, a multidisciplinary board will discuss viable treatment options whilst giving consideration to a multitude of variable factors: the condition of the patient, what has been the treatment thus far and is there room for (another) chemotherapy or second radiotherapy treatment, perhaps after (second) surgery. Chemotherapy treatment in this setting may consist of a rechallenge with TMZ for astrocytomas and PCV for oligodendrogliomas, even if they were used before.

## 15.5    Nursing Management Issues

### 15.5.1 Patient Education

Oncology nurses work closely together with glioma patients receiving chemotherapy to evaluate the process and initiate supportive therapies when necessary. Chemotherapy may consist of oral and intravenous agents. Of the previously described alkylating agents, only vincristine (as part of the PCV schedule) is administered intravenously, every 3 weeks. Orally administered chemotherapy (such as TMZ) is hence more convenient for the patient and also has less severe side effects as compared to PCV.

At the beginning of a chemotherapy treatment, the responsibility of the oncology nurse is to inform the patient about the efficacy and potency of the specific treatment, which safety precautions need adhering to, how to manage side effects and how and when to report them. Treatment adherence or compliance is affected by the patient's knowledge and understanding of the specific regimen [14]. Patients with a glioma may suffer from cognitive problems, resulting in difficulties adhering to chemotherapy schedules. Thus, it can be a challenge to arrange for adequate support when a patient is not able to understand correct dosages: oncology nurses need to check the ability of the patient to follow the prescribed regimen and ascertain if there is supportive care at home or otherwise arrange for active home care [15].

Effective education of the patient and his/her caregiver promotes patient safety, optimal dosing and accurate assessment of side effects and toxicities [16]. Therefore, patients and their caregivers need to receive verbal and written instructions on how to take medication and which measures to take to prevent side effects such as nausea and vomiting and in which circumstances there is a need to contact the acute oncology nurse (e.g. in case of fever, haematoma, insufficient oral intake due to vomiting). Fever may be suppressed in patients using corticosteroids (such as dexamethasone), which necessitates nurses' awareness of other signs and symptoms of infections during evaluation.

Dosages of chemotherapy depend on body surface, and the patient often needs to take multiple capsules of varying strength. For example, TMZ is administered over 5 days every 4 weeks. The PCV schedule is even more complicated: once every 6 weeks, lomustine is given orally on day 1 and procarbazine from day 8 to 22; and every 3 weeks vincristine is given intravenously (Fig. 15.2). Both TMZ and lomustine have to be taken on an empty stomach, due to the reduction of the rate (and extent) of absorption otherwise cause by the consumption of food. Because the peak plasma concentration of TMZ after oral intake occurs within 1 h and TMZ enhances the effect of radiotherapy, TMZ has to be taken an hour before the scheduled time of radiation during the concomitant radiation phase and on days without radiotherapy in the morning (Fig. 15.2).

Patient education is an ongoing process during the treatment period. A dedicated key worker (normally a specialist nurse) is allocated to patients receiving chemotherapy. This allows for adequate nurse-led follow-up and guidance during treatment, with regard to (dis)continuation and adherence of medication. These nurse-led clinics can be undertaken either within an outpatient setting or via telephone [17, 18]. Supportive tools developed by the Multinational Association of Supportive Care in Cancer (MASCC)—for example, the MASCC Oral Agent Teaching Tool (MOATT) [19]—consist of written information of the correct dosage and schedule, a patient's diary and medication accountability form. Nurses need to stay informed and educate themselves about chemotherapy and other new agents and their side effects and toxicity, to be able to perform and understand the challenges of good patient education [20].

## 15.5.2 Management and Nursing Implications of Side Effects

Alkylating chemotherapy agents are fairly myelosuppressive (reduced bone marrow function) and require careful monitoring of complete blood counts to prevent complications associated with anaemia, neutropenia, thrombocytopenia and lymphopenia. During the concomitant radio-chemotherapy period, a weekly blood count is required. During the adjuvant phase of TMZ and PCV, there will be a blood count on the day of the expected 'nadir' (lowest amount of blood counts) and the day before the start of the next cycle, when recovery of the nadir is expected and required, to start the next cycle. Treatment delay will lead to recovery of the blood counts, and subsequent dose adjustments (as required by protocol) will allow the patient to continue chemotherapy treatment (see Table 15.2). Despite the fact that myelotoxicity is relatively uncommon in patients using TMZ, there are case studies of severe toxicity resulting in treatment delays or even myelodysplasia resulting in death [21, 22].

**Table 15.2** Management of chemotherapy toxicity

| Toxicity | Interruption of chemotherapy | Discontinuation of chemotherapy |
|---|---|---|
| Absolute neutrophil count | Neutropenia CTCAE grade II $\geq 1.0$ and $<1.5 \times 10^9$ L$^{-1}$ CTCAE grade III $\geq 0.5$ and $<1.0 \times 10^9$ L$^{-1}$ | Neutropenia CTCAE grade IV $<0.5 \times 10^9$ L$^{-1}$ |
| Platelets | Thrombocytopenia CTCAE grade I $\geq 75$ and $<100 \times 10^9$ L$^{-1}$ CTCAE grade II $\geq 50$ and $<75 \times 10^9$ L$^{-1}$ CTCAE grade III $\geq 25$ and $<50 \times 10^9$ L$^{-1}$ | Thrombocytopenia CTCAE grade IV $<10 \times 10^9$ L$^{-1}$ |
| CTC non-haematological toxicity (except for alopecia, nausea and vomiting) | CTC grade II | CTC grades III and IV |

In trying to identify factors leading to severe myelotoxicity after a first course of TMZ, several variables were analysed. It appeared that women experienced more myelotoxicity than men. In men with a body surface area $\geq 2$ m$^2$ and in women who did not have prior chemotherapy, the occurrence of toxicity after the first course of TMZ was higher. Additionally, looking at age, older men did not have an increased risk; however for women there was a trend for an increased risk in those 31–40 years of age and for those older than 60 years [23]. Although rare, renal or hepatic functions may be disturbed by the use of chemotherapy, which may necessitate dose adjustment. Besides evaluation of blood counts (and once per cycle a full biochemistry panel), it is important to evaluate other side effects and how the patient tolerated the chemotherapy treatment. The nurse needs to be aware of the impact on patients and caregivers of a dose delay or reduction. These interventions often temper the hope for tumour response in patients with gliomas, necessitating adjustment of perspective and goals for the future.

### 15.5.3 Nausea and Vomiting

A patient commencing chemotherapy will be prescribed anti-emetic drugs *to prevent* nausea and vomiting. For patients with a GBM during the concomitant radiotherapy phase, it is advised to take ondansetron (or granisetron) for the first 3 days only. One of the side effects of ondansetron is constipation, when taken longer than prescribed. In case of persistent nausea, the advice (besides changing the anti-emetic drug to metoclopramide or domperidone) is to take laxatives. Nausea, however, can also mask more serious problems such as raised intracranial pressure (ICP). Other signs alerting to raised ICP are (besides nausea) headache, drowsiness and worsening of pre-existing focal deficits. In such cases an increase in oedema around the radiated brain tissue might be responsible, and dexamethasone could be added to the prescribed drugs. During the adjuvant TMZ and PCV cycles, anti-emetic drugs are again prescribed before taking the oral chemotherapy drugs. However, despite these precautions, nausea and vomiting still occurs in some patients. A reduced quality of life might interfere with adherence to treatment and subsequent success. Despite the fact that TMZ and PCV regimes have a low emetic profile, it is best to change or add another anti-emetic drug when continuing nausea and vomiting becomes apparent and raised ICP has been ruled out. A combination of metoclopramide, dexamethasone and lorazepam can be added to the prescribed anti-emetic drug if required for persistent cases of nausea and vomiting.

It is not uncommon for patients receiving oral chemotherapy to experience a loss of appetite, especially if cycles are continued for a longer period. However, in most patients with a glioma, loss of appetite does not often lead to involuntary weight loss. If this is the case, it is possible to support the patient with high-caloric drinks to prevent losing too much weight. In addition, other causes of loss of appetite and subsequent weight loss (mucositis, gastrointestinal infections, fatigue, depression) need to be considered and treated if necessary.

## 15.5.4 Thrombocytopenia

For patients with a GBM, TMZ is administered daily with radiation therapy during 6 or 7 weeks. During this period, they may develop a significant thrombocytopenia. Thrombocytopenia is a severe complication manifesting itself with an abnormally low platelet count (see Table 15.2), necessitating discontinuation of TMZ treatment and often limiting the administration of further chemotherapy. It can also necessitate frequent platelet infusions and places the patient at risk of bleeding.

Therefore, blood counts are monitored weekly and are intensified if the thrombocyte count is rapidly decreasing. Patients with thrombocytes $<10 \times 10^9 \, L^{-1}$ will require a platelet infusion, because of the risk of (intracranial) haemorrhages even without trauma. The infusion may lead to increased platelet counts; however, dose adjustment or discontinuation of TMZ is still recommended for some patients, depending on the moment of the occurrence, its severity and its recovery period. In some cases, the thrombocytopenia is prolonged, not recovering in weeks or even months [24], which means that the patient is not allowed to start adjuvant treatment. Myelotoxicity in patients receiving PCV chemotherapy is more common than in patients receiving TMZ or lomustine monotherapy. In the described trial in patients with anaplastic oligodendrogliomas [25], 33% of the patients ($n = 161$) receiving PCV needed to discontinue treatment due to haematological toxicity (e.g. grade III/IV toxicities: neutropenia 32%, thrombocytopenia 21%). In cases of severe thrombocytopenia, adjustment of anti-epileptic drugs might be considered to help recover the number of platelets, because they potentially contribute to myelosuppression (valproic acid).

### 15.5.4.1 Case Study

A 51-year-old male patient with a history of alcohol abuse resulted in an amnesic (Korsakov) syndrome and forced institutionalisation in a nursing home. He underwent a resection for an anaplastic astrocytoma in 1995 and received radiotherapy afterwards. In 2006 his tumour recurred, and it was decided to commence TMZ treatment. The patient was referred to the nurse practitioner to discuss and start treatment and follow-up; however baseline lab results showed a pre-existing thrombocytopenia grade II (platelet counts $54 \times 10^9 \, L^{-1}$). A diagnostic abdominal ultrasound was ordered and revealed a splenomegaly, responsible for the low platelet count. There was an absence of portal hypertension (e.g. oesophageal varices), which would have been a contra-indication for the start of TMZ. The patient was put on a regimen of TMZ 100 mg *per day*, as opposed to the normal regimen of 150–200 mg/m², because of his ongoing thrombocytopenia. The patient successfully received 12 cycles of TMZ for 5 days every 4 weeks, without irreversible toxicity (platelets remained between 41 and $92 \times 10^9 \, L^{-1}$), with a response of the tumour on MRI follow-up.

## 15.5.5 Neutropenia

Neutrophils are the most important defence mechanism of the body against acute bacterial infections and certain fungal infections. Patients receiving PCV have a greater risk of neutropenia (an abnormally low level of neutrophils), as compared to patients receiving TMZ. The risk of developing a fever whilst having a neutropenia (see Table 15.2) increases with age and, for those with a lower KPS, a worse nutritional status and a pre-existing pancytopenia (reduction in the number of red and white blood cells, as well as platelets), before the start of chemotherapy [26]. An infection due to severe neutropenia (neutrophil count, $0.5 \times 10^9$ L$^{-1}$) might be life-threatening, and if necessary, a patient is admitted to the hospital to treat the infection with intravenous antibiotics.

The neutrophil count is monitored as frequently as the thrombocyte count in patients using both PCV and TMZ—at the day of the expected nadir, the day of the expected recovery and the day before commencing the next cycle. Dose reductions and/or treatment delays will be carried out according to protocol Common Toxicity Criteria Adverse Events (CTCAE) grade II, neutrophil count $<1.5 \times 10^9$ L$^{-1}$ (see Table 15.2). Patients and their caregivers need to be alert for signs and symptoms of infections and report these to their oncology nurse (key worker). Supportive care with the injection of neutrophil growth-stimulating factors is an option to be able to continue chemotherapy treatment in patients with persisting grade III toxicity, despite dose reduction.

## 15.5.6 Lymphopenia

Lymphocytopenia, or lymphopenia, is the condition of having an abnormally low level of lymphocytes in the blood. Lymphocytes are part of our immune system and consist of white blood cells with important functions in helping to prevent opportunistic viral infections from setting in. In cases of chemotherapy-induced lymphopenia (where more specifically a reduction in T lymphocytes or CD4 count is noted), these white blood cells are lacking, giving rise to opportunistic infections. Long-term use of corticosteroids may have the same severe side effect, causing a reduction of lymphocytes ($<0.8 \times 10^9$ L$^{-1}$).

Lymphopenia is putting the patient at risk for immunosuppressive infections such as pneumocystis carinii pneumonia (PCP), herpes simplex, herpes zoster and fungal infections. Because of an earlier finding in a clinical trial [27] of the occurrence of PCP in patients using TMZ and corticosteroids in the chemoradiation phase, patients treated for GBM are prescribed prophylactic antibiotics (trimethoprim-sulfamethoxazole) in this phase. In case of lymphopenia occurring in concomitant phase, the lymphocyte subpopulation—CD4 count—is determined to address the necessity of prolonged use of prophylactic antibiotics (CD4 count $<0.2 \times 10^9$ L$^{-1}$). Some patients show an allergic reaction (rash) when prescribed trimethoprim-sulfamethoxazole. An alternative for PCP prophylaxis is inhalation of pentamidine, every 4 weeks. If there is no lymphopenia after the concomitant phase, antibiotics can be stopped; however, CD4 deficiency can persist for months after completion of concomitant TMZ, necessitating monthly CD4 counts and continuation of prophylactic antibiotics. When lymphopenia occurs during the adjuvant TMZ phase (which is less common), the same prophylactic antibiotics are prescribed in case the CD4 count drops to $<0.2 \times 10^9$ L.

### 15.5.7 Fatigue

Fatigue is a commonly reported symptom in patients with all types of glioma throughout the disease trajectory, which can decrease quality of life, particularly by the effect of fatigue on neurological deficits. The causes for fatigue in glioma patients can be multiple, such as the treatment of the tumour by radiotherapy and chemotherapy, the use of anti-epileptic drugs, focal deficits and sleep disturbances and depression. A review of exercise interventions in adults with advanced cancer showed that exercise maintained or improved fitness and physical function and may diminish fatigue and enhance quality of life [28]. There are multiple strategies for managing fatigue. The oncology nurse can ask glioma patients about their daily activities and how fatigue affects them. Educating patients regarding which interventions are suitable for their specific situation, and early referral to rehabilitation services, may help the patient in obtaining appropriate resources and support for fatigue management.

### 15.5.8 Neuropathy

Neuropathy is a specific side effect of vincristine (which forms part of the PCV schedule). Symptoms of neuropathy may include loss of sensitivity of hands or feet, loss of sense of touch, pain, tingling and burning sensations and balance disorders. Neuropathy can make walking more difficult and occur within weeks after the start of vincristine and may necessitate dose reductions or discontinuation, depending on the severity of the neuropathy. Educating patients about reporting this side effect to be able to intervene is important: at some point neuropathy can be irreversible, with a major impact on quality of life.

### 15.5.9 Fertility

All chemotherapy used for the treatments of adult gliomas may affect the male and female reproductive cells. For that reason, women starting chemotherapy treatment are advised not to become pregnant, and male patients are advised not to cause pregnancy. This advice relates to the treatment duration and also the 6-month period after treatment. Male patients may be advised and counselled about cryopreservation of semen prior to treatment commencing, due to the possibility of irreversible infertility. For women, it is more difficult to preserve reproductive cells, and these little applied procedures are often not carried out successfully. It is the responsibility of the prescribing physician to discuss these issues with patients and their partner, although it is a difficult subject to bring up, and it is often also brought up during consultation with the oncology nurse. When women with a glioma become pregnant, treatment interventions are discussed in a multidisciplinary team, including a gynaecologist. Case series of women with gliomas indicate that all types of antitumour interventions have been applied during pregnancy. The timing of chemotherapy treatment should preferentially be deferred until the second or third trimester because of the risks on congenital malformations when applied in the first trimester. In case series of women who became pregnant during or after using TMZ or PCV, healthy newborns are described; however, there is a paucity of information on the long-term development of the newborns [29].

### 15.5.9.1  Case Study

A 35-year-old male patient living in the Netherlands, originally from Turkey, was diagnosed with a GBM. The patient and his spouse were referred to the oncology nurse to discuss the start of concomitant chemo-radiation treatment. Because of their age, they were asked if they had a child wish, and they did. The oncology nurse informed them about the possibility of semen preservation before the start of the chemotherapy treatment. The spouse was asked if she used any birth control—it transpired she was diagnosed in Turkey (and subsequently in the Netherlands as well) with infertility; she could only become pregnant with the help of egg donation.

Guidelines on cryopreservation suggest that male patients need to freeze their sperm before commencing chemotherapy. This implies that the couple has to consider thinking about having children before the start of the therapy, in a situation in which both the present and future remain uncertain. From research it is known that couples could experience cryopreservation with a positive attitude: there is a future, a life after the cancer, a chance of recovery and a long-term outlook. The chances of becoming infertile after oncological treatment are dependent on the type of malignancy and the intensity of treatment duration. Even with a limited life expectancy, cryopreservation needs to be considered [30, 31].

The oncology nurse realises that she needs to sensitively approach the subject around cryopreservation with this couple. However, past experiences have taught her that couples facing an incurable disease are in a difficult position when they try and effectuate the cryopreservation by in vitro fertilization (IVF) or intracytoplasmic sperm injection (ICSI). In this particular case, there is also the need for an egg donor (given her infertility diagnosis), which will likely complicate the process further. There are cases described of male and female patients being able to have a child after treatment with temozolomide; infertility does not have to emerge [32, 33].

During the consultation the oncology nurse listens empathetically and guides the patient and his wife during the discussion. They had received an enormous amount of information in a language they did not understand that well. Nevertheless, the oncology nurse reflected on their feelings towards children and towards the diagnosis and shared the information she had on fertility, guidelines and procedures. The couple was on an emotional roller-coaster, meandering between good treatment outcomes from a glioma perspective and the hope for becoming parents. Ultimately, the patient and his wife decided that it would be more appropriate to start the necessary treatment for the glioblastoma as soon as possible, rather than wait for an appointment in the fertility department at the nearby academic hospital, which would have likely delayed his treatment start. They left with the hope that it still might be possible in the future to further explore their wish for a child.

# References

1. Armstrong TS, Gilbert MR. Chemotherapy of astrocytoma: an overview. Semin Oncol Nurs. 1998;14(1):18–25.
2. Graham CA, Cloughesy TF. Brain tumor treatment: chemotherapy and other new developments. Semin Oncol Nurs. 2004;20(4):260–72.
3. van den Bent MJ, Brandes AA, Taphoorn MJ, Kros JM, Kouwenhoven MC, Delattre JY, Bernsen HJ, et al. Adjuvant procarbazine, lomustine, and vincristine chemotherapy in newly diagnosed anaplastic oligodendroglioma: long-term follow-up of EORTC brain tumor group study 26951. J Clin Oncol. 2013;31(3):344–50. https://doi.org/10.1200/JCO.2012.43.2229.
4. Gorlia T, Delattre JY, Brandes AA, Kros JM, Taphoorn MJ, Kouwenhoven MC, Bernsen HJ, et al. New clinical, pathological and molecular prognostic models and calculators in patients with locally diagnosed anaplastic oligodendroglioma or oligoastrocytoma. A prognostic factor analysis of European Organisation for Research and Treatment of Cancer Brain Tumour Group Study 26951. Eur J Cancer. 2013;49(16):3477–85. https://doi.org/10.1016/j.ejca.2013.06.039.
5. Cairncross G, Wang M, Shaw E, Jenkins R, Brachman D, Buckner J, Fink K, Souhami L, Laperriere N, Curran W, Mehta M. Phase III trial of chemoradiotherapy for anaplastic oligodendroglioma: long-term results of RTOG 9402. J Clin Oncol. 2013;31(3):337–43. https://doi.org/10.1200/JCO.2012.43.2674.
6. Stupp R, Mason WP, van den Bent MJ, Weller M, Fisher B, Taphoorn MJ, Belanger K, et al. European Organisation for Research and Treatment of Cancer Brain Tumor and Radiotherapy Groups; National Cancer Institute of Canada Clinical Trials Group. Radiotherapy plus concomitant and adjuvant temozolomide for glioblastoma. N Engl J Med. 2005;352(10):987–96.
7. Pignatti F, van den Bent M, Curran D, Debruyne C, Sylvester R, Therasse P, Afra D, et al. European Organization for Research and Treatment of Cancer Brain Tumor Cooperative Group; European Organization for Research and Treatment of Cancer Radiotherapy Cooperative Group. Prognostic factors for survival in adult patients with cerebral low-grade glioma. J Clin Oncol. 2002;20(8):2076–84.
8. https://ctep.cancer.gov/protocoldevelopment/electronic_applications/docs/ctcaev3.pdf.
9. Perry JR, Laperriere N, O'Callaghan CJ, Brandes AA, Menten J, Phillips C, Fay M, et al. Short-course radiation plus temozolomide in elderly patients with glioblastoma. Engl J Med. 2017;376(11):1027–37. https://doi.org/10.1056/NEJMoa1611977.
10. Buckner JC, Shaw EG, Pugh SL, Chakravarti A, Gilbert MR, Barger GR, Coons S, et al. Radiation plus procarbazine, CCNU, and vincristine in low-grade glioma. N Engl J Med. 2016;374(14):1344–55. https://doi.org/10.1056/NEJMoa1500925.
11. Rogers TW, Toor G, Drummond K, Love C, Field K, Asher R, Tsui A, et al. The 2016 revision of the WHO classification of central nervous system tumours: retrospective application to a cohort of diffuse gliomas. J Neurooncol. 2017; https://doi.org/10.1007/s11060-017-2710-7.
12. van den Bent MJ, Baumert B, Erridge SC, Vogelbaum MA, Nowak AK, Sanson M, Brandes AA, et al. Interim results from the CATNON trial (EORTC study 26053–22054) of treatment with concurrent and adjuvant temozolomide for 1p/19q non-co-deleted anaplastic glioma: a phase 3, randomised, open-label intergroup study. Lancet. 2017;390(10103):1645–53. doi: https://doi.org/10.1016/S0140-6736(17)31442-3. Epub 2017 Aug 8.
13. Wick W, Hartmann C, Engel C, Stoffels M, Felsberg J, Stockhammer F, Sabel MC, et al. NOA-04 randomized phase III trial of sequential radiochemotherapy of anaplastic glioma with procarbazine, lomustine, and vincristine or temozolomide. J Clin Oncol. 2009;27(35):5874–80. https://doi.org/10.1200/JCO.2009.23.6497.
14. Hollywood E, Semple D. Nursing strategies for patients on oral chemotherapy. Oncology. 2001;15(1 Suppl 2):37–9.
15. Bordonaro S, Raiti F, Di Mari A, Lopiano C, Romano F, Pumo V, Giuliano SR, et al. Active home-based cancer treatment. J Multidiscip Healthc. 2012;5:137–43. https://doi.org/10.2147/JMDH.S31494.

16. Hartigan K. Patient education: the cornerstone of successful oral chemotherapy treatment. Clin J Oncol Nurs. 2003;7(6 Suppl):21–4.
17. Zwinkels H. The developing role of the neuro-oncology nurse: a Dutch perspective. Br J Neurosci Nurs. 2008;4:390–3.
18. Zwinkels H, Roon K, Jeurissen FJ, Taphoorn MJ, Hop WC, Vecht CJ. Management of temozolomide toxicity by nurse practitioners in neuro-oncology. Oncol Nurs Forum. 2009;36(2): 225–31. https://doi.org/10.1188/09.ONF.225-231.
19. MASCC Oral Agent Teaching Tool. 2009. http://www.mascc.org/MOATT. Accessed 8 Aug 2017.
20. Bedell CH. A changing paradigm for cancer treatment: the advent of new oral chemotherapy agents. Clin J Oncol Nurs. 2003;7(6 Suppl):5–9.
21. Noronha V, Berliner N, Ballen KK, Lacy J, Kracher J, Baehring J, Henson JW. Treatment-related myelodysplasia/AML in a patient with a history of breast cancer and an oligodendroglioma treated with temozolomide: case study and review of the literature. Neuro Oncol. 2006;8(3):280–3.
22. Natelson EA, Pyatt D. Temozolomide-induced myelodysplasia. Adv Hematol. 2010;2010:760402. https://doi.org/10.1155/2010/760402.
23. Armstrong TS, Cao Y, Scheurer ME, Vera-Bolaños E, Manning R, Okcu MF, Bondy M, et al. Risk analysis of severe myelotoxicity with temozolomide: the effects of clinical and genetic factors. Neuro Oncol. 2009;11(6):825–32. https://doi.org/10.1215/15228517-2008-120.
24. Gerber DE, Grossman SA, Zeltzman M, Parisi MA, Kleinberg L. The impact of thrombocytopenia from temozolomide and radiation in newly diagnosed adults with high-grade gliomas. Neuro Oncol. 2007;9(1):47–52.
25. van den Bent MJ, Carpentier AF, Brandes AA, Sanson M, Taphoorn MJ, Bernsen HJ, Frenay M, et al. Adjuvant procarbazine, lomustine, and vincristine improves progression-free survival but not overall survival in newly diagnosed anaplastic oligodendrogliomas and oligoastrocytomas: a randomized European Organisation for Research and Treatment of Cancer phase III trial. J Clin Oncol. 2006;24(18):2715–22.
26. Lyman GH, Djulbegovic B. The challenge of systematic reviews of diagnostic and staging studies in cancer. Cancer Treat Rev. 2005;31(8):628–39.
27. Stupp R, Dietrich PY, Ostermann Kraljevic S, Pica A, Maillard I, Maeder P, Meuli R, et al. Promising survival for patients with newly diagnosed glioblastoma multiforme treated with concomitant radiation plus temozolomide followed by adjuvant temozolomide. J Clin Oncol. 2002;20(5):1375–82.
28. Dittus KL, Gramling RE, Ades PA. Exercise interventions for individuals with advanced cancer: a systematic review. Prev Med. 2017;pii:S0091-7435(17)30262-1. https://doi.org/10.1016/j.ypmed.2017.07.015.
29. Zwinkels H, Dörr J, Kloet F, Taphoorn MJ, Vecht CJ. Pregnancy in women with gliomas: a case-series and review of the literature. J Neurooncol. 2013;115(2):293–301. https://doi.org/10.1007/s11060-013-1229-9.
30. Dohle GR. Male infertility in cancer patients. Int J Urol. 2010;17:327–31.
31. Naysmith TE, Blake DA, Harvey VJ, Johnson NP. Do men undergoing sterilizing cancer treatments have a fertile future? Hum Reprod. 1998;13(11):3250–5.
32. Ducray F, Colin P, Cartalat-Carel S, et al. Management of malignant gliomas diagnosed during pregnancy. Rev Neurol (Paris). 2006;162(3):322–9. (in French)
33. McGrane J, Bedford T, Kelly S. Successful pregnancy and delivery after concomitant temozolomide and radiotherapy treatment of glioblastoma multiforme. Clin Oncol (R Coll Radiol). 2012;24(4):311. https://doi.org/10.1016/j.clon.2012.01.005.

## Sara Robson and Louisa Gilpin

**Abstract**

Allied Health Professionals (AHPs) in the United Kingdom (UK) work across all healthcare settings including acute hospitals, rehabilitation wards, community teams, social care teams and voluntary sectors and within private healthcare.

Within any of these settings, AHPs provide rehabilitation to enable and support recovery for the patient and facilitate independence and activity, as much as possible. Rehabilitation for the brain tumour patient involves a combination of surgical, cancer, neurological and palliative rehabilitation principles as a result of the complex and varying symptoms that fluctuate throughout the cancer journey—all of which will be explored in this chapter. Allied Health Professional rehabilitation can include many varied interventions from the AHPs involved and can include education about deficits; symptoms and impairments; a patient-centred approach to reducing dysfunction caused by impairments; involvement of family and friends; common goal setting; and, most importantly, multidisciplinary working to achieve individual rehabilitation goals.

In this chapter, the varying professions that make up the term AHP are explored and how in turn each one has a pivotal role in supporting the glioma patient through their treatment pathways. This chapter also aims to give a basic knowledge of how rehabilitation interventions can help a person with glioma and their families, friends and carers with the aim of improving understanding of rehabilitation and making appropriate use of the rehabilitation services in your area.

**Keywords**

Allied Health Professional · Rehabilitation

S. Robson (✉)
Neuro-Oncology AHP, The Christie NHS Foundation Trust, Manchester, UK
e-mail: sara.robson@christie.nhs.uk

L. Gilpin
Neuro Oncology AHP, London, UK

© Springer Nature Switzerland AG 2019                                                    245
I. Oberg (ed.), *Management of Adult Glioma in Nursing Practice*,
https://doi.org/10.1007/978-3-319-76747-5_16

**Learning Outcomes**
- To gain deeper knowledge and insight into the varying professions that make up the term AHP (allied health professional) and how each one individually, and as a whole, has a role to play in supporting the glioma patient through their disease trajectory.
- To gain a deeper understanding of the term rehabilitation and how AHPs apply this in the clinical setting to glioma patients both pre- and post-surgery to enable them to achieve their full potential.
- To gain insight into how healthcare professionals (not just AHPs) are responsible for providing daily rehabilitation to the patient and how part of this journey is to enable the patient to self-manage their disease trajectory.

## 16.1   AHP Rehabilitation and Brain Tumours

The title "Allied Health Professional" or AHP refers to a group of non-medical professions who hold a professional registration in the UK with the Health and Care Professions Council. For the purposes of this chapter, the focus will mainly be on the four professions more commonly associated with rehabilitation:

- Dietitians
- Occupational therapists (OT)
- Physiotherapists (physio)
- Speech and language therapists (SLT)

Later in the chapter, the roles of some other AHPs are introduced, whose titles and roles are less frequently associated with rehabilitation but are equally as important in managing some of the symptoms, especially those experienced by people with glioma:

- Orthoptists
- Orthotists
- Therapeutic radiographers
- Diagnostic radiographers

Rehabilitation is a broad and nebulous concept—encompassing more of a philosophy than a specific health intervention. It aims to maximise quality of life and enable the recipient to gain as much independence as possible. The interventions provided by AHPs to facilitate rehabilitation will be varied and diverse, but the overall aim should be to help the person achieve a goal, or a functional gain, regardless of their underlying disease and prognosis.

The fact that rehabilitation can be provided by different professions in different locations through a variety of interventions makes defining "rehabilitation" difficult. The chartered society of physiotherapists [1], for instance, defines rehabilitation as a process, "...*enabling and supporting individuals to recover or adjust, to achieve their full potential and to live as full and active lives as possible. Rehabilitation should start as soon as possible to speed recovery".*

NHS Choices website [2] also tries to define rehabilitation from the point of view of the patient: *"Rehabilitation aims to improve your ability to carry out the everyday activities that have been affected by illness, injury or surgery".*

The document published by the National Health Service (NHS) Improving Quality titled "Improving Adult Rehabilitation Services" [3] defines rehabilitation as: *"...the restoration, to the maximum degree possible, of an individual's function and/or role, both mentally and physically, within their family and social networks and within the workplace where appropriate".*

All are valid definitions, the final one being more holistic by including the ideas of addressing mental health and social care needs. These rehabilitation interventions will also incorporate treatment of symptoms, such as pain, changes in muscle tone and breathlessness, as well as interventions aiming to improve (or adjust) a deficit, which helps the person with a glioma adapt to life with a neurological deficit, for example.

The interventions offered by rehabilitation professionals may be implemented in various settings and by many different teams. These will differ depending on how their rehabilitation services have been established, funded and developed within their geographical area. This will also differ greatly in different countries, depending on the health economy of the country. Rehabilitation interventions in the UK commonly occur:

1. Within an acute hospital environment, e.g. chest physiotherapy interventions following a glioma resection to prevent chest infections/complications after anaesthetic.
2. Within an acute or subacute settings in a specifically designated rehabilitation institution, e.g. a neuro-rehabilitation centre.
3. In a community rehabilitation facility (inpatient or outpatient), e.g. an intermediate care facility. (These settings usually provide generic rehabilitation rather than specialising in a disease group, i.e. stroke or spinal injury.)
4. In the patient's own home.
5. In a hospice as either a day-patient or inpatient.

The variety of and disparity between the types of rehabilitation services available throughout the UK and also individual team's referral criteria and service provision make negotiating your way through these services difficult.

If you are able to provide your patient and their carers with examples of how each profession will work *with* them, it will help them gauge their expectations around their rehabilitation potential. Some people with high-grade glioma may misunderstand the meaning of "rehabilitation" and think it is only for people who are going to fully recover and get back to their previous level of function; hence they might refuse a physiotherapy referral, for example. If you are able to explain to them *how* a physiotherapist might help them regain their balance or learn to walk independently with a walking stick, this might help the patient both in terms of understanding what can be offered and of motivating them to partake in activities and help themselves.

A person with a glioma may present with varying complex symptoms depending on where the tumour is situated in the brain, what type of surgery they may have had (e.g. debulking or biopsy) and how much oedema surrounds the tumour. The symptoms for one individual may fluctuate throughout their disease trajectory depending on the treatment they have had, the nature of the glioma and the presence or absence of symptoms such as seizures. This drives the need for a very person-centred approach to rehabilitation for this group of people and makes a prescriptive or inflexible approach inappropriate for most neurosurgical patients [4].

This next section will describe in detail three distinct types of rehabilitation that a person with a glioma may experience in isolation or in combination: surgical, oncological/palliative and neurological rehabilitation.

*Surgical rehabilitation*: It occurs immediately before or after a surgical intervention. Not all people diagnosed with a glioma will have a surgical intervention; others may have more than one intervention. The type of rehabilitation provided prior to and after surgery will be taken from a different model than the rehabilitation interventions provided later in the patient's journey [5, 6]. Increasingly the role of rehabilitation within any acute hospital in the UK is one of assessment and discharge planning. Therefore a rehabilitation intervention in an acute hospital setting will be more focused on facilitating a safe discharge, rather than obtaining longer-term rehabilitation goals.

When caring for a patient following surgery, there are certain symptoms which should prompt the neurosurgical nurse to consider a referral to the rehabilitation team within your institution. Below are examples of symptoms you may see post-surgery and examples of which AHP the patient should be referred to, in conjunction with their medical team:

*Breathing difficulties (physio)*: A physiotherapist will have skills in treating breathing and chest problems with manual techniques and the use of equipment if required. A physiotherapist might be involved in acute and emergency treatment of chest problems on an "on-call" basis.

*Slurred speech, difficulties in communication (SLT)*: A speech and language therapist would assess for problems with communication and offer exercises or strategies to reduce the impact of the communication difficulty.

*Confusion/disorientation (OT/psychology)*: Neuropsychologists, psychologists or occupational therapists may be involved in addressing neurocognitive dysfunction and may use a combination of specialist tools to assess the cognitive functioning of a person with a glioma [7].

*Difficulty eating and drinking (SLT)*: A speech and language therapist would assess a person's ability to swallow different textures and consistencies of food and drink and may suggest a specialist diet or thickened fluids.

*Need for a feeding regime to be established (dietitian)*: If a person's ability to take nutrition orally has been temporarily or permanently affected by surgery or the presence of a glioma, it may be necessary for a dietitian to establish a feeding regime with an alternative route, i.e. percutaneous endoscopic gastrostomy (PEG) or nasogastric (NG) tube feeding.

*Difficulties in personal care (OT)*: An occupational therapist may assess a person with a glioma prior to discharge from hospital to ensure they are independent in personal care. If they are not, they may introduce aids and adaptations in the home to assist or even refer for a carer to be enlisted to help the person with personal care.

*Motor weakness (OT and physiotherapist)*: Occupational therapists and physiotherapists may aim to improve a weakness by introducing certain exercises or by encouraging the normal use of a limb within activities of daily living.

*Tonal changes, either high or low tone (OT and physiotherapist)*: Occupational therapists and physiotherapists will have skills in managing changes in tone through therapeutic handling, splinting or positioning.

*Double vision, nystagmus or altered visual fields (orthoptics)*: An orthoptist may introduce specialist lenses to reduce the impact of visual disturbances.

These issues should be discussed at the ward multidisciplinary team meeting (where available) and inpatient referrals made to the appropriate rehabilitation professionals. Similarly there may be specific circumstances where a rehabilitation assessment may be required before a surgical intervention. One example of this is a speech and language assessment before an awake craniotomy so that a baseline has been recorded for the patient prior to the intraoperative assessments taking place.

In some circumstances, AHPs may be involved in monitoring a patient intraoperatively when an asleep/awake craniotomy is carried out in order to try and reduce neurological deficit from surgery. Speech and language therapists or neuropsychologists can be involved in language assessments to try and preserve language function during surgery [7]. Physiotherapists may be involved in the assessment of motor functions intraoperatively to try and preserve function and reduce motor weakness caused by surgery.

Ideally, a newly diagnosed glioma patient will be assessed by an appropriate AHP to gauge their level of rehabilitation needs whilst still in hospital. This may require a period of inpatient rehabilitation on a designated ward in order for the patient to regain sufficient function or learn adaptive strategies to be able to manage outside of a care environment. Sometimes, the rehabilitation professionals are instrumental in making decisions about the longer-term future of the patient with a glioma, i.e. whether they require care within a residential or nursing home to fully manage their needs. Post-operatively a patient may only require a short intervention from the ward-based AHPs in order to facilitate a discharge home. Although, as is mirrored throughout the rest of their journey, patients with a glioma will have very specific and individual rehabilitation needs and should be assessed accordingly, it is not possible to be prescriptive about individual interventions that may be required at this stage.

At the surgical phase of treatment, the complete histology and diagnosis of the person with a glioma may not be known, so all patients should have equal access to rehabilitation regardless of whether a low-grade or a high-grade tumour is suspected. Access to rehabilitation should be based on need not on diagnosis. All patients with a confirmed or suspected diagnosis of glioma will be anxious and unsure about their future and will need emotional as well as psychological support. As AHPs are central to the patient's care, they may be expected to provide a certain level of psychological support in keeping with assessments from other key members of the local multidisciplinary team (MDT) and their own level of psychological training. AHPs who have undertaken specialised training at a postgraduate level will be able to provide a higher level of emotional and psychological support than those who are newly qualified [8].

*Cancer rehabilitation*: It is an area which has developed greatly within the last 10 years in the UK. AHPs who have chosen to specialise in this way and who have completed the required postgraduate training will provide interventions and therapies fitting into the four stages of cancer rehabilitation:

- Preventive (reduction of the scale of expected disability).
- Restorative (facilitation of the patient's return to their previous level of functioning without disability).
- Supportive (limitation of functional loss, provision of support).
- Palliative (compensation and symptom management to reduce complications associated with illness) [4].

Specialist AHPs working in cancer rehabilitation and palliative care have an in-depth understanding of the nature and impact of the problem (such as the presence of a glioma) on the individual and, in addressing the impact of the problem, simultaneously prioritise the patients' choices. Thus, rehabilitation interventions which result in goal achievement may not be implemented if this is not in line with the individual's choice.

AHPs without specialist postgraduate training will have the basic skills to rehabilitate someone with cancer, but not at a complex level or in a case with a high level of risk [8]. The reasoning used by the AHPs in cancer and palliative rehabilitation is broader than just clinical, it encompasses other types of reasoning such as social, emotional, economic, etc. It is a mature and sophisticated reasoning allowing specialist practitioners to tackle complex situations. It allows the specialist AHP to know when to incorporate an active intervention and when not to intervene, driven by sensitivity to individual's choices about rehabilitation goals and outcomes.

Specialist AHP interventions within palliative care are not rooted in the medical model, thus making them inherently different to interventions that may be carried out by nurses or other healthcare professionals. Often AHP interventions are carried out in the recipient's own home or in a hospice, so are not directed by a medical practitioner. These interventions may also be offered as part of a multidisciplinary approach to the total care of the palliative patient [9].

As suggested, non-AHPs may conduct "prescribed" rehabilitation interventions under supervised direction. However it is the AHP who should conduct the initial assessment and plan any rehabilitation interventions. Furthermore, the specialist AHP is the one who recognises the need to change or adapt the rehabilitation goals in an appropriate and timely manner. Function and ability can change quickly for a person with a glioma, and their rehabilitation needs require adaptation in order to successfully cope with their fluctuating needs.

The assessment conducted by a specialist AHP working within cancer care or palliative care identifies the individual's ability, limitations and potential; they then use the individual's attitudes and beliefs about the impact of these issues to negotiate the goals of rehabilitation.

*Neurological rehabilitation*: Like cancer and palliative rehabilitation, this is another individual area where a specialist AHP practitioner will have carried out extra postgraduate training to enable them to provide specific interventions relating directly to the neurological function of an individual. The science upon which neurological rehabilitation is built is that of neuroplasticity which involves retraining of skills and strategies to compensate for impaired skills [10]. A specialist in neurological rehabilitation will have advanced skills in assessing the extent of damage caused by the presence of a glioma or surgery carried out to debulk the glioma. In some cases, there may be permanent neurological damage (in which case rehabilitation will not help), but equally there are circumstances where the damage is deemed reversible and neurological rehabilitation can assist with neuroplasticity and any associated improvement in function.

Each profession (physio, OT, SLT, etc.) will have a specific set of core skills and approaches by which they choose and structure their rehabilitation intervention. These will be guided by the type of rehabilitation they aim to carry out, the environment in which this is provided, at which stage of the disease trajectory the individual is at and how their disease is expected to progress. The patient should be at the centre of all of these choices, and rehabilitation should be guided by their own goals and aims. For example, a physiotherapist with a specialist neurological background and postgraduate training may follow a normal movement approach [10] to treating a patient with a glioma, whereas a cancer rehabilitation physiotherapist may adopt a more functional and compensatory approach.

To illustrate the aforementioned points, a patient with a motor weakness of the lower limb which is affecting their mobility can be used as an example. A rehabilitation approach aiming to regain motor activity through neural plasticity may use lots of therapeutic handling to promote increased synaptic activity to occur around the damaged area of the brain [11]. This may involve preventing the patient from trying to walk unaided if a correct gait pattern cannot be achieved without therapeutic intervention. The oncology-trained therapist, however, may allow the same patient to adapt their gait with the use of a quad stick to enable the patient to be more functional and mobile even though their gait pattern would not be ideal. Both are examples of rehabilitation, but they are from different theoretical models (*normal movement* versus *compensatory*). Neuro-rehabilitation aiming for improvement through neural plasticity can be a long and tiring process for a patient often requiring inpatient rehabilitation for a number of months. As such, a patient with a high-grade glioma with a short prognosis may choose not to spend such a long time in rehabilitation and may prefer a compensatory approach even if their walking never returns to normal. There is evidence to suggest that allowing a patient to compensate with increased use of the unaffected limb may impair or delay recovery of the affected limb, so as with any approach, the best long-term interests of the patient need to be taken into consideration [11].

Any person with a glioma is at risk of having seizures, and some rehabilitation interventions can help manage symptoms and reduce the risk of injury occurring to a person during a seizure. Occupational therapists would be involved in educating a patient about safety within the home and how they affect activities of daily living [12]. Furthermore, they may advise ways of reducing the risk of, for example, scalding or burning by adapting kitchen tasks to avoid carrying hot food, should the patient be at risk of seizures.

Fatigue can be difficult to quantify and difficult to treat. Some causes of fatigue such as anaemia and endocrine dysfunction can be treated medically. Other causes, such as the fatigue caused by radiotherapy to the brain or fatigue caused by the presence of a tumour, are more difficult to treat. An occupational therapist would be involved in fatigue management by teaching methods of conserving energy possibly through the use of adaptive equipment, such as sitting down to do meal preparation rather than standing up. A physiotherapist would treat the symptom of fatigue by introducing appropriate gentle exercises, and a dietitian may treat fatigue by ensuring that a patient is receiving sufficient nutrition to meet their energy requirements.

People with glioma can often experience varying degrees of sleep disturbance at points throughout their disease trajectory. This may be due to fatigue causing them to sleep more during the day, subsequently making sleep at night time less forthcoming. Sleep disturbance can also be caused in some individuals by the use of steroids or anxiety about what the future may hold. Occupational therapists can offer advice on sleep management techniques, relaxation and possibly the introduction of sleep hygiene [13]. A physiotherapist may offer advice on appropriate exercise to try and promote restful sleep, and a dietician may give advice on avoidance of stimulants in the diet, such as excessive caffeine.

## 16.2  Types of Allied Health Professionals in the UK

### 16.2.1  Occupational Therapy

"Occupation" refers to practical and purposeful activities that allow people to live independently and have a sense of identity such as essential day-to-day tasks including self-care, work or leisure [14]. Occupational therapists aim to maintain a person's independence and quality of life, through taking a holistic, person-centred approach to both mental and physical health and well-being and providing rehabilitation to enable individuals to achieve their full potential at all stages of illness.

Symptoms of cognitive impairment (e.g. memory, attention, organising thoughts, concentration and safety awareness), mobility issues, fatigue and difficulties managing day-to-day activities are frequently seen in people with brain tumours [15]. Occupational therapists assess and provide rehabilitation to individuals using purposeful activity, strategies and occupation to prevent further disability, facilitate recovery, promote health and independent function and enable individuals to overcome barriers that prevent them from doing the activities (occupations) that matter to them [15].

*An example of a rehabilitation intervention* by an occupational therapist would be a kitchen assessment, where a person with a glioma (following surgical intervention) is brought to a kitchen with an occupational therapist to see how they can manage a routine task of making a cup of tea and toasting a piece of bread whilst assessing cognitive processes and motor function. The occupational therapist throughout this process assesses the patients' cognitive abilities of planning, organising, remembering location of items, safety awareness with hot water and electricity, completion of the required task and how they problem-solve if something isn't working. In addition, motor processes are assessed, such as how they reach into cupboards and balance, whilst they complete tasks. More subtle things are also observed such as if the person with a glioma is using both hands appropriately. Based on these findings, an occupational therapist can extrapolate what function is likely to be when the patient is discharged from hospital, and they may also identify new cognitive, motor or sensory disturbances.

Rehabilitation by an occupational therapist can also include the following:

- Provides assessment, advice and rehabilitation in activities of daily living, such as bathing, dressing, eating, gardening, working and learning.
- Provides assessment, rehabilitation and strategies for cognitive impairment including memory, personality, attention, safety awareness, etc.
- Provides assessment and advice on capacity and safety of an individual in the home environment, including falls risk.
- Provides assessment and rehabilitation for fatigue management.
- Assesses and recommends equipment, such as mobility aids, wheelchairs (alongside physiotherapy) and special devices to help around the home or workplace.
- Offers advice and support to adapt the home or workplace to meet a person's needs.
- Provide vocational rehabilitation through working with organisations to improve employees' ability to perform their job.

## 16.2.2 Physiotherapy

Physiotherapists provide rehabilitation through movement and exercise, manual therapy, education and advice. Loss of muscle strength and use, loss of sensation, impaired balance and coordination and changes in muscular tone are frequently seen in people with brain tumours [4].

A physiotherapist aims to optimise patient function and well-being, through rehabilitation of these physical impairments as a result of neurological damage caused by the brain tumour. Rehabilitation by the physiotherapist focuses on retraining and establishing functional strategies for impairments based on the patient's goals, their prognosis and their stage of illness.

*An example of a rehabilitation intervention* by a physiotherapist is a person with a brain tumour is helped to mobilise from the bed in the days following surgical intervention. Physiotherapists use specific moving and handling methods to mobilise patients in these acute stages aiming to optimise return of function and prevention of secondary musculoskeletal and respiratory complications. This is done through the provision of advice, information and training about positioning, patient moving and handling techniques and the role of multidisciplinary team members and relevant carers. Physios also assess for falls and the safety of the patient mobilising once they are discharged home.

Rehabilitation by a physiotherapist can also include the following:

- Provides assessment, advice and rehabilitation to muscular paralysis and weakness.
- Assesses and recommends equipment, such as mobility aids and wheelchairs (alongside occupational therapy).
- Assesses and recommends exercise and activity programmes based on impairments, level of fatigue and stage of illness.
- Assesses, advises and provides rehabilitation for changes to balance and posture, including managing falls risk.
- Assesses and manages changes to muscle tone and spasticity in collaboration with specialist neurology teams.
- Provides pulmonary/chest physiotherapy, assessment and rehabilitation. This includes management of tracheostomies in collaboration with speech and language therapy.

### 16.2.3 Speech and Language Therapy

Communication and swallowing difficulties as a result of a brain tumour are assessed, diagnosed and treated by a speech and language therapist. Communication difficulties such as language (aphasia), speech (dysarthria) and cognition and language impairments (cognitive communication disorder) are seen in people with brain tumours as well as swallowing difficulties (dysphagia) [11]. Through taking a whole-person approach, relearning of skills and providing educational and functional alternatives (e.g. communication picture board, hand gestures or electronic devices with communication software), a speech and language therapist aims to optimise a person's ability to communicate effectively and eat and drink as safely as possible whilst maintaining quality of life throughout all stages of the illness.

*An example of a rehabilitation intervention* by a speech and language therapist is the assessment of swallowing, language, speech and cognitive communication skills following surgical intervention. They assess how safely the person can swallow their diet and if they can maintain a good nutritional status are assessed during a meal time. During conversation, the patient's ability to understand words, sentences and questions and subsequently being able to respond appropriately is assessed, alongside their ability to physically produce speech. A speech therapist will look at the level, type and severity of impairment and suggest immediate day-to-day communication strategies to facilitate the patient's ability to get their needs and wants met (e.g. use pictures to help understanding, only ask short questions with one piece of information) and reduce frustration, alongside longer-term plans to establish the best method of communication for that patient once they go home. This can include the use of technology (picture symbols producing words/sentences or text-to-speech technology), communication books and carer and multidisciplinary team training and education.

Rehabilitation by a speech and language therapist can also include the following:

- Provides assessment, advice and rehabilitation of communication impairments.
- Provides assessment and advice on capacity in collaboration with multidisciplinary team.

- Assesses and recommends augmentative and alternative communication (AAC) devices to facilitate communication (e.g. gestures, sign language, picture boards, speech-generating devices, buttons to call for attention).
- Provides assessment, advice, rehabilitation and long-term management of swallowing impairments (e.g. difficultly chewing, difficulty starting the swallow and difficulty clearing food residue from the mouth and throat).
- Assesses, advices and manages swallowing and communication in patients with a tracheostomy. This includes weaning off a tracheostomy management in collaboration with physiotherapy and the multidisciplinary team.

### 16.2.4 Dietitian

The consequences of malnutrition which significantly impact on the brain tumour patient's well-being include decreased performance status, muscle function, quality of life and increased fatigue [16]. Despite rates of malnutrition in the overall brain tumour population being low, there is a significant association recognised between increased weight loss and malignancy [17] indicating the importance of nutritional screening throughout the patient journey.

Dietitians specialise in nutritional assessment of brain tumour patients, which is used alongside clinical information to prescribe dietary treatment. They aim to assess for malnutrition and restore optimum nutritional status and minimise side effects of oncological and surgical treatments.

Rehabilitation by a dietitian can include the following:

- Calculating an individual's nutritional requirement using standard equations based on assessments of blood chemistry, temperature, stress, mobility and other relevant factors.
- Providing assessment, advice and rehabilitation for patients who have oral, enteral (e.g. nasogastric tubes) or parenteral nutrition requirements (e.g. intravenous administration of total parenteral nutrition).
- Providing assessment and advice on food intake requirements, eating habits and diet textures of meals in collaboration with the speech and language therapist.
- Educating and advising patients, family and carers as well as other professionals on how therapeutic diets and dietary therapy can improve the management of their conditions.

### 16.2.5 Neuropsychologist

A neuropsychologist is a psychologist who specialises in understanding the relationship between brain structures and systems and subsequent behaviour and cognitive function as a result of the brain tumour. The site of the brain tumour and its growth typically determine the neuropsychological and neurocognitive impairment seen in the patient.

Through neuropsychological evaluation, the neuropsychologist can acquire data about a patient's cognitive, motor, behavioural, linguistic and executive functioning—they are able to assess for levels of impairment at both a domain-specific and a global level. Brain tumour patients present with significant neuropsychological impairment when matched with controls, which has been shown to be a key factor in determining overall quality of life [14].

The occupational therapists and speech and language therapists work in collaboration with the neuropsychologists to assess cognition and communication impairments and how this, in turn, impacts on their daily function and communication. In addition, other AHPs involved in the rehabilitation process also liaise closely with the neuropsychologist on managing impairments impacting on function. Rehabilitation by a neuropsychologist can include the following:

- Provides assessment, advice and rehabilitation of cognitive, motor, behavioural, linguistic and executive abilities from a domain-specific (and a global neuropsychological) functioning level.
- Provides neuropsychological evaluation to further localise organic abnormalities within the CNS and aid in confirming diagnosis.
- Provides assessment and advice on capacity in relation to cognitive functioning.
- Provides assessment and rehabilitation for mood disorders.
- Provides vocational rehabilitation alongside occupational therapy through working with organisations to improve employees' ability to perform their job.

## 16.2.6 Broader Multidisciplinary Team Members

As previously mentioned, there are a number of AHPs that feature in the wider multidisciplinary team caring for a person with a glioma, and some AHPs will only be required if a person is experiencing specific deficits. Orthoptists, for example, diagnose and treat defects of vision and abnormalities of eye movement. They usually form part of a hospital-based team, and they look after people with eye problems [15, 18].

At present there are no accurate numbers available to suggest how many people with gliomas experience visual problems, but symptoms such as homonymous hemianopia (visual field loss on the same side of both eyes), double vision and blurred vision are common amongst this group of patients. Therefore a referral to an orthoptist should be considered if a visual problem is identified. Some people have visual disturbances as their presenting complaint prior to the diagnosis of the glioma and may have visited their optician complaining that their glasses weren't strong enough. Sometimes the optician may even be the person who identifies the presence of the tumour during an assessment, as they may identify papilloedema (swollen optic discs).

Another AHP who may be involved in the care and rehabilitation of a person with a glioma is an orthotist—unsurprisingly people may get these two professions confused because of their title, but their roles are very different. An orthotist is the person responsible for the provision or construction of orthosis; these may include foot drop splints, neck collars, spinal braces or upper limb splints. In some areas, these services may also cover specialist wheelchair and seating provision in collaboration with occupational therapy and physiotherapy.

## 16.3    Rehabilitation Pathway and Allied Health Professionals in the UK

Emerging evidence and best practice guidelines recognise that rehabilitation should start at the point of diagnosis and continue through all stages of the patient pathway through to end of life. As rehabilitation is an essential component of anticipating problems caused by the disease and subsequent treatment(s), as well as maximising outcomes along the patient's cancer journey, it is vital that the medical and rehabilitation pathways are integrated at all key stages (Graph 16.1).

### 16.3.1  Key Points/Takeaway Learning

– Rehabilitation is an intervention carried out by Allied Health Professionals (including dietitians, physiotherapists, occupational therapists and speech and language therapists) which aims to enable and support individuals to recover and adjust to impairments as a result of a brain tumour.
– Rehabilitation in people with brain tumours includes a combination of the principles of neurological rehabilitation, cancer rehabilitation and palliative rehabilitation.
– The medical and surgical pathway and the rehabilitation pathway should be integrated through all stages of the patient journey.

There is no doubt that people with glioma (regardless of the WHO grading of their tumour) have specific rehabilitation needs, and in some areas of the UK, this has been acknowledged by NHS services, and specialist AHPs have been employed to ensure that this small patient group are receiving appropriate rehabilitation interventions [19]. Macmillan Cancer Support in the UK has acknowledged the role for both specialist and generalist workers within cancer care [5] and suggests that the "*specialist role is critical to the quality of services but should enhance and not undermine the skills of the generalist*" [15].

This reinforces the idea that all UK-based AHPs will have the basic skills to treat a person with a glioma, upon completion of their undergraduate courses. However, in order to manage complex cases, they would require the support of a more highly specialist AHP with relevant postgraduate training. In the UK, the National Institute for Health and Care Excellence (NICE) Guidelines for Improving Outcomes for People with Brain and CNS Tumours introduced the idea of a specialist AHP being involved at multidisciplinary level to help streamline and guide appropriate rehabilitation provision for people with gliomas [16, 19].

*Specialist AHPs – Representatives of the allied health professions, including occupational therapy, physiotherapy, speech and language therapy, dietetics and others as appropriate, who have knowledge and experience of dealing with this patient group, with responsibility for education and liaison with other local specialist AHPs* [19].

The professions providing rehabilitation have been in existence for varying amounts of time; therefore some are more widely acknowledged and familiar than others.

| Medical and surgical pathway | | | AHP rehabilitation pathway<br>*Reasons for referrals and key interventions* |
|---|---|---|---|
| *AHP referral red flags – Changes to mobility, independence, cognition, communication, swallowing, nutritional status, vision* | | | |
| **Diagnosis and care planning** | Presenting symptoms. Patient scanned and referred to neuro oncology MDT | Hospital admission, clinic appointment, Oncology planning, treatment appointments | • Pre intervention/diagnosis risk Ax AHP<br>• Cognitive impairment OT<br>• Mood/psychological factors affecting function OT<br>• Speech, language, voice, cognitive communication SLT<br>• Falls risk assessment PT<br>• Exercise and physical wellbeing OT/PT<br>• Information/support AHP<br>• Nutritional support including swallowing and alternative feeding SLT/DT<br>• Pre-treatment rehabilitation referral/liaison with community AHP<br>• Changes in respiratory function PT<br>• Work, leisure and ADL's OT |
| **Treatment** | For surgery | Biopsy and diagnostic histology<br>Debulking and diagnostic histology<br>Radiotherapy and chemotherapy | • Motor, sensory and mobility Ax PT<br>• Cognitive functioning OT<br>• Mood/psychological factors affecting function OT<br>• Speech, language, voice, cognitive communication SLT<br>• Equipment Provision and seating assessment OT/PT<br>• Exercise and physical wellbeing OT/PT<br>• Information/support AHP<br>• Nutritional support including swallowing and alternative feeding SLT/DT<br>• Quality measures, goals AHP<br>• Rehabilitation referral/liaison with community and palliative AHP services AHP |
| | No surgery | Radiotherapy and chemotherapy<br>Symptom management | • Respiratory function PT<br>• Work, leisure and ADL's OT<br>• Fatigue management and support OT<br>• Home discharge risk assessment and planning AHP |
| **Post treatment** | Clinic review<br>Repeat scans | | • Motor, sensory and mobility Ax PT<br>• Cognitive Ax and rehabilitation OT<br>• Mood/psychological factors affecting function OT<br>• Speech, language, voice, cognitive communication SLT<br>• Exercise and physical wellbeing OT/PT<br>• Information/support on impairments AHP<br>• Nutritional support including swallowing and alternative feeding SLT/DT<br>• Rehabilitation referral/liaison with community and palliative AHP services AHP<br>• Work, leisure and ADL's OT<br>• Fatigue management and support OT |
| **Monitoring and survivorship** | Acute and community team, consultant, GP, Nurses and AHP follow up | | • Motor, sensory and mobility Ax PT<br>• Cognitive Ax and rehabilitation OT<br>• Mood/psychological factors affecting function OT<br>• Speech, language, voice, cognitive communication SLT<br>• Exercise and physical wellbeing OT/PT<br>• Information/support on impairments AHP<br>• Nutritional support including swallowing and alternative feeding SLT/DT<br>• Rehabilitation referral/liaison with community and palliative AHP services AHP<br>• Work, leisure and ADL's OT<br>• Fatigue management and support OT |
| **Palliative care and end of life care** | Acute and community team, consultant, GP, Nurses and AHP follow up<br>Advice to colleagues on managing symptoms by nurses, consultants. | | • MDT and patient centred goal planning AHP<br>• Support for mood/psychological factors affecting function and wellbeing AHP<br>• Cognitive Ax, capacity and strategies OT<br>• Speech, language, voice, cognitive communication and capacity education SLT<br>• Communication aid provision SLT<br>• Information/support on impairments AHP<br>• Fatigue management and support OT<br>• Motor, sensory and mobility Ax to optimise and enable mobility PT<br>• Respiratory function PT<br>• Nutritional support, education and QoL for swallowing and alternative feeding SLT/DT<br>• Rehabilitation referral/liaison with community and palliative AHP services AHP<br>• ADL's, leisure and lifestyle adjustments OT |

**Graph 16.1** Describes the integration of the medical and rehabilitation pathways including the outline of AHP key referral triggers and interventions at each stage based on the National Cancer Action Team Brain CNS Rehabilitation Care Pathway [16]

As such, some areas of medicine have closer links with rehabilitation than others. The links between medicine and neuro-rehabilitation are strong and well established, whereas the links between oncology and rehabilitation are still in their relative infancy; the discipline of neuro-oncology rehabilitation lies somewhere between the two.

# References

1. Rehabilitation [Internet]. The Chartered Society of Physiotherapy. 2017. http://www.csp.org. uk/your-health/conditions/rehabilitation
2. Rehabilitation [Internet]. nhs.uk. 2017. https://www.nhs.uk/conditions/occupational-therapy/ rehabilitation/
3. NHS England. NHS England improving rehabilitation service programme regional report – London. 1st ed. London: NHS England; 2017. https://www.england.nhs.uk/london/wp-content/uploads/sites/8/2016/09/rehab-leads-report-london.pdf
4. Rankin J, Robb K, Murtagh N, Cooper J, Lewis S. Rehabilitation in cancer care. John Wiley & Sons; 2009.
5. Hagedorn R. Occupational therapy foundations for practice: models, frames of reference and core skills. London: Churchill Livingstone; 1992.
6. Anderson C, Van der Gaag A. Speech and language therapy "issues in professional practice". Whurr, Hoboken, NJ; 2005.
7. Dwan TM, Ownsworth T, Chambers S, Walker DG, Shum DH. Neuropsychological assessment of individuals with brain tumor: comparison of approaches used in the classification of impairment. Front Oncol. 2015;5:56.
8. Macmillan Cancer Support. The Macmillan allied health professions competency framework. London: Macmillan Cancer Support; 2018.
9. Doyle D. Oxford text book of palliative medicine Oxford University Press 1993 speech and language therapy in palliative care. Oxford Author(s): Tim Luckettand Katherine L.P. Reid. Oxford: Oxford University Press; 1993.
10. Bobath B. Adult hemiplegia: evaluation and treatment. 3rd ed. Oxford: Heinemann; 1990.
11. Cauraugh JH, JJ Summers Neural plasticity and bilateral movements: a rehabilitation approach for chronic stroke. Prog Neurobiol 75(5):309-320.
12. National Cancer Action Team (NCAT). Rehabilitation pathway for brain and CNS tumours. London; 2009.
13. Pergolotti M, Williams GR, Campbell C, Munoz LA, Muss HB. Occupational therapy for adults with cancer: why it matters. Oncologist. 2016;21(3):314–9.
14. Schutte-Rodin S, Broch L, Buysse D, Dorsey C, Sateia M. Sleep: clinical guidelines for the evaluation and management of chronic insomnia in adults. J Clin Sleep Med. 2008;4(5):487–504.
15. Royal College of Occupational Therapists. https://www.rcot.co.uk/. Accessed 1 Oct 2017.
16. Ching W, Luhmann M. Neuro-oncologic physical therapy for the older person. Topics Geriatr Rehabil. 2011;27(3):184.
17. Van Cutsem E, Arends J. The causes and consequences of cancer-associated malnutrition. Eur J Oncol Nurs. 2005;9:51–63.
18. British and Irish Orthoptics Society. https://www.orthoptics.org.uk. Accessed 1 Sept 2017.
19. McCall MI, Leone A, Cusimano MD. Nutritional status and body composition of adult patients with brain tumours awaiting surgical resection. Can J Diet Pract Res. 2014;75(3):148–51.

# Teenagers and Young Adults/Transition Services: Implications for Nurses

# 17

Jane Robson

**Abstract**

Cancer care for teenagers and young adults (TYAs) is increasingly being recognised as a speciality in its own right due to the complexities involved of caring for this group of patients at such a significant developmental stage in their lives. Nurses caring for these young patients need to develop enhanced communication skills and knowledge in order to promote the best outcomes for these young people and their families.

This chapter outlines the developmental stages of adolescence and young adulthood and what impact a cancer diagnosis can have on the young person and their family and helps to explain some of the stereotypical adolescent behaviours young people may display at this stage of their lives. Key recommendations are suggested to promote therapeutic working with this age group, and opportunities for professional development are suggested to support the professional in working with TYAs.

**Keywords**

Teenagers · Adolescence · Cancer · Developmental stage · Transition · Palliative care

**Learning Outcomes**
- Gain a deeper understanding of the developmental stages (domains) of adolescence and young adulthood.
- Understand how a glioma diagnosis and the social stigma surrounding this can impact on a young adult in their adolescent years, and gain deeper insight into why typical adolescent behaviour is often displayed during this time.

J. Robson (✉)
Teenage Cancer Trust Lead TYA Nurse (East Anglia), Addenbrookes Hospital, Cambridge University Teaching Hospitals Foundation Trust, Cambridge, UK
e-mail: Jane.robson@addenbrookes.nhs.uk

© Springer Nature Switzerland AG 2019
I. Oberg (ed.), *Management of Adult Glioma in Nursing Practice*,
https://doi.org/10.1007/978-3-319-76747-5_17

- Gain deeper insight into your role as a health-care professional caring for this transitional age group, and recognise how you can promote therapeutic working with them to help achieve the best outcomes.

## 17.1   Introduction

Each year there are approximately 2400 new cases of cancer diagnosed in young people aged between 15 and 24 years in the UK (United Kingdom) [1]. This accounts for only 1% of cancer diagnoses and is rare in this age group, yet it is increasingly recognised that teenage and young adult (TYA) cancer is a distinct speciality in its own right due to the complexities of the cancer types and their behaviour and the particular challenges a cancer diagnosis in this age group presents.

Of the 2400 new cases of cancer diagnosed in young people every year, approximately 300 of these will be new diagnoses of tumours of the central nervous system, accounting for approximately 14% of overall cases, the fourth most common type of cancer diagnosis in young people [1].

A distinct group from those with a new diagnosis are those treated for brain tumours in childhood who transition into adult services and who may have significant morbidity from late effects of their cancer treatment (e.g. neurosurgery, radiotherapy, chemotherapy) which impacts on their physical or cognitive function and psychosocial development.

Young people who have a poor prognosis and need palliative care may have additional challenges because of the inconsistent structure of local palliative care and community services within the UK.

Nurses working within adult cancer care rarely come into contact with TYA patients because of its low incidence and therefore can feel particularly challenged when caring for the patient and their family.

This chapter will introduce the key concepts of caring for TYAs with cancer and explore how developmental stage can influence adjustment to a cancer diagnosis and how health professionals can interact with the patient to promote the best outcomes.

## 17.2   Adolescent Developmental Stage and the Impact of a Cancer Diagnosis

Adolescence is a time of massive change and readjustment as the young person attempts to make sense of themselves in the adult world and evolve an independent identity within complex modern society. Adolescence is a transitional period between childhood and adulthood where the young person develops characteristics and skills to enable them to adopt adult roles in society [2].

This transition involves significant changes spread over several years in multiple domains which will be explored below.

- Biological
- Cognitive
- Psychological
- Psychosocial
- Spiritual

## 17.2.1 Biological

The onset of puberty results in massive physiological changes in the adolescent body with development of primary and secondary sexual characteristics. It is not unusual for the young person to become increasingly self-conscious and sensitive to their appearance. Embarrassment and a heightened need for privacy are common as they compare themselves to their peers, and they can become hypersensitive to any deviation from what they identify as 'normal'. Anything that distinguishes them from their peers can have huge psychological implications as it can undermine self-confidence and the ability to interact positively with their social group, leading to isolation and withdrawal and subsequent mental health problems [3].

## 17.2.2 Cognitive

Another significant biological change occurring in the adolescent is changes within the structure and function of the brain, impacting on cognitive and behavioural development [4]. Studies of adolescent brain functioning by MRI have identified significant changes in the grey matter in the frontal lobe which is largely responsible for impulse and emotion control. During this time the brain rewires itself to enable better control of emotions and allow higher executive functioning [5]. Increased control and co-ordination of thoughts and behaviours are noted, working memory increases and improved reasoning and problem-solving skills can be identified. At the same time, there is an increased ability to explore hypothetical and abstract thinking which allows the young person to revaluate their own thoughts and spiritual beliefs and their place in wider society. They may take on others' opinions and views as they test out their own and challenge the parameters set by those previously with influence over their thoughts and feelings. The need for immediate gratification together with feelings of invulnerability may foster risk-taking behaviour with drugs, alcohol, sex and adrenalin highs.

Sleep patterns change as the sleep-inducing hormone melatonin peaks in this age group at 0100, as opposed to 2200 in adulthood, altering their natural body clock. Changes in sleep behaviour enable the TYA to stay up until the early hours and lie in late in the morning, often interpreted as 'laziness' by adults rather than a natural state for the adolescent [5].

Changes in the brain are a gradual process and are accompanied by the increasing impact of sex hormones in puberty, (testosterone and oestrogen), which can impact on emotional responses and make behaviour inconsistent and unpredictable [6].

### 17.2.3 Psychological

Psychological development in adolescence is focused around formation of a sense of identity and self-esteem and developing the emotional resilience needed in adulthood. It is heavily influenced by social factors, predominantly relationships with peers, sexual identity and other important relationships. It encompasses an emerging ideology of the world and the young person's place in it and is inherent in the personality development of the young person [6]. Young people tend to internalise thoughts and feelings and struggle to differentiate other people's thoughts and feelings from their own [6]. If they are preoccupied by a particular issue, they will assume everyone else shares the same thought and feeling. Therefore a negative thought about appearance can quickly develop into a problem with body image as the young person believes everyone else is fixated on the issue which is dominating their thoughts [6]. Hence, young people can be particularly sensitive to changes in appearance due to treatments such as scarring, hair loss, weight changes and disability. Young people may act out their frustrations and fears through classic adolescent behaviours such as mood swings, inconsistency, egocentricity and stretching boundaries which can be challenging to manage.

Mental health problems can emerge in adolescence, and if there is concern that the behaviour of the young person may be due to an underlying psychiatric disorder, rather than development norms exacerbated by emotional distress, prompt referral to psychiatric or psychological services should be made.

### 17.2.4 Psychosocial

As the young person is adjusting to the evolving physical and cognitive self, they are simultaneously trying to make sense of the society in which they live and how they fit into the world. Young people often receive bad press through the media and are constantly exposed to information and influence over social media. This can impact on how they view themselves and interact with those identified as in authority (e.g. parents, teachers, doctors, nurses). It can also influence how people in positions of authority stereotype the TYA and interact with them. Health professionals working with young people need to be mindful of how the young person may view their professional role and how this may impact on interactions with health professionals and the influence the health professional may have on the young person's behaviour. Young people reject paternalistic advice and do not like being told what to do as is often the approach in health care. TYAs respond much more positively to open, frank, non-judgemental communication, using information to enable them to make informed choices and produce their own solutions to the problems with which they are faced [7].

Human beings are social animals, and young people particularly need reinforcement of their acceptance from their social groups and judge their own value on how they identify and interact with peers. Peer relationships tend to be their major support structure. Anything that disrupts these relationships will have a negative impact on the young person's psychosocial wellbeing, and a cancer diagnosis causes major disruption in opportunities to socialise with peers due to interruptions in school/ college, work and social activities [6]. This can lead to the young person feeling isolated and lonely and exacerbate feelings of loss as they can miss out on shared experiences with their friends and major life events, e.g. university graduation or 'the prom'. The importance of these milestones must not be underestimated.

Adolescence is a time for exploring one's sexual identity and exploring intimate relationships. Healthy development of sexual identity impacts significantly on high self-esteem, and a cancer diagnosis which interrupts this phase of development can have a negative impact on self-esteem. Reduced engagement in social activities may reduce the young person's exposure to opportunities to develop the interpersonal skills necessary to foster development of intimate relationships in the future [8].

Early intimate relationships are tested by a cancer diagnosis as the young couple try to make sense of what it means to their burgeoning relationship and are unable to deal with the intense emotions, leading to feelings of rejection and isolation. Those in more established relationships may question their longer-term life plan including children as fertility may be compromised and they and their partner are faced with the anxiety and uncertainty of what the long-term prognosis means in terms of health and lifestyle expectations. Parents and partners may come into conflict as to who should be the primary carer for the young person as they attempt to juggle their feelings and combine the practicalities of caring for a young person with cancer with work and financial commitments, leading to feelings of confusion and resentment [6].

Close family relationships can vary within this age group from the child/parent dynamic to those who are parents themselves. A diagnosis of a life-threatening illness affects the whole family, impacting on parents, siblings and extended family members, and will depend upon the pre-existing dynamics in that particular family unit. Whatever relationships are important to the young person must be acknowledged and respected, and be mindful these relationships will be evolving as the young person moves along the treatment pathway through the developmental stages of adolescence. Where once a young person may be happy to share all information with their parents, for example, it is natural as they mature to have increasing independence and wish to discuss sensitive issues in private and they need to be given the opportunity to do so. Sense checking what the wishes of the young person are to ensure their wishes are met and confidentiality maintained is vital to enable these sensitive conversations to occur [7]. This can be challenging when the parent does not recognise how their child is developing into an autonomous young person and needs to be handled sensitively. This can be further complicated by the young person's inconsistency, moving along the developmental continuum in both directions, sometimes regressing to a greater level of dependency and childlike behaviour whilst at other times exhibiting a very independent autonomous self [6]. Regression is often seen in times of great stress such as when diagnosed with a life-challenging disease, and levels of independence can vary along the treatment pathway. Younger siblings can become resentful of the attention and time spent on the young person as they struggle to understand what is happening and the distress expressed by those close to them. They can blame the young person as the source of this distress, leading to feelings of guilt within the family.

In an attempt to protect their child, parents may wish to withhold distressing information or create dependency. The young person forced to become more dependent on parents after establishing some financial and social autonomy can become resentful and angry that their independent lifestyle is curtailed and opportunities lost. Young people are forced to spend far more time with parents than is normal for their age group which can inhibit further social interactions with peers and intimate partners. Parents should be supported to give their child time and space to engage in normal adolescent socialisation.

TYAs with gliomas may be more at risk of increased dependency on family members to carry out aspects of care or make decisions on their behalf not normal for this age group due to physical or cognitive impairments, making them particularly vulnerable. Safeguarding concerns for this age group may include inappropriate treatment decisions made by parents (e.g. forcing the TYA to proceed with further or alternative treatments with no proven benefit, withdrawing treatments, physical or emotional abuse by parents or partners or online abuse) [9]. Nurses working with the age group must ensure they receive appropriate safeguarding training for both children and adults as the age group straddles both children and adult safeguarding legislation (see Chap. 13).

It is important to remember that in today's society there are many complex family situations with multiple parents and grandparents. Parents may be estranged; new partners on the scene may have difficult relationships. It is helpful to understand how these relationships work, how the adults surrounding the TYA interact and how they support the young person in difficult times to avoid being caught up in confusing family situations/conflicts. Occasionally family conflicts can play out in the health-care setting as anxious family members are brought closely together at a time of great emotional stress.

A small proportion of TYAs will be young parents themselves. This adds additional pressures as they struggle with the uncertainty of their future and the additional pressures of being a parent and concern about being there to support the child emotionally and financially. Periods of separation from their child can be particularly traumatic as they struggle with not being able to care for their child as they would like. For those who need to attend hospital regularly, the need for additional childcare is a major concern and can have huge implications on the extended family emotionally, practically and financially.

A recent report on the costs of cancer in the UK by the charity CLIC Sargent [10] demonstrated that a cancer diagnosis in a young person adds an additional £600 to the family budget per month, putting families under huge financial and subsequent psychological strain.

## 17.2.5 Spiritual

It is usual through adolescence for young people to develop a sense of purpose and meaning of life, within or without a religious ideology, as their ability to assimilate ideas and experiences becomes more abstract and analytical. Young people facing a cancer diagnosis often are forced to reflect on issues not normally within the radar of young people and for which they may not have the intellectual or emotional maturity to process. Reflecting on the meaning of life and death at a time when their peers are focussed on what may be regarded as superficial life-style choices sets them apart from their peers [6]. They may question 'why me?' and may question any existing religious or spiritual beliefs as they face the uncertainty of their future. Their cancer experience can distinguish them from their peers and leave them feeling isolated in their beliefs, thoughts and feelings.

Adolescence is a time of major change which involves negotiating significant life milestones (e.g. leaving school, starting work, living independently). Such significant change can lead to considerable stress and, due to the limited emotional maturity of the young person, can lead to behaviours stereotypically labelled as adolescent which can be difficult to manage or understand without insight into adolescent development. Many young people negotiate these challenges in a positive way, but it is recognised that a cancer diagnosis at this crucial developmental stage can severely impact on the young person ability to develop a positive sense of self which can have lifelong implications on their quality of life [6].

## 17.3 Nursing Considerations in Caring for TYAs with Cancer

Developing and maintaining a therapeutic nursing relationship with the TYA patient are the bedrock of promoting positive outcomes in these patients [7]. Through understanding the stages in adolescent development, it is easier to explain why young people may exhibit behaviours which may be viewed as difficult and overcome the barriers to effective communication with this patient group, fostering self-engagement in their care.

### 17.3.1 Newly Diagnosed TYA Patient

Recognising the individuality of the young person, allowing them to tell their story in their words and demonstrating active listening skills foster a feeling of being valued and understood. Time is one of the most valuable resources within the health service and is constantly rationed as health professionals struggle to balance the demands of the job. However, investment in time with a young person at the start of their cancer journey results in much greater engagement and understanding, improved concordance with treatment regimens and better relationships with members of the health-care team [7]. This ultimately results in less reactive crisis management along the pathway and improved outcomes for the patient and their family.

Consent for treatment can pose challenges as, as long as the young person has capacity, they are able to consent to treatment (see Chap. 16). The health professional must ensure that the information given to ensure informed consent is in a way that can be understood by the young person and issues need to be addressed that may not normally be of concern in an older population, e.g. fertility. Parents often wish to be involved in the consent process, and if the young person wishes for their involvement, then it is helpful so they can support the young person in their decision. Occasionally, challenges arise when the young person's wishes differ from that of the parent. The parents may argue that their 'child' is too young and doesn't understand the implications of their decisions. This can be more complex if the young person has a degree of cognitive impairment due to surgery or treatment. The health team need to assess capacity and, if the young person has capacity, must honour the TYAs decision and support discussions between the family to reach a consensus where possible. It is important to remember that young people's view on the world and motivating factors can be considerably different to older adults and influence their decision-making in ways older adults may not understand. Because other adults think the decision is unwise does not mean that the young person lacks capacity. Inconsistency is also a feature of the adolescent brain so decisions may change rapidly as the TYA processes the information over time and perspectives change on the situation [5]. The role of the nurse as an advocate for the patient is paramount here to ensure the TYA's wishes are respected.

Holistic needs assessment (HNA) tools are employed as it is increasingly recognised that managing a disease in isolation of other aspects of a person's life does not result in good outcomes in terms of quality of life. TYA-friendly HNA tools do exist [11]. The differing focus of the TYA HNA tool is that it looks further into the future with a greater psychosocial focus, as well as dealing with immediate concerns, to look beyond the cancer diagnosis and at longer-term aspirations. It is used to start a conversation to build up the therapeutic relationship between the young person and health-care professional and identify actual or potential concerns which can be addressed to promote positive outcomes.

Opening up conversations about all aspects of the young person's life recognises the universal impact of a cancer diagnosis on them and their world and legitimises non-medical conversations around the topic so that the TYA is not reluctant to raise a concerns thinking that it may be outside the remit of the health professional. TYA's limited experience of the world may inhibit their willingness to ask questions about non-medical-related topics, but these may be of the greatest concern to the individual. TYAs should be offered to complete the HNA in private as parents/partners/peers may inhibit honest responses in some of the domains as the young person attempts to protect those they care about; alternatively family members may try to answer questions on the young person's behalf.

Some young people may be very reluctant to engage with the health professional and may be very introverted and reluctant to speak. The nurse should develop a relaxed, less formal style of communication whilst maintaining a professional manner [7]. Gentle encouragement and understanding and a willingness to approach them using an alternative tactic may be useful. For example, starting a conversation discussing what they are interested in socially, rather than their medical or psychological needs, can be a more effective way of facilitating a conversation to allow the TYA to begin to trust and open up to the professional. This may then lead on to more intense topics which the TYA finds more difficult to discuss, e.g. sexuality and fertility. Allow the TYA to lead the conversation at their pace; if the young person feels pushed or rushed, they may raise barriers which will inhibit future conversations. Sometimes it is easier for the young person to break the conversation down into bite-size chunks to allow them to process one issue before moving onto another aspect of their life. Again, let the TYA lead to encourage further disclosure. Also, acknowledge that at times the TYA may not be ready to discuss some aspects of their life with a relative stranger and this must be respected and revisited at a future date when the TYA is more confident in the relationship.

In order to build a therapeutic relationship with a TYA, consistency is vital as TYAs tend to be less willing to trust health professionals up front and need time to build the relationship. Therefore, avoiding multiple staff changes is advisable, but this must be balanced with creating an over-reliance on individual health-care professionals. The balance between maintaining professional boundaries and promoting a therapeutic working relationship can be particularly challenging for this age group. Due to the more relaxed communication style needed to interact with young people, it can be easy for the young person to misinterpret professional friendliness for friendship, and the nurse must be vigilant for signs of crossing boundaries and inappropriate interaction [12]. It is natural for adolescents to challenge boundaries so the nurse must be careful not to overreact but to re-emphasise the professional nature of the relationship.

The most important factor in these assessments is allowing the TYA to guide the conversation. At a time when they feel disempowered over an uncertain future, it reinforces a sense of control lost in the crisis of diagnosis [7].

It must be born in mind that due to the nature of a diagnosis of glioma, the young person may have neurological deficits as a direct result of the tumour or surgery which interrupts the development continuum and forces significant re-evaluation of the young person's future aspirations. These deficits may be cognitive or physical and care must be titrated to individual need. The important factor is that the TYA remains a unique individual with unique needs. The presence of cognitive or physical limitations has huge implications on the long-term impact on the individual and their immediate family, and they must be supported and signposted to agencies that can provide ongoing support.

## 17.3.2 Transition: Survivors of Childhood Cancer

Brain tumours are the second most common cancer type in children accounting for 26% of childhood cancers [1]. Many of these tumours occur in early childhood and are treated aggressively with a combination of surgery, radiotherapy and/or chemotherapy. Whilst survival rates have improved, significant late effects have been demonstrated in this population who are now growing up and transitioning to adult services.

The main late effects are endocrine (43%) [13] and neurocognitive sequelae [14], though cardiovascular late effects have also been reported [13]. Endocrine late effects are directly related to cranial radiation +/− chemotherapy and include hypothyroidism, growth hormone deficiency, osteoporosis and delayed puberty. Prepubescent referral to an endocrinologist for supplementation is essential to promote normal growth and development in the child, and the young person needs to remain under the care of specialist endocrinology teams for monitoring as function can continue to deteriorate over time.

In recent years, clinical trials have focused on reducing late toxicity whilst maintaining cure rates, but there remains a significant proportion of young people who will transition into adult services who were treated with more toxic regimens but will survive into adulthood. It has been demonstrated that children treated with cranial radiation who experience neurocognitive sequelae have a poorer quality of life than their sibling controls [14].

In addition to the potential developmental challenges posed by physical causes, there may have been significant interruptions in schooling and social interactions which have impacted on the development of the young person's social networks and self-identity. It may be that the young person will never have the capacity to live independently from family members and the family unit, and long-term future planning to allow the young person to meet their full potential involving external agencies that can support the young person and family to achieve this may be the ultimate goal.

Successful transition from children to adult services requires involvement from professionals from both disciplines. It should be a planned supportive process in partnership with the patient and parents. The TYA team may support this process by attending clinics with the patient in both settings to ensure continuity of staff throughout the transition process. TYAC (Teenagers and Young Adults with Cancer) charity has produced 'transition best practice statement' which can provide guidance on how to manage this emotionally challenging time to promote best outcomes for the patient and their family [15].

### 17.3.3 Palliative Care

Some young people will be diagnosed with a high-grade glioma which will shorten their life expectancy and will need involvement of palliative care to optimise their quality of life and promote a peaceful death. Conversations around palliative care and end of life can be particularly challenging with the young as they struggle to come to terms with the reality of their own mortality. Even when young people openly talk about dying, the ability to accept that this is inevitable for them is counterbalanced with a hope that somehow a cure will be found. It is not unusual in conversations for young people to demonstrate inconsistency, one minute appearing to accept their fate whilst the next planning a holiday with family and friends many months into the future. Planning for the future helps the young person to process the concept of a limited life expectancy and maintain hope in a crisis situation.

Ideally, the health professional giving bad news should be known to the patient, and they should already have a trusting professional relationship in which open communication is embedded. Though this is not always possible, employing effective age-appropriate communication techniques will promote therapeutic conversations around this difficult subject [16].

It is important that the health professional that introduces the poor prognosis has skills in communicating effectively with young people, using language that is not ambiguous or misleading. Most young people prefer honesty and openness and wish to be involved in these conversations from the start. Sometimes the health professionals feel it easier to talk to family members before the young person, but this should only be done if the young person expressly wishes it. If the young person finds it too difficult to discuss end of life issues, they may abdicate this responsibility to family members, and this wish must be respected. Sometimes family members ask health professionals to withhold information from the patient to 'protect' them, but collusion should not be encouraged as it will undermine trust between the health professional and the young patient. Supporting open and honest communication between the family members is challenging as often they may be anxious about displaying fears and anxieties in order to protect other family members, including the young person, from their own fears and witnessing their own distress.

Conflict may arise between the young person, partner and family where their wishes differ, e.g. preferred place of care for end of life. A young person may wish to die at home, but the parents may feel unable to cope and are too frightened at this prospect; a partner may wish to be primary carer for their loved one, but the family may wish to take them 'home' to die. These complex scenarios require sensitivity and diplomacy, and it is often useful to involve another member of the multidisciplinary team, e.g. chaplaincy, who can support these very difficult conversations. They may also be able to help with practicalities such as writing wills and planning funeral arrangements.

A practical consideration in palliative provision in the UK is where the most appropriate community support available is in their locality and will be dependent on age. In many areas of the UK, children's hospices support young people and families up to the age of 19, with adult hospice services accessible from age 16 years (though this can vary between regions). Children's hospices focus on supportive care for children and young people mainly with degenerative progressive conditions, and it can be challenging to deliver end of life care to young people requiring unfamiliar medication in relatively high doses which need to be reviewed and reassessed regularly by an expert in palliative care. The environment is often designed with very much younger children in mind. Adult hospices on the other hand are set up to manage complex end of life symptoms and may have 24-hour expert medical cover. However, the environment is provided for adults at a much later age in life, and young people may not find it an appealing place to receive care. Services are constantly evolving and improving, and designs for new services are considering the needs of the younger patient, but provision is variable throughout the UK.

Provision of community nursing support can also be inconsistent, particularly for those aged 17 as often children's community services are commissioned up to age 16, whilst adult do not begin until 18 years of age. Specialists in TYA care will be aware of where these local disparities occur and should have strategies to work around them.

Encouraging early engagement with local services to promote building therapeutic relationships and normalising the hospice experience are recognised as best practice [17]. However, young people and families are often reluctant to engage with hospice services as they feel this is tantamount to accepting the inevitability of the end which conspires against their need for hope.

NHS England [17] advocate that every young person should have a key worker who can co-ordinate end of life care. Each region in the UK has a principal treatment centre for TYA care, and the most appropriate individual to take on this complex role on may be the TYA clinical nurse specialist who should have a pre-existing relationship with the patient and their family and will be familiar with local services provision appropriate to this age group.

When a young person dies, the loss is not only felt by the family and staff caring for the individual but also by the other patients and families who may have travelled with them on their cancer journey. The same rules of open honest sensitive communication apply whilst at the same time respecting the privacy of the young person who has died. Often, young people find out about the death of a fellow patient through social media and will be aware of the loss before contact with a health-care professional. Exploring how this has impacted on the young person can facilitate conversations not previously explored on philosophical and practical discussions around the meaning of life and mortality.

## 17.3.4 TYA Specialist Multidisciplinary Team

TYA care is recognised as a speciality in its own right in the UK and services are structured around a specialist TYA multidisciplinary team. Members of the TYA multidisciplinary team can help support treating teams in the care of TYAs in non-specialist TYA areas. Each region in the UK has a specialist TYA service which can help to provide support for this age group.

TYA services in the UK are based on a structure of a TYA principal treatment centre (PTC) and a number of designated TYA centres which feed into the PTC and have a TYA specialist support team including medics, clinical nurse specialists, youth workers and AHPs [18]. The actual configuration of this service differs from region to region, depending on the local configuration of children and adult oncology and haematology services. The regional team is there to support the care of TYA patients wherever they receive their care and can be called upon as an expert resource to support the local treating teams manage their young patients. The TYA team has access to specialist services and resources and will refer on to other support services external to the NHS such as social services and charities providing psychosocial support and practical assistance to young people. Building relationships with the TYA support team locally can facilitate access to their support when facing a challenging TYA patient and open gateways to additional support services which can facilitate optimal outcomes for the young person and their family.

TYA services support young people in a multitude of different ways including the novel approach to delivering activities and events which bring groups of young people together. It has been previously noted that cancer can be an isolating experience for a TYA due to its rarity. By encouraging networking of patients, and their families, the young people can share their experiences with others who understand what it's like to have cancer at an early age, likewise with family members. The therapeutic impact of these social opportunities should not be underestimated, and conversations can vary from the intensely serious to the extremely superficial within the same forum. Engaging with TYA services facilitates access to such activities and can help the young person process their experience through social interaction with other young people who can empathise as they have shared the same experience.

### 17.3.5 TYA Professional Development

The challenges of caring for a young person with cancer have been noted above and can discombobulate even the most experienced health-care professional. Professional development opportunities exist which can help develop the skills and attributes needed to care for this complex group. Education varies from single study days for those who encounter young people irregularly in their area of work to master level postgraduate courses for those working consistently with young people with cancer. Undertaking training specific to TYA care can demystify this complex patient group and facilitate developing skills to deliver expert nursing care to the young people and their families.

Advanced communication skills training is well recognised as a core requirement for senior nurses working with cancer patients as it enables difficult and challenging conversations to take place with patients at a time of great stress and emotion whilst managing one's own emotional response to distressing circumstances.

The impact on the professional of caring for these young patients along the cancer pathway should not be underestimated. This can be particularly profound when a young person dies. It is important that the nurse has insight into the impact of a death of a young patient on themselves and colleagues, and debriefs and clinical supervision can be useful in managing these emotions and promoting resilience when working with this challenging patient group.

A competency framework exists to support nurses working with TYAs to assist in delivering excellent care and identifying areas for professional development [19].

### 17.4 Conclusion

This chapter has outlined the particular challenges in caring for a young person with a malignant diagnosis. By understanding the developmental challenges of adolescence and how these impact on the various domains in adolescent development, the nurse can adapt her care to optimise a successful outcome for the young patient.

**Key Recommendations**

- Treat every young person as an individual and respect their attitude and beliefs; do not make assumptions on what they think and feel.
- Adopt a flexible, less formal communication style to allow time to build trust and confidence with the young person.
- Allow some flexibility in ward routines, visiting times and treatment plans to enable the young person to have appropriate support from family, facilitating attendance at important events, and to continue socialising with peers to maintain some semblance of normality.
- Support the family to give some space to their child to allow time with partners and friends.
- Be aware of the sensitivities of body image issues and do not be dismissive of their concerns.
- Ensure the TYA has privacy, provide a single room if possible when inpatient, facilitate access to the Internet so they can stay in touch with friends and allow family to stay if requested.
- Understand how the changes in adolescence can drive behaviour to promote innovative ways of engaging the young person whilst ensuring unacceptable behaviour is not tolerated and boundaries maintained.
- Understand the importance of family in a young person's world and offer the family support so they have the resilience to cope with their distress.
- Be aware of the difficulties in caring for this patient group and engage in opportunities to increase resilience.
- Involve the specialist TYA services locally to help support care of the young patient and to facilitate access to the specialist resources available to support them through their cancer journey.

# References

1. Cancer Research UK. http://www.cancerresearchuk.org/health-professional/cancer-statistics/teenagers-and-young-adults-cancers/incidence#heading-Seven. Accessed 11 Aug 2017.
2. Larson R, Wilson S. Adolescence across place and time: globalization and the changing pathways to adulthood. In: Lerner R, Steinberg L, editors. Handbook of adolescent psychology. New York: Wiley; 2004.
3. Taylor RM, Pearce S, Gibson F, Fern L, Whelen T. Developing a conceptual model of teenage and young adult experiences of cancer through meta-synthesis. Int J Nurs Stud. 2013;50:823–46.
4. Coleman C. Thinking and reasoning. In: Coleman C, editor. The nature of adolescence. 4th ed. London: Routledge; 2011. p. 40–55.
5. Morgan N. Blame my brain – the amazing teenage brain revealed. London: Walker Books Ltd.; 2013.
6. Finch A, McCann B, Ingram B, Poole J, Knott C, Newton C, Cable M. Development and the impact of cancer. In: Smith S, Mooney S, Cable M, Taylor R, editors. The blueprint of care for teenagers and young adults with cancer. 2nd ed. London: Teenage Cancer Trust; 2017. p. 17–46.

7. Morgan S, Davies S, Palmer S, Plaster M. Sex, drugs and rock 'n' roll: caring for adolescents and young adults with cancer. J Clin Oncol. 2010;28:4825–30.
8. Zebrak B, Bleyer A, Albritton K, Medearis S, Tang J. Assessing the health care needs of adolescent and young adult cancer patients and survivors. Cancer. 2006;107:2915–23.
9. Cable M. Staffing considerations. In: Smith S, Mooney S, Cable M, Taylor R, editors. The blueprint of care for teenagers and young adults with cancer. 2nd ed. London: Teenage Cancer Trust; 2017. p. 53–61.
10. Clic Sargent. Cancer costs. The financial impact of treatment on young cancer patients and their families. 2016. http://www.clicsargent.org.uk/sites/files/clicsargent/cancer-costs-report-2017rebrand.PDF. Accessed 11 Aug 2017.
11. Cargill J, Cheshire Jand Hewett-Avison S. Holistic needs and supportive care. In: Smith S, Mooney S, Cable M, Taylor RM, editors. Blueprint of care for teenagers and young adults with cancer. 2nd ed. Teenage Cancer Trust: London; 2016. p. 63–76.
12. Royal College of Nursing. Adolescence: boundaries and connections. An RCN guide for working with young people. London: Royal College of Nursing; 2008.
13. Gurney JG, Kadan-Lottick NS, Packer RJ, Neglia JP, Sklar CA, Punyko JA, Stovall M, Yasui Y, Nicholson HS, Wolden S, McNeil DE, Mertens AC, Robison LL. Endocrine and cardiovascular late effects among adult survivors of childhood brain tumours. Atlanta, GA: American Cancer Society; 2003.
14. Mulhern RK, Merchant TE, Gajjar A, Reddick WE, Kun LE. Late neurocognitive sequelae in survivors of brain tumour in childhood. Lancet Oncol. 2004;5:399–408.
15. TYAC. Teenagers and young adults with cancer. Transition TYAC best practice statement for health professionals. 2016. https://www.tyac.org.uk/transition-tyac-best-practice-statement-for-health-professionals. Accessed 6 Aug 2017.
16. Bates AT, Kearney JA. Understanding death with limited experience in life. Dying children's and adolescents understanding of their own terminal illness and death. Curr Opin Support Palliat Care. 2015;9:40–5.
17. NHS England. NHS cancer services for teenagers and young adults. London: NHS England; 2015. https://www.england.nhs.uk/commissioning/wp-content/uploads/sites/12/2015/nhs-canc-serv-tya.pdf. Accessed 10 Aug 2017.
18. National Institute for Health and Care Excellence. Guidance on cancer services: improving outcomes in children and young people with cancer. London: NICE; 2005.
19. Teenage Cancer Trust/Royal College of Nursing. London. London: Teenage Cancer Trust/Royal College of Nursing; 2014.

## Suggested Reading

Smith S, Mooney S, Cable M, Taylor RM, editors. The blueprint of care for teenagers and young adults with cancer. 2nd ed. London: Teenage Cancer Trust; 2016.

# 18

## Zara Lorenz

*Suddenly we're shaken*
*To our very core*
*A family we stand the tide*
*But the wind still howls*
*The wind still howls*

(Sophie, my daughter *The Wind, It Howls*)

**Abstract**

When Chris was diagnosed with a brain tumour in early 2005, it changed our lives, a rug pulled sharply from under our feet. Thirteen years on we have dealt with the reality of the symptoms, the grief of having our future expectations shattered and the anticipatory grief. With the constant awareness also comes appreciation and extraordinary joy in everyday life, which can't be taken for granted in the context of the uncertainty of the prognosis.

Being a carer wasn't what I had expected, but it is what has happened. Our experience has evolved over time, with distinct phases, from the adjustment and acceptance of the diagnosis through the crisis periods, treatments and cycles of scans and now a normality that exists whilst also being constantly aware that the brain tumour is impacting in very many ways. Together we are continuing on this journey, a journey I would like to be able to stop at times, but also one that I don't want to end, as I do not want my partner to die—it is such a complex dilemma.

**Learning Outcomes**
- To gain a deeper understanding and insight into how a glioma diagnosis not only affects the patient but their loved ones and family members too.

Z. Lorenz (✉)
Department of Neurosurgery, Addenbrooke's Hospital, Cambridge University Hospitals NHS Foundation Trust, Cambridgeshire, UK
e-mail: ingela.oberg@addenbrookes.nhs.uk

© Springer Nature Switzerland AG 2019
I. Oberg (ed.), *Management of Adult Glioma in Nursing Practice*,
https://doi.org/10.1007/978-3-319-76747-5_18

277

- To better understand the burdensome role a carer takes on and acknowledge the impact (financial, emotional, physical, etc.) this subsequently has on them.
- To gain first-hand insight into issues experienced by a carer and understand what we can do as healthcare professionals to holistically support them better.

My daughter (20) uses her song writing and music to express and process her emotional responses to significant life experiences. She wrote 'The Wind, it Howls' after hearing our recent news that Chris needs further treatment. I'm struck by how well she captures so much of what I've been hoping to say, with considerably more ease, in so few beautifully chosen phrases and eloquent words.

Yesterday we had our scheduled oncology appointment. We have a well-established routine—we walk to Queen's Square from King's Cross, familiar streets. Chris says *aren't we going to the tall building*? I say *no, we never have appointments there*; he's confused as he had his last scan there. Chris jokes that I'm his 'satnav' and only need to come to get him there. The previous evening, Chris said I didn't need to come, and I said I did, as one day he will have news and have to make decisions and then won't fully remember what's discussed, and that's more stressful for me.

As we walk we recap with each other what we would like to discuss. Chris wants to ask about prognosis; I notice my irritation; he always wants to know what's going to happen. I explain that at some point the tumour will change, he will have treatment and then another interval of active surveillance, which will be shorter than this one, and then treatment again. I reassure him he won't be dying very soon. None of this is unusual conversation on route to the appointment.

We walk in and sit down and are called through more or less immediately. Today's the day when the game changes again: the oncologist quickly tells us the scans show change. We are all a little surprised, numb even, had become accustomed to stable scans and hoped this might have continued for longer. I like to see the scan as it helps me to visualise and process the news: seeing is somehow believing. Contemplating sharing the news is difficult, and we debate and agree on how to explain it to our 13-year-old son and Chris's 90-year-old mother. We both cry on the train on the way home. Here we are, heading into active treatment.

I have attended almost all of the oncology appointments with him: he has had over 50 MRI scans. Therefore, over 50 cycles of anticipating, waiting and assimilating news have been our main overriding experience.

Thirteen years on my family and I have dealt with the reality of the symptoms, the grief of having our future expectations shattered, and the anticipatory grief. This has now become our normality. With the constant awareness also comes appreciation and extraordinary joy in everyday life, which can't be taken for granted in the context of the uncertainly of the prognosis. Our experience has evolved over time, with distinct phases, from the adjustment and acceptance of the diagnosis through the crisis periods, treatments and cycles of scans and now a normality that exists whilst also being constantly aware that the brain tumour is impacting in very many ways. This can be an isolating experience.

Being a carer wasn't what I had expected, but it is what has happened. When Chris was diagnosed with a brain tumour in early 2005, it changed my life, a rug pulled sharply from under my feet. As a family, this moment became our reality, our daily life. Together we are continuing on this journey, a journey I would like to be able to stop at times but also one that I don't want to end, as I do not want my partner to die, but at times I do wish for the caring, accommodating, compromising part of my life to end. It is such a complex dilemma.

I chose to be engaged and informed, educating myself and facing it head on. I became my partners advocate. For me it was important to acknowledge what I was frightened of, which was quite a lot of things, not least expecting my partner to die and being left alone with young children. To prepare myself and understand the situation as best I could, I sought out good information and found knowledgeable people to speak to, including charities and organisations.

I also learnt how to slide, between being partner, lover, advocate, carer, parent and breadwinner. Sometimes, inevitably, I slip up and am in the wrong mode at the wrong time, which is tough. Mostly I'm very positive and well-adapted to our circumstances, engaged with life, my family and work and my sense of a future. I also know that I can cope with the unexpected, and even manage a crisis well, and I find that not much phases me. But this has taken a long time; I'm grateful that we have had the time to allow our circumstances to feel normal.

I have also learnt to look after myself, which is sometimes exceptionally hard to do. Even though it's become easier to pay attention and listen to what my mind and body need, it's still a struggle to respond to these needs, particularly in the context of the competing needs of my family, partner and children.

## 18.1  Our Story

When Chris was diagnosed, it happened to me too. It's like 'we' have the brain tumour. It's residing in and is part of his body, but it affects us both and affects how we interact with each other and the world we live in, impacting daily in one way or another. It is, of course, more his, but it is also ours.

Our experiences are very different. This was apparent from the outset: he was the one having the seizures, but retained no conscious memory of them, whilst I was witness to the vivid detail of it all. This gave me the capacity to process what might be happening, whilst Chris could only remember fleeting details. Chris's ability to process the situation and any new developments was impacted in the early days by seizures, by the tumour itself, surgery, medication, memory loss, fatigue and simply not feeling well. His experience is different and he would be writing a very different account.

Through the years we have also been witness to and part of a change in how brain tumours are understood. The original diagnosis and prognosis were given in terms of grade and cell type, but these are no longer considered so predictive. The shift has been to genetics and biomarkers giving greater stratification and providing more clarity around disease progression and prognosis. This is reflected in how we first understood Chris's tumour and how right now we are waiting for its methylation status (referred to as MGMT) to be clarified, as this test wasn't available at the last point of treatment 8 years ago. This marker predicts how well Chris's tumour is likely to respond to chemotherapy.

As we have moved through different phases of this journey, there are a variety of themes and experiences that have emerged. Whilst some of these would be familiar, everyone will experience them differently at different times and in the context of their individual social and family circumstances.

This is my personal account, of living with my partner with a brain tumour; others will and do experience this differently and want to cope, live and manage very differently from how we have chosen to. There is no one way to do this. It is individual. A compassionate and kind experience of the healthcare service makes a significant difference to how this diagnosis and reality impacts on lives.

## 18.2    Pre-diagnosis Symptoms

The first day that we knew something was not right, but only with the benefit of hindsight, I was 4 months pregnant and we were walking on the beach. Chris was suddenly overcome by an urgent need to leave and go home, saying the inspectors were coming. I went along with it, putting it down to stress, as there were no inspectors anywhere in sight.

Again, with the benefit of hindsight, Chris was likely having an absence seizure and over the coming months between seven and ten partial seizures a day, with a distinctive facial drop on one side, like an emotional yawn. All of these things were just a bit odd, and didn't really add up until Chris started to have regular seizures in his sleep, and then the epilepsy was both undeniable and unmissable.

It was the early hours of Sunday morning in late November 2004, when the distinctive roar of Chris's breath being forced from his lungs as his muscles constricted startled me awake. His unconscious jerking movements followed and continued for what felt like forever, in reality only a matter of minutes. Adrenaline flooded my body and our rollercoaster ride began.

Regaining consciousness, Chris was very confused by the presence of two men in green suits, amulance crew, in our bedroom. This was the frightening bit for him: who were they? Why were they there? His complete lack of knowledge of his seizure added to the dynamic: he didn't think there was anything else wrong.

We had been to Chris's cousin's funeral the day before, and when in A&E I was asked about alcohol consumption, I'd said he had a few. I literally meant a few! We had a small baby and were not big drinkers anyway, so I was talking about a beer and a couple of glasses of wine over an afternoon and evening. I believe now the team we saw assumed it was considerably more and therefore treated it as an isolated seizure. An urgent referral to a neurologist was made, but when it came through, it was for March which was 4 months away. Unfortunately, he didn't have a CT scan, which would have identified the tumour there and then.

Chris then went on to have one complex night-time seizure a week for a further 6 weeks. I could feel them build, almost sense them coming. We went to the GP three or four times; desperate for clarity, they chased the referral. Sometime between Christmas and New Year, Chris had a seizure at 12.30 am; I felt relieved I could now rest as I had no need to be in a heightened state of alert. However, at 4 am I was woken by the roar of his breath being forced from his body once again.

By now I was documenting exactly what was happening: how long the convulsions lasted, how long he lay recovering with jagged breath and how long it took for him to regain consciousness. This second seizure really tipped my stress levels over the edge. Who do you call at 4 am? I debated calling an ambulance, but how would that help? It hadn't last time; it had only resulted in a referral that was still being chased. I thought of my children sleeping and the disruption and distress it would cause them. I eventually called the out of hours GP and spoke with a very lovely GP who listened and helped me personally and urged us to see a neurologist.

## 18.3  Diagnosis

We saw a neurologist soon after the night of two seizures. He said it was very likely a brain tumour and arranged a scan. Chris was halfway down the stairs to the kitchen where I was standing, when he received the phone call from the neurologist confirming the scan had identified a brain tumour. I felt relieved, pleased even. We knew the cause of the epilepsy, and it could be fixed; Chris would have surgery. All the people I knew of who had brain tumours had had them removed, so that's what would happen. A year later we could expect this to be behind us.

On the Monday, we attended hospital with Alex in a sling. What happened next was so unexpected and incomprehensible. Chris's tumour was in a tricky place and could not be completely removed. This was a game changer and very shocking news. Chris was booked in for a biopsy a week later. This is still invasive brain surgery and carries risks. Our son was just 3 months old at the time, and my partner's first child, and we were full of excitement with our expanding family and new life together. Three nail-biting weeks later, we learnt it was a grade 2 (diffuse) astrocytoma. We moved to 'watch and wait', as it was then called (now, normally referred to as 'active monitoring'). At the time it felt like doing nothing, just looking again in 3 months' time.

The early years were very hard on Chris; denial played a big part. The seizures were under control and he was back driving a year later. He felt well and functioned normally; we had the cycles of scan and stress to remind us and tell us otherwise.

## 18.4  New Diagnosis, New Prognosis

Chris continued under 'watch and wait' for 3.5 years, having 3-monthly scans with the results appointments to follow. During this time, he was reviewed by a neurosurgeon. At each 3-monthly appointment, we would ask the same questions, seek impossible clarity, long for some certainties and were left with a sense that the tumour was highly unpredictable, that things, the tumour and Chris could change at any moment. Our lives were punctuated by these 3-monthly scans creating a rhythm of joy, relief and anxiety with waves of fear. The concept of time is very interesting, as it goes at quite a different pace when waiting for scan results. The institution's sense of reasonable time was not the same as ours, and the knowledge that someone else already knows something that you don't yet was hard to live with.

We had an early spring holiday in Spain, and Chris was feeling particularly well, and then on our return, we had an appointment that showed that the tumour was showing signs of change. There was no correlation between how he felt and what the scan showed. Chris's tumour had grown and showed enhancement, a fairly small white spot to my untrained eye. He had de-bulking surgery, a craniotomy which is a big deal. I knew this was a turning point, and whilst Chris was undergoing surgery, I waited and was overcome with a sense and a knowing that our lives, and Chris, were changing, being changed, and that things would never be quite the same again. And they weren't.

This surgery did move the goal posts, in a few ways. An important one was it led to a new more nuanced diagnosis and prognosis, grade 3 (anaplastic) oligodendroglioma. We had surgical and oncology second opinions early on, and we did not go with the initial chemotherapy and radiotherapy treatment offered, but with the recommendations from the second opinion (not an easy thing to do), offering chemotherapy only. This second opinion led to further molecular testing which gave us the valuable information that the tumour was also 1p19q co-deleted (see pathology chapter for further details on molecular diagnostics). We hadn't considered that his diagnosis and prognosis could change. We had understood it was all about grade, so this was a big thing to take in and confusing: grade 3 was not good news, whilst a co-deleted 1p19q was better news. Just how good was not clear at the time.

Chris went on to have PCV chemotherapy in Brighton, with delays to chemotherapy cycles due to liver problems. The treatment makes the person with the brain tumour feel unwell, my caring role more physically demanding and what I'm juggling all the more complex.

Soon after Chris's PCV chemotherapy treatment ended, his oncologist moved hospital. It was planned well; we were told personally, had notice and were able and supported to consider our options. After a period of time, we decided to move hospitals as there was no new neuro-oncologist in sight. This has been positive: the oncologist from whom we had sought our second opinion was now Chris's oncologist. She was really engaged with research, which was reassuring, and she was confident with 1p-19q factor, which gave us confidence. The sense of new prognosis grew as we had more and more stable scans. We had more time and began to believe we could expect to have much more. We changed oncologists again, this time with an unexpected departure, yet again leaving for a professorship elsewhere. We were not told, even by letter, which was deeply disappointing. It was pretty difficult to be faced with number four in such a short period of time.

The relationship feels so important, and all these changes, which were outside of our control, added stress. Each oncologist has a different style, in particular around how they share information, and this shapes the relationship and the power balance between Chris and the tumour in impacting upon and shaping our lives. The difference in culture between the two hospitals is subtle; the new one suited us, the tone of the appointments was different, they were timed at our convenience, and there was a sense of hope, but not false hope, optimism and a sense of possibility.

Since the surgery and chemotherapy, Chris has had regular stable scans, despite experiencing considerably more symptoms. Chris has had significant fatigue, pain and memory difficulties, mood swings and difficulty concentrating for sustained periods. Maintaining family life to the best of our ability, and planning so that he can participate as fully as possible, is an ongoing work in progress, requiring flexibility, resilience and compassion and a huge amount of love. Managing extended family has in our case been an additional strain at times. Our acceptance that there is not a 'cure' can be perceived as appearing to give up hope, which is not the case, but living in ignorance is most definitely not an option.

## 18.5   Cycle of Scans

### 18.5.1  Scans and Waiting for Results

Why you're having a scan shapes the experience: diagnoses, monitoring treatment and active surveillance are all very different, with different motivations and desired outcomes and therefore different experiences. I was so relieved, even pleased, when Chris's tumour was diagnosed, as it made sense of sudden-onset epilepsy in his mid-40s, which was a welcome explanation from a hard-to-get scan.

Chris finds the scan experience challenging, not the scanning process, noise or clostrophobia some people feel, for him its being passive, having things done to you, he will wondering how easily the cannula will get put in, will there be any staff there he is met before, what are they like? Then there is the knowledge that they see his tumour there and then, and yet give nothing away, no infomation. Then several weeks would follow waiting for the results, with increasing anxiety and living with the knowledge that someone knows something about you or your loved one that you do not, which he finds is really challenging. Please bear this level of anxiety in mind when communicating the results with patients and relatives.

Scans and the appointments following them punctuated our lives. There is a rhythm to the cycle of scans and results appointments. Planning more than 3 months ahead was almost tempting fate, and in hindsight, it was protective to think like this, as having plans for 6 months or a year's time ahead that you might not be able to do would create even more loss and grief.

How the clinical team present and share the information, judging how to deliver information on individual basis is also key to the experience, as the same truth can be presented in many ways. We have had bad news presented in such a way we have left feeling positive and hopeful, whilst good news badly presented has left us feeling anxious and scared.

At first, active surveillance feels like you're doing nothing, and then you come to realise it's not; it's more proactive monitoring. Whilst we came to understand fairly quickly that this is a good thing, it was very hard for extended family to understand, which is part of what we had to deal with.

For about the first 4 years, these appointments were planned absolutely to the clinician's time frames, and the preference, as in clinical trials, is to have regular data with imaging at 12-week intervals. This meant that scans and associated appointments results fell with no regard to our life, heightening the emotion and sense of importance, falling on our wedding anniversary and on or very close to family birthdays. We had entered a system that came first, was inflexible and that we had to comply with: it couldn't accommodate our requests. It emphasised that the tumour came first, rather than Chris as a person. I didn't feature anywhere, nor did our family. We became wiser and did manage to move scans so sometimes it was as short as a 5-day wait until the appointment, which was much better.

The 3-month cycles actually go very quickly, as in fact it's 9/10 weeks between the appointment and next scan. Immediately after the scan results, we often experienced initial euphoria, an extraordinary sense of being alive, intense gratitude, then a crash and several weeks of recovering and assimilating the news that it, the tumour, was still there. I would often experience a heightened sense of gratitude for stability, along with a desperate isolation as my fears and concerns would often go unspoken or rarely spoken. I've felt euphoric with relief after scans that showed 'no significant change' or 'stable' depending on the clinician, when they coincided with significant life events and changes for my children, such as moving school or important exams that impact their future. I'm ever conscious of how all this impacts on them.

In the earlier years, each scan and subsequent results appointment provided an opportunity to ask questions, to understand a bit better. It helped to keep asking the same questions a slightly different way and hearing very similar answers and explanations, as this was helpful, part of assimilation and acceptance. The scan and appointment were also a stark reminder of the massive presence inside my partner's brain, changing how he feels about himself and acts in the world and how he relates to me and our children. He was in denial at first (for at least a year), and then he began to believe it, accept it and feel sad, angry and at times depressed, and he would also dip into feeling guilty about how this impacted us all. Guilt was not something I could indulge: Chris hadn't chosen or imposed it, it had happened and we would deal with it together.

Scans can be enormously reassuring, especially during treatment as you're hoping for particular news, confirmation that the treatment is effective, shrinkage or even the possibility that what remains might be operable. After two cycles of PCV, both Chris and I, as well as the oncologist, needed to know if chemotherapy was working, to keep going, to frame our outlook and to gain strength: hope is so difficult to balance alongside preparing for seeing no change or even disease progression. That first scan after two cycles of PCV chemo was really important. The shrinkage was amazing, and we felt that our oncologist wanted it as much as we did. He admitted he was a little nervous too, and it felt very human, which really helped.

Chris often pays considerably more attention to how he is feeling in the weeks leading up to the appointment. The one time he was feeling really brilliant and well, and we were just back from a holiday to Spain, was when we had the appointment that the upgrade was suspected and de-bulking surgery and chemotherapy and radiotherapy were proposed. This mismatch between Chris feeling really good, not anxious and looking fantastically healthy with a light tan and the disease progression was so hard to make sense of. He had no obvious symptoms to suggest change. This was also when the diagnosis and prognosis changed.

Now many years later, we have a 6-month interval, which is so different. Scans are also digital, viewed on a computer screen, smaller as a result, emailable and something you can take home via a photo on your phone. Every 6 months really allows you to get on with living in between; it feels like a long time in a good way. I don't go along to scans anymore, mostly due to it taking all day and wanting to be able to do the school run and be home for the children. So, I hear about them: did they get the cannula in easily, what were the scan people like, he often falls asleep during them now, and maybe something else about the day. We have the 2 weeks' wait, which we accept, and then the appointment. We worry less and almost forget about it; it finally has become routine. We have conversations the day of the appointment or the night before, but it doesn't run our life. The conversations are comfortable and practised; we can talk with ease about Chris's fear that he will get bad news and die quickly. I assure him that's most unlikely; we will have to face more treatment, which will be the consequence. Scans and appointments are also planned to fit in with our life, not the other way around, so not the week of family birthdays or the first week back after summer holidays. We know who we will see, and our oncologist knows us.

It is hard sharing news from scans and appointments, especially for Chris's mothers, as there is nothing acceptable or right about the possibility that her son may predecease her, no matter how well he has been for so long. She is now 90 and this remains the case. Sometimes, she thought that I wasn't fighting hard enough for him, seeking out the right person, considering all the options. To appease her, we had Chris' scans sent to an American doctor/magician, and the latest were sent to a proton centre. It was not easy to be the bad guy, constantly delivering negative information, as I endlessly explained why X wouldn't work or Y wasn't suitable for his tumour type or size. My mother-in-law would send newspaper cuttings about any brain tumour treatment innovation or treatment expecting them to work for Chris, refusing or not being able to believe that we had explored all avenues. She wanted to believe that if I just tried harder, we could find a cure and Chris would be better. This dynamic created so much stress. What I desperately wanted and needed was to be supported, as well as some compassion and understanding.

What Helps:

- Minimising the wait for scan results and test results as much as possible
- Being genuine
- Respectful communication
- Providing quality evidence-based information
- Listening to what we feel is important, our values
- Building relationships with key clinicians and continuity
- A supportive team

The experience of time when waiting for results is important to highlight, and how the personal experience intersects with the institutional systems. It's a real emotional balance of preparing for the worse and hoping for the best. There is also increased interest and focus from extended family, so it's also a time of managing their anxieties and interest. Whilst anticipating results, thoughts on the other hand pick up a pace, fuelled by concerns about preparing on some level for the possibility of news that might be bad or difficult, trigger treatment and confirm disease progression whilst also really hoping desperately for good news. We try to make a rational assessment of how Chris has been, but this is so confusing as memory, mood and fatigue have impacted our daily lives and this hasn't correlated with the disease progressing.

The time frames that seem acceptable to the hospitals systems have an entirely different and variable sense of what's reasonable. There is so much variation in the UK on how quickly scans can be reported, from the same day up 2–3 weeks. It's crucial to know when to expect the results and not have extra anxiety born out of poor communication. Like with many aspects of this journey, time has helped it become easier. I guess we are resigned to it, but it is eased by having an oncologist with whom we have a good relationship and a clinical nurse specialist which has been built over the years.

## 18.6    The Consultation

The appointment where we find out about the results of the latest scan – Chris always refers to it as 'scan results' or 'meeting', like its being jointly organised. I have a friend who had his GMB grade 4 surgically removed, followed with chemotherapy and radiotherapy; 7 years on he remains clear of visible tumour and calls them his 'all clear meeting'.

One challenge is managing the differences between my needs and my partner's. This can cause tension between Chris and I at times: my partner processes things more slowly, and my mind jumps ahead. It's very difficult to hold back to allow the information exchange at appointments to go at his pace. Sometimes Chris just wants to get out of there really quickly; he's so relieved to discover he's not dying imminently, as he was beginning to believe he might be. Whereas I feel we have a precious and limited opportunity to ask questions we need to ask, or as is often the case, ask the questions that run through his mind in the run up to the appointment. Is there anything new, are there any trials, could X work and how long might it stay the same? We are desperately hoping for answers whilst knowing there's no crystal ball, just data. But there is no data specifically on Chris, how his body and his immune system will work alongside the cells that make up this tumour.

## 18.7    Our Relationship with the Clinician

It was very important to us to navigate this relationship and to decide what would be right for Chris. Chris has had four oncologists, each with their own style and differing interpersonal skills, with two moving on to become professors elsewhere. I do feel, however, that this has enhanced my understanding of how important this relationship is, and when it is working well, it can fundamentally improve one's outlook and ability to lead a full life. Chris has also been a patient in two hospitals, each with its individual and differing culture, and currently has his oncology care in London, whilst he sees a neurologist and endocrinologists locally in Brighton. He has also been an outpatient at the local hospice and attended the pain clinic. What has been very important throughout is the relationship with the practitioner, the rapport, trust and honesty whilst seeking support for what is right for us and for Chris on an individual basis, with an optimistic but realistic outlook.

During appointments, we dislike being interrupted by people walking in with notes, assuming it's OK to stay without asking, and not introducing themselves whilst sitting behind you is even worse! Not having control of the space is difficult: it's the practitioner's work space, but during the consultation, it is our private space but one where seemingly anyone can walk in.

During Chris's recent pre-radiotherapy mask making, there were three people in the room with one person teaching the student, and the other completely focused on Chris, making him comfortable and explaining everything. As the mask was moulded to his head and bolted to the table, there was a 5-min countdown, with Chris being told at minute intervals how long was remaining. During this time more and more people joined us from the room next door, just voices to Chris, and it suddenly felt like the staff room with warm chatty banter, but not appropriate. Chris couldn't see who was there, or why they were there, lying with his head bolted to the hard couch.

In our first hospital, after some appointments on a one-to-one basis, we then had results in a room that included the neurosurgeon, Chris's regular oncologist (for a few years two oncologists), the specialist nurse and typically three more staff, either junior doctors or students. This is intimidating and much more formal. The power was in the suit sitting behind the desk; the opening questions would always be, How are you? Any seizures? Are you working? Chris would be answering these whilst waiting to find out what the scan showed, and felt like he had to prove his wellness in court, answering to the judge and jury, at least that's how it felt to him.

What works well is respectful communication, where all that can be done is done to make us feel comfortable, to meet us where we are with kindness, warmth and compassion, as well as clarity with information. Medical staff need to be clinically good, that's a given, but also genuine, accessible, human. Good ones can give you news you don't want to hear but leave you feeling engaged with life. We have had appointments that are with the lead clinician, neurosurgeon or oncologist on their own with us. These are my favourite, followed by those with a trusted specialist nurse.

## 18.8  After the Appointment

Immediately after appointments we go somewhere to assimilate the news, sigh an enormous amount of relief and congratulate Chris (knowing he has very little control over the facts) on being well and of course to talk. Usually I send a whole number of joyful text messages. We feel extraordinarily alive, really bright, engaged and have a disproportionate sense of joy. We sit, take it in and prepare for normality again. Then I just want to get home, the empty post-adrenalin feeling of tiredness hits along with a desire to minimise disruption for my children.

We often had opportunities to talk with the specialist nurse following news that lead to treatment, but rarely after stable scans. For me, this is where the system and professionals are determining my/our need at what may look like trigger points. We would have benefited from more opportunity to talk in the earlier years, to help us make sense of the situation and to deal with the desperate sense of isolation. I found this help in national as well as local charities. When you're in a period of treatment, there's a lot of support, and it's also a time when friends offer help and you can more easily engage your community networks.

## 18.9   Impact on the Children

The experiance for a child living with a parent with a brain tumour varies depending on their age, personality, and the timing with other important life and events, including key educational periods and the usual frendship situations. There is the significant differences between the often more hidden longer term implications and the crisis periods, where both needs and impact are often more apparent.

My daughter Sophie (from a previous relationship) was 7 when Chris was diagnosed. An example of the impact on her of the big things, like treatment. When Chris came home from surgery with his shaved head, Mickey Mouse-shaped scar from ear to ear and bruised eyes, Sophie vomited within the hour and was off school in bed for 24 h. I'm sure it was a visceral response to the horror of the image, slightly Frankenstein-esque. The other parts are the facts that I met my partner when she was nearly 5; we had a baby when she was almost 7, and within 3 months, Chris took centre stage as the person who needed my attention. It was very hard for her during that period.

Many other parents were amazing and so accommodating, having Sophie to play when we had appointments and even doing shopping for me. I will always be grateful. I also think it is tremendously helpful to have meals delivered: it's what I always encourage other people to accept. It's so much more than putting dinner on the table. I felt cared for, and it also allows people who feel helpless to have a role. It ensures we eat well, rather than a ready meal or another bowl of pasta, when I'm ragged from juggling work, family and caring commitments.

Gaps between scans and apparent stability are another matter entirely, as support falls away, and you appear to be coping, but there are good days and bad ones. It's hard when you ask for help, like looking after a child for an appointment and the person says no or changes their mind at the last minute: some people just aren't flexible. Sophie at age 10 had to walk home to an empty house, knowing we were at an appointment in London and I wasn't able to pick up at the agreed time due to the trains running late. This felt very unkind at the time, and the lack of compassion and thought was really difficult, neither she nor I have forgotten this occasion.

Because Alex was so young, it is really all he's ever known. As a young child, he understood not to make lots of noise because his dad would likely be resting in the afternoon, and not to disturb him in the bedroom. This was all normal and Alex was able to accommodate these needs. It also meant his dad was in the house, around more than he would have been when we didn't know about the tumour. Chris reduced his work, letting go of a charity he had established and moving his office into our home.

Alex turned 5 during the first period of Chris's treatment, surgery and chemotherapy. It was a tricky time as it was also during the transition from nursery to school. Alex found the school noisy and struggled with separation. The school were inflexible and didn't seem to grasp what was going on, how distressed we all were and how anxious we were not knowing for some considerable time whether the treatment would be effective. We eventually decided to move him to a new, much smaller school, where compassion was central to its ethos.

Telling Alex aged 13 and 1 month, about the change and need for treatment, was difficult. He didn't ask when we came home from the appointment, which is unusual; he was thinking about food and wanting to know what we were going to eat. Chris and I had spoken on the train and Chris wanted some time to process the news. He was feeling very angry and upset. This was hard for me, to hold back information, but I could see Chris needed a little time. It felt difficult to me, as I wanted our children to be the first to know, so I too had to hold it. I was tense and found the sound of Alex's bouncing basketball really challenging. I could have snapped, but I didn't. Instead I went to yoga that first night.

There was a point when not telling Alex also meant that Chris could hide, feeling angry and wishing it wasn't true. As the half-term holiday approached, I could see the value of telling Alex, so he had some privacy and time with us to ask questions and adjust to the idea. We agreed I would tell him.

I told him in his room on Saturday morning; I explained that his dad's tumour had changed, and he needed more treatment. He sobbed and sobbed and couldn't look me in the eye. I desperately wanted to understand, but despite my best efforts, he was unable to verbalise his thoughts and fears. He knew a boy at school, whose Dad had died within the year of a GBM grade 4. I don't know, but I wondered if this is what Alex thought would now happen; it must have looked likely in his eyes, but I didn't want to make the connection unless he had.

I tried to reassure him that the treatment had worked before so we could expect it to work again, but his distress continued; I had a photo of the scan and told him I had it and he could see it if he wanted to. He did want to see it and studied it with great interest. I explained that he could come and see the radiotherapy department, that they were used to showing children around and that we could visit his dad in London. Going on holiday the following Monday proved a very good distraction and gave us processing time. We all felt close, and Chris made the effort to do things with Alex.

There is a lack of good resources for teenagers with a parent with a brain tumour. When Chris was first diagnosed, this was also the case for younger children, but it has improved, thanks to the brain tumour charities. I'm frustrated yet again at the lack of helpful information—the clinical nurse specialist had had nothing to offer and asked me to let her know if I had any suggestions.

## 18.10  Loving and Caring for a Changed Person

Chris and I hadn't been together for many years when he was diagnosed. It really helped that we were in the new intense love period.

Sophie's dad had left me when she was a small baby, which had been devastating. Here I was again with another small baby and now anticipating losing this man too; I just didn't know when. My grief was immense. Oddly, the one comfort was that there was no betrayal. Dying was easier to deal with than unexpected rejection and another woman. This lovely kind man who was the father of my second child did not want to leave me. I also felt the loss of the hope, dreams and excitement we had shared, meeting after previous relationships and feeling like we could both be our best selves by being together. I was now anticipating being a widow, once again a single parent, this time with two young children. My life felt shattered; I had questions such as would my son have memories of his dad?

I wish I had known then that we would have time and lots of it. Time has been amazing; my feelings have changed so much. I probably grieved quietly for 4 years, on more than one occasion tears overwhelming me in the supermarket. I think it's the anonymity, and it being a brief moment away from young children. In tandem I felt very alive, very present and experienced great joy in the simple things in daily life. Young children help with this too, and it coincided with Alex's pre-school years. My children brought me a lot of joy and as their needs were intense and pretty constant that was very helpful.

Now this has changed into dealing with the unexpected: about managing symptoms and a long-term chronic condition, building resilience and making as good a life as I can for us, given Chris's abilities and limitations. I have to create and maintain continuing threads of my life, moving forwards regardless of what's happening with Chris. Much of this is about the work I do. It provides me with income, companionship, purpose, identity and a sense of myself and creating a future that is not dependent on Chris.

This has been a hard paragraph to write. Grumpy is an understatement, but I love him dearly.

The diagnosis of a major illness, disease or cancer is life changing, and it changes people, sometimes fleetingly and sometimes permanently: the impact of the news, the vulnerability, facing mortality and the reality of symptoms. The word cancer is loaded with expectations. What's different with brain tumours is the location, even the idea of something growing in your brain, the part of your body that defines who you are. And you can't remove it like cancers in other parts of the body, as you need your brain. So, it's not just the experience, but it's also the tumours' physical presence that changes the person. Where it's located can have so many different effects, some physical and dramatic like seizures, but it also affects the person's thinking, their memory, mood, cognitive function, energy levels, the sense of who they are and their personality. These effects and changes are deeply felt in the privacy of your home whilst seemingly invisible to your community and extended family.

My experience is that this fluctuates. Sometimes Chris is Chris; other times he's having 'brain tumour moments' as I call them. Sometimes he's so tense and irritable being around him and interacting with him is challenging, hurtful even, sometimes especially if I feel my resilance is low, I can feel attacked and sad, and sometimes tearful. This is the most difficult thing I face, the bad days of mood swings and irritability and grumpy interactions. I feel I am so stretched on these days and often very alone. I do all I can to buffer the children from this. Doing too much physically and being with people, especially those who are more demanding or challenge him, are also triggers. I also know that getting the balance right between giving into fatigue and engaging with life is tricky and that sometimes there are costs and consequences: sometimes these are worth it.

What triggers these 'brain tumour moments' is varied. When the children were younger, he would be irritated by the sounds of them playing; happy noises were disturbing to him when he was exhausted or in pain. Often, he would want to sleep at 3 pm when they would soon be coming home from school, so he was disturbed by their home coming. Fatigue is a big one, how to manage rest to enable the person to live well, but not so much that the person becomes withdrawn and disengages with life. Chris isolates himself and needs to decompress—he shuts doors and retreats to the room called his office. We have to plan, and pacing is key. If we have friends over in the evening, or are planning a family trip, Chris needs a quiet day with an afternoon nap and then can emerge on really good form. I then hear everyone saying how well he looks and seems, which though great to here also sometimes painfully highlights the difference between the private family expertance and the more public one that can be pulled off for short periods acter careful planning and managment of his fatigue.

Chris has the capacity to fall asleep mid-sentence, to sleep anywhere. A recent example of his confusion was on going to see his sister: he'd slept all the way there, almost 6 h drive in terrible traffic, we arrived and ate dinner and then he very politely said we should leave them to their evening and that it was time to go home. I had to explain that we had come a long way and that we were staying, as he was fairly determined to leave, and we were expected to stay. He was very confused, but eventually he agreed to stay. After a night's sleep, he was himself again.

## 18.11  Helping Chris to Make Sense of Things That Have Happened

This is twofold: there's the element of memory, losing sense of his journey's chronology, and the history being muddled or even absent, so this is where I fill in gaps retell the story providing clues like coat hangers to place his memories on. This is also true of our personal life, when we last saw X or went to visit Y. Photographs help and so does describing events until there's something from which Chris can hook out the memory. Sometimes he just pretends to remember.

What is also worth explaining is how I have helped Chris accept what's happened when he's lost consciousness and has no memory, usually seizures. This is very difficult, as in part he thinks I'm making it up, being overdramatic. When he had seizures with one rolling into the next, he didn't know this had happened. Chris was cross; his clothes had been cut up and didn't understand why the paramedics had done that—he couldn't grasp that it was an emergency situation.

The goalposts have kept moving and we keep adjusting, and re-calibrating our expectations. Both together and seperatly, all the harder for Chris with the tumours imact on his thinking. Chris sometimes wants me to help him re build the narative, events get muddled, the what and when all jumbled, bits missing or remenbered out of context, sometimes getting these details straight in his mind are important. We both have different ways of managing the uncertainty, conversations are helpful.

We do however openly acknowledge I am likly to live longer than he is. I also have a sence of my future that would be richer should he be part of it, but its also possible to imagine another version on my own, having this rather important thread of an idea of a life beyond.

## 18.12 Life on Hold, Decision to Go Alone When Needed

Living with someone with fatigue is complicated, as for many years I used to wait for Chris to feel able to go out, and often this energy didn't happen. I'd wait all day, with the children hoping, and then we didn't go. This was frustrating, but I wanted to include him as I felt loyal to him and wanted him to be a part of the family. It was hard to work out how to include him in the family, make memories and respect him as a partner and father.

This has changed: we don't plan much together. But I do make plans; I'm no longer waiting and hoping, I'm doing and sometimes he comes, he's included, but mostly not. Sometimes I encourage him, and sometimes I push him. Sometimes I'm so frustrated. Sometimes it works out just wonderfully, especially when Chris has planned and had a rest before, rather than a demanding day from which he's still recovering.

## 18.13 Steroids and Long-Term Use

We didn't really know the implications and risks when Chris was continuing on dexamethasone through his chemotherapy: he underestimated its impact on his body. It's actually really rubbish. He didn't manage to come off it. He often felt it gave him a boost, and he had a lot of headaches through his chemotherapy, so staying on them seemed a good idea at the time. He ended up with losing his natural ability to produce cortisol. Chris started to have problems with his skin, armpits and face mostly, and he feels very self-conscious of the facial sore areas and rashes. The armpits were more painful. Chris's appetite increased, especially for midnight snacks, leading to weight gain. The body dysmorphia was distressing as he changed from his lifelong skinny form to a round moon-faced man with a bloated, distended belly. He also felt uncomfortable and became less mobile as his legs were increasingly painful.

The summer of 2016 was too hot for Chris. With his swollen legs, walking was very painful, but I couldn't tempt him to the cool breeze at the beach. He had just changed steroid to hydrocortisone, to see if we could reduce side effects. It was a year ago that we first showed the oozing ulcers to the oncologist: Chris's skin had turned to filo pastry. It took months to get an appropriate diagnosis of gravitational oedema and leg ulcers in part as a result of long-term dexamethasone usage. I had to really focus on helping Chris, improve his comfort, mobility and reduce what felt like an additional complication and risk we really didn't need. My practical role was significantly increased: months of compression bandages, weekly trips to the GP and practice nurse, some diuretics, resting legs up and short periods of exercise, a little walk, and a year later and three stones lighter it's a totally different situation, legs are healed and not at all swollen, Chris is more mobile, and happier as a result. I'm very glad as facing active treatment for a changing tumour this time last year would have been very different.

## 18.14  Public Face and Private World

This is one of the most persistent and challenging dilemmas I face and continue to face. No one really walks alongside me or witnesses my hard moments and it is deeply isolating. In a way, time has made this more so, as we appear to be coping well, and in many ways, we are and I do manage. But the toll is mostly hidden: when Chris's not feeling great, when he is particularly tense and grumpy, unable to engage or is in significant discomfort, this all takes place mostly within the privacy of our home.

There's a really stark contrast between the public Chris and the private Chris. What's not seen by others is how our lives actually are. Chris will rest in the afternoon and have a quiet morning before meeting friends for dinner and then will mostly be on good form and seem extremely on the ball and well. Then he might withdraw when we get home and need time to decompress and retreat the next day. The more public signs are around memory, which are not quite so hidden. He will often forget previous conversations, arrangements or shared experiences.

Chris attended rehabilitation at UCH (University College Hospital, London) and has also had a number of neuropsychological assessments and has seen the neuropsychologist several times to review the situation. These assessments have provided really useful information about Chris's processing difficulties, which have helped us to plan and develop our strategies.

I have personally received counselling over the years since Chris's diagnosis, with the intention of giving me some support and avoiding crisis and with a focus on building my resilience. This has provided me with an invaluable safe space and allowed me to reflect on our journey. It's not a weekly requirement but fulfils the need in me to have someone who understands, someone whom I can share the most challenging days with and who does not judge me or Chris. This is so important and has really helped me to be who I want to be, and not just defined by my role as a carer.

## 18.15  The Language Around Brain Tumours

A brief dip into social media and the language of living with a brain tumour has much fighting talk, the hero or warrior, dying described as 'a battle lost'. This language is still prevalent, perpetuated in these online communities and not really helpful; I find this very difficult to relate to. It is so opposed to how we have approached living with this tumour. We have taken a different approach, of acceptance integrating the changing Chris and the tumour into our lives. We are not fighting, or battling. We are doing our best to be engaged with life, be present in what we do and how we function and engage actively on a day-to-day basis, living life as best we can.

## 18.16  The Rollercoaster Analogy

We heard it used in brain tumour and other cancer conversations; I even used it myself. Then in the summer of 2016, I went to a theme park with my daring and brave boy who, then aged 11, wanted to go on all the rollercoasters on offer, so we did! Yes, there are similarities: what struck me was that whilst you can see before you the entire experience, you can't anticipate how the experience will be, but you know where it starts and stops, and you have a pretty good idea what's involved. It's over in about three minutes, just three minutes! My rollercoaster has been running for 13 years, that's no funfair ride. The only similarity is the stomach churning moment when you're heading into the unknown. It's endurance, a test of resilience. I'm acutely aware of the long-term effects of the sustained role and the endurance required for the reality we live.

When Chris is having a really bad time, and he's lashing out or withdrawn, I feel hurt, attacked and sad. For years I have managed these times by recognising that it's a brain tumour moment and that it's not about me or him. I find this is the hardest thing to deal with and it impacts on my resilience. This is the thing that has meant I have cried at my desk at work and just felt beaten. I made a shift a few years ago: I'm now extra kind to Chris when he's cranky, tense and snappy, and I name it, *"I say you don't seem to be feeling well"*. Breakfast in bed or his favourite dinner of pea and leek risotto helps.

## 18.17  Managing My Needs: Who Am I in This?

We have been fortunate to have had many years since the initial diagnosis, which has allowed time for me to develop my sense of expertise, both as an advocate for my partner and as a carer. This is a role that I adopt in daily life, for example, in dealing with day-to-day memory issues, how to get somewhere and which train to catch, as well as when we attend medical appointments. I am aware that I know my partner's history very well and can join up the dots. I am able to articulate calmly for the human, lived experience of dealing as a family with the situation where the husband and father has a brain tumour. One of the first things we realised was that I, as the carer, and Chris, as the person with the brain tumour, may be in very different places and have different experiences with differing needs at different times. A big lesson I've learnt is it's one thing recognising what you need, listening to your own internal voice and body, and it's entirely different to be able to act on this, as it is constrained by so much.

I have been Chris's advocate, protector and researcher and also his partner. It's not always easy to know which one to be at which precise moment. I am also a mother and have developed a new career since his diagnosis. Good information has been a key part of my coping strategy and has enabled us to make fully informed choices, at our pace, whenever we have had the option to do so.

Living with a loved one with a brain tumour brings particular challenges, due to the complexity of the disease. I have focused on my personal resilience to deal with the intensity of the situation and crisis avoidance, and I have wanted help to do this as well as I possibly could. Counselling has provided me with an invaluable safe space and allowed me to reflect on our journey. It also fulfils the need in me to have someone who understands, someone whom I can share the most challenging days with, who does not judge me or Chris. This is so important and took time to find; having had support has really helped me to be who I want to be, and not just defined by this role and identity.

I have also found yoga invaluable, this community of people were part of my life before and it helps me notice how I hold tension in my body and how I feel. It nurtures me, along with my work as a breastfeeding advocate, providing education, training and support. I am passionate about this work in its many forms and work with lovely people which provide a welcome respite.

One of the challenges in my role is that when Chris has to go into hospital, I have on occasion found it difficult to get good information about what is going on. At home, I am in control. At outpatient appointments I am involved in supporting and advocating for Chris. In hospital, I am usually disempowered. Recognising this and ensuring good communication would really help (as would having visiting hours during the school day). I'm quite assertive and so have got around these barriers, but it could have been made easier.

With the recent news, and imminent radiotherapy, there's been a big difference in how I share the news and seek support. The network is tighter and smaller; it has shrunk in part due to no longer having primary school-aged children and the other factors being that networks take time to maintain, time I have had less and less of it, and I also sense compassion fatigue. It's been going on a long time, hard for people to understand, and I know quite what this now means.

## 18.18   My Own Health

As a parent, and as the expected surviving parent, it feels very important to be well, healthy and not do anything to risk this. I couldn't afford for anything to happen to me, it's unthinkable and the responsibility is great. I felt this particularly acutely when my children were younger.

It became clear as the years went on that being a carer was a risk to my health. I knew in theory that this was the case, but I hadn't felt it. It crept up on me. I think the sustained low-level but long-term stress with its fluctuations is significant, and the acute periods are more obvious.

So how has this manifested in me? I've had repeated shoulder injuries: it's where I hold my stress. It started with the first known seizure; I pulled my shoulder stopping Chris from falling out of bed and ended up with a frozen shoulder. It is hard to keep up with routine appointments like dentist, smear test, etc. It rarely feels as important as everything else, and with competing priorities, I cancel my appointment.

I'm rarely unwell, but I am usually really unwell by the time I seek help needed from a GP: I've had a couple of urinary tract infections (UTI), a kidney infection and a chest infection that left me in bed and unable to properly look after myself. There was no one to bring me hot drinks, make lunch and let alone take care of my family. Being unwell as a parent and carer is very difficult. For many years I had a brilliant GP who had known me since I was 18—he was my family GP; he knew me, my children and my history; we had a good relationship; and this made me feel safe. He also understood the complexity and potential impact of the caring role. It was a great loss to me when he retired.

When I have a medical appointment, being a carer is vital information to share, as it's an opportunity to help me more broadly when I need to seek help, give me more time and really listen. Don't underestimate how unwell I might be feeling. I've not been anxious about my health, but had I been, I would want to be met with appropriate investigations and understanding.

What has helped is when I've received proactive care, such as the follow-up phone call when I had a UTI to find out how I was, to make further positive suggestions, being signed off sick from work when needed. I felt cared for and it was much easier to ensure I was receiving appropriate treatment and management.

A more direct relationship between Chris's health and mine can occur. When Chris was in intensive care, I developed an UTI. In hindsight it's easy to see how: I was subconsciously restricting what I drank, so I didn't have to leave him to go to the loo as it was difficult on to get back on the ward.

Chris and I have together and separately had counselling over the years, at first through the cancer centre, and then Chris saw another counsellor there. I do think counselling has enormous potential in supporting people living with a brain tumour; it's really very good to have help making the constant adjustments. I also think it's important that the counsellor or practitioner understands the nature of the disease, and its effects on mood, cognition, memory and sense of self. Any therapeutic work always has to go through this lens. The safe place and ongoing relationship with my counsellor is crucial for me: it is where I can share my darkest thoughts and my deepest frustrations, as well as ensuring I'm living life to the full as best I can as much of the time as I can.

The relationship with the practitioner, whoever it may be, is really important. Kindness and compassion go a long way, along with the appropriate clinical skills. When you need to seek help for yourself, you are also acknowledging yourself, putting your needs in the mix, first even, in a way that you're not very often able to in your daily life.

## 18.19  Learning to Live with Uncertainty

This has actually happened as a result of time, conversation, experience and more time. I now have an inner sense that no matter what, I'll be OK, and I'll do my best. I cope well in a crisis, and whilst I've run many scenarios through in my head, and none may happen, they do serve as preparation. Resilience is key, my ability to bounce back, to recover, and whilst this is not perfect, it couldn't be, it's what I work on, focus on and hold in mind.

> *Unease settles round my panicked heart*
> *I hold my mother's hand*
> *As all the trouble starts*
> (Sophie, my daughter, "*The Wind It Howls*")

Love for each other, our friends and family helps a lot.
Compassion experience of life makes all the difference.
I would like to thank my partner for supporting me in telling my story and my children for being my constant reminder of joyfulness and the love we share.

# End of Life Care for the Glioma Patient

## 19

Roeline Pasman, Hanneke Zwinkels, and Lara Fritz

**Abstracts**

The definition of palliative care is explored in this chapter—it includes 'end of life' care, which is defined as care that is given in the last months of life of a patient. End of life care is of great importance for patients with a glioma since the disease trajectory is often accompanied with burdensome symptoms. Survival after diagnosis is relatively short, and the disease can influence patients' decision-making capacity. Above that, the disease often also has a major impact on relatives of the patient.

In this chapter we will describe the most common physical symptoms in the last months of life of patients with a glioma, and the impact the disease can have on daily life including the psychosocial and spiritual part of life. We will focus on the role of specialist nurses in the last months of life, illustrating the many challenges a nurse can face when caring for a patient with a glioma.

**Keywords**

Palliative care · End of life care · Neuro-oncology management · Advance care planning · Terminal care · Dying

R. Pasman (✉)
Department of Public and Occupational Health, Expertise Center for Palliative Care,
Amsterdam Public Health Research Institute, Amsterdam UMC, Vrije Universiteit Amsterdam,
Amsterdam, The Netherlands
e-mail: hrw.pasman@vumc.nl

H. Zwinkels · L. Fritz
Department of Neurology, Haaglanden Medical Center, Antoniushove,
Leidschendam, The Netherlands
e-mail: h.zwinkelsvan.vliet@haaglandenmc.nl; l.fritz@haaglandenmc.nl

© Springer Nature Switzerland AG 2019
I. Oberg (ed.), *Management of Adult Glioma in Nursing Practice*,
https://doi.org/10.1007/978-3-319-76747-5_19

**Learning Outcomes**

- To understand the difference between palliative care and end of life care.
- To recognise signs and physical symptoms that a patient is entering the end of life phase and know how to manage each symptom individually and expectantly.
- To know the processes involved in advance care planning and how this can help reduce patient and carer stress in the end of life phase.
- To learn how to mentally prepare patients for ethical issues and discussions around palliative care, end of life care and cessation of active treatment, in a sympathetic, open and honest way.

## 19.1    Introduction

Care for patients with a glioma is of a palliative nature, because cure cannot be obtained. Palliative care is defined by the World Health Organization (WHO) as 'an approach that improves the quality of life of patients and their families facing the problem associated with life-threatening illness, through the prevention and relief of suffering by means of early identification and impeccable assessment and treatment of pain and other problems, physical, psychosocial and spiritual'. Palliative care is applicable early in the course of a life-threatening illness, in conjunction with other therapies that are intended to prolong life, such as chemotherapy or radiation therapy [1]. In glioma patients these therapies are administered to delay tumour growth. Palliative care such as good symptom management and supportive care throughout the disease trajectory improves the quality of life of the patient and their relatives.

Palliative care includes 'end of life' care, which is defined in this chapter as care that is given in the *last months of life* of a patient. End of life care is of great importance for patients with a glioma since the disease trajectory is often accompanied with burdensome symptoms. Survival after diagnosis is relatively short, and the disease can influence patients' decision-making capacity. Above that, the disease often also has a major impact on relatives of the patient.

In this chapter the most common physical symptoms in the last months of life of patients with a glioma are described, and the impact the disease can have on daily life including the psychosocial and spiritual part of life. Particular focus will be on the role of specialist nurses (also referred to as a key worker) in the last months of life.

This chapter will start with a first-hand case description of Mrs. Murdock (fictional name), illustrating the many challenges a nurse can face when caring for a patient with a glioma. This case description was written by Hanneke Zwinkels, and part of it was previously published in the European Association of Neuro-Oncology (EANO) open access Journal Issue 2, 2013 [2].

Mrs. Murdock, 49 years of age, married, two children of 16 and 18 years old.

I first met Mr. and Mrs. Murdock 3 years ago when she presented to our hospital with a suspected high-grade glioma of her left frontal-temporal lobe. She had complained of a loss of sensation in her right hand and she had experienced an episode of speech arrest. When I first met her, we spoke about her planned operation the following day. She was full of hope, of recovering after the operation and returning to everyday life. At some point during our conversation she understood the seriousness of her illness. Several weeks later she told me she had been crying the whole evening before the operation, being aware of her changed future perspective.

During treatment with radiotherapy and chemotherapy (in accordance with the Stupp protocol [3]), we got to know each other quite well and I was able to support Mrs. Murdock in her way of coping. Because she also participated in a clinical trial, we kept seeing each other on a more regular basis than she otherwise would have. After every MRI we discussed the results and implications in regards to possible future treatment options. We also discussed how she and her family (she has two teenage children) were doing. She was managing quite well, with subtle speech disturbances when she was tired, as well as some reduced or altered sensory feelings in her right hand.

'My life is of good quality, but when I am thinking of the fact it will not last long enough to see my children grow older, to see them go to university and graduate, start a relationship, marry, to see them become parents, to become a grandmother...then I become very upset, very sad, very angry and I regret the fact this disease is my fate....and the fact I am empty handed....'

By giving Mrs. Murdock and her husband the opportunity to talk about their fears and hopes for the future, by listening to their grief of lost health, their bereavement on powerlessness, on their mourning over the inescapable outcome, they were able to adjust to both the current situation and future outlook. Receiving reassurance and support was essential in helping them to cope with the illness, and allowed them both to hope for a period of stable disease. But the balance between maintaining realistic hope and their bereavement was fragile. Each time a new MRI was performed and results had been discussed, they again asked for support in regaining this balance.

Mrs. Murdock was employed in her husband's company as a secretarial administrator, but because of her language problems, she was unable to work a year after her initial treatment. Mrs. Murdock and her husband regained a sort of balance after the children moved out of the house to attend college, but then the tumour recurred—her only option was to participate in another clinical trial. Every 6 weeks an MRI was performed, and we spoke about the tension and fear of MRI results, future treatment options and her anticipatory grief over her future prospects. Every next step was a step closer to losing the ability of taking any step, as she said.

The last time I met Mr. and Mrs. Murdock, she was wheelchair bound because of a hemiparesis and she was unable to speak. We discussed the implications of her diagnosed recurrence and her subsequent focal deficits. Mr. Murdock told me how they were doing at home: she needed help with daily activities, could speak a few words like 'yes' and 'no', but most of the time couldn't find the right words; she needed to rest with increasing frequency, was only up for about 4 h/day, and didn't suffer from headache or nausea. Resulting from these conversations, a hospital bed was arranged for their home, help from friends was available, the general practitioner was informed and home care was implemented.

Mrs. Murdock tried to understand what we were talking about, but it was difficult for her to respond to questions. I asked them if they wished to hear about what could be expected for the last phase of her life, and Mrs. Murdock looked questioningly into the eyes of her husband. After a few seconds, he told me he would be glad to listen, and she agreed by nodding her head. Hence, I carefully and sensitively talked about what to expect. Tears fell (not only from the eyes of Mr. and Mrs. Murdock), and after ending our conversation, we said our goodbyes. I wished her a valuable time surrounded by lots of love, care, understanding and the hope for a good and beautiful completion of her life.

Since the last visit to the outpatient clinic, the husband and I had contact by phone during her end of life phase. Within a week, Mrs. Murdock deteriorated; she suffered from less energy, slept for prolonged periods and had worsening speech disturbances; and she 'had given up', as stated by her husband. There was a possibility of re-challenging her with temozolomide (TMZ), but the treatment could not start because of on-going thrombocytopenia. Therefore, we simply checked her blood counts a few times.

Mrs. Murdock experienced a seizure and anti-epileptic drugs (AEDs) were commenced and dexamethasone was started (8 mg/day). A week later I contacted Mr. Murdock who informed me she had not shown any improvements in her symptoms after the start of the dexamethasone, so it was stopped. We also decided to drop the option for re-challenge TMZ, because of her clinical deterioration and lasting thrombocytopenia. Mrs. Murdock did not show lots of emotions (as she had done previously), and was not able to use her right arm and leg at all anymore.

A week later, Mr. Murdock told me, that after stopping dexamethasone, she had recovered somewhat, suggesting that it took some time for the corticosteroids to show an effect. Mrs. Murdock was able to speak better and gained some kind of balance again and hoped for the start of TMZ. We decided (treating physician and nurse practitioner) to check her blood counts again and re-commence high dose dexamethasone to see if there would be any further improvement, given her previous delayed positive response to them.

Although she continued to be wheelchair bound, she enjoyed life a bit more, understood her situation, was supported by her husband, children, family and friends, and the GP was a frequent visitor. We decided to slowly decrease the dose of dexamethasone.

This status-quo situation lasted a few weeks, but then Mrs. Murdock deteriorated once again, slowly loosing awareness of her surroundings and situation. Whilst eating and drinking was no problem at the beginning, it became more difficult to swallow thin liquids. Home care was started two months after the last visit to the hospital. Her speech disturbances worsened, communication was no longer possible, there was no movement in the right side of her body, and a final seizure led to a change in AEDs from tablets to buccal clonazepam. This was sufficient to prevent any further seizure. Two days later there were signs of increased intracranial pressure and she received midazolam subcutaneously (via infusion pump) to keep her comfortable. Mrs. Murdock died peacefully at home 3 months after the last visit to the outpatient clinic.

### 19.1.1 Symptoms and Symptom Management in the Last Months of Life

Most patients with a glioma present with neurological deficits and burdensome symptoms relating to the tumour location, impacting their daily lives.

Mrs. Murdock exhibited several of the most common symptoms in the last phase of life of patients suffering with a glioma [4]. When the nurse saw her for the first time, she only had minor complaints, such as a subtle loss of sensation in one of her hands and a few episodes of speech arrest. The deficits worsened as the disease progressed; she became wheelchair bound and unable to speak. She also suffered from fatigue. When the disease progressed further she developed seizures, and slowly loses awareness of her situation and gets swallowing problems.

In the section below, emphasis is placed on a selection of the most common symptoms that were also presented in the aforementioned case description: neurological deficits, fatigue, cognitive disturbances, swallowing problems and seizures. For management of other symptoms, such as pain, headache, nausea and delirium, we refer to the European Association of Neuro-Oncology (EANO) guidelines for palliative care in adults with glioma [4].

Good symptom management is an important part of end of life care and can improve the quality of life of patients with a glioma. Nurses have an important role to play in symptom management by monitoring and discussing strategies with the treating physician, as well as in informing patients and relatives about symptom management and control alongside coping strategies.

#### 19.1.1.1 Neurological Deficits

Neurological deficits often occur in patients with a glioma and are directly caused by the size and location of the tumour and its surrounding oedema, which in turn leads to raised intracranial pressure. Common neurological deficits at the end of life include lowered or altered consciousness and worsening of pre-existing focal deficits, such as unilateral weakness and speech disturbances, as highlighted in the case report.

These focal deficits may disappear entirely or improve after the intracranial pressure is decreased by surgical resection and further treatments, such as chemotherapy. However, at tumour recurrence and/or in the end of life phase, these focal deficits may return or even worsen. Dexamethasone (a type of steroid) is often prescribed in case oedema is partly responsible for the neurological deficits. Physiotherapy can also be helpful in maintaining neurological functions, or help the patient adjust to his/her situation and limitations as long as possible [4]. It is important to monitor and record the neurological deficits and discuss the impact it has for the patient and relatives. Guidance towards adequate tools and support may be given by a nurse specialist (or key worker) who coordinates the care at the outpatient clinic. Please see the Chap. 11 on holistic needs assessment for further details.

### 19.1.1.2  Fatigue

Fatigue is a frequently reported symptom in patients with a glioma. A systematic review of the literature showed that between 25% and 90% of all patients with brain tumours report fatigue, which can occur at any time during the disease trajectory [5], but it is most prevalent at the time of radiation therapy [6] and in the end of life phase.

Mrs. Murdock suffered from fatigue. As her disease progressed she needed to rest more and more. When the nurse saw her at the time of her disease recurrence, she was only up for about 4 h/day. Fatigue often has a major impact on daily life activities; it actually disturbs and disrupts daily life, when you only are up for a couple of hours per day.

Unfortunately, fatigue is hard to prevent. There are general strategies described to manage fatigue, such as finding a good balance between activities, resting and relaxing and prioritising activities [7]. There is also evidence that exercise for cancer-related fatigue (not specifically glioma related) can result in clinically relevant improvements and might be effective in treating fatigue. However, these therapies often include walking or resistance training and due to the neurological deficits (such as those exhibited by Mrs. Murdock) may therefore not be applicable to many glioma patients in the end of life phase [6].

Fatigue management needs an individually tailored approach, and a nurse specialist can help support patients by discussing the impact of fatigue on aspects of their daily living and can help set individual priorities for the patient and his/her relatives. Goals are aimed at finding a good balance between activities and rest/relaxation is aimed at minimising the adverse effects of fatigue [7].

### 19.1.1.3  Cognitive Disturbances

Cognitive deficits such as memory loss, personality change, apathy and problems in executive functioning and understanding occur in about one third of patients with a glioma and often increase as the disease progresses [8]. Also mood and behavioural disorders frequently occur in patients with a glioma. It is found that a clinical depression occurs in about 20% of patients and personality changes can affect up to 60% of patients [9]. These deficits can impact greatly on daily living and functioning of the patients and subsequently affect the relationship with their family members and other loved ones.

Due to cognitive disturbances and diminished awareness of the situation in the end of life phase, it may be difficult to judge the patient's ability to help decide what is best for him/her. In this difficult period of the disease, partners need all the support they can get, from their relatives, treating physician and if possible their specialist nurse (key worker), who is well known to them.

A key worker has an important task in informing and monitoring patients with these symptoms, discussing their condition with the treating physician as well as their relatives, either within a hospital setting or in the community.

### 19.1.1.4  Swallowing Problems

In the last weeks or days of life, patients with a glioma often have difficulty swallowing (also known as dysphagia) and decreased levels of consciousness [8]. Losing the ability to swallow might hamper nutrition, hydration and oral administration of drugs. Since most patients are cared for at home or at another institution other than a hospital, it is important that healthcare professionals in these settings are aware of this. Key workers can prevent problems by pre-emptively informing professionals about anticipated symptoms in the last days of life and how to manage them successfully. For swallowing problems, interventions such as a change of oral drugs to injections, nasal spray, patches or suppositories can be discussed. When the patient is entering the last few days of his/her life, it is possible to withdraw medication—even dexamethasone—to ensure comfort in the process towards imminent death.

### 19.1.1.5  Seizures

Seizures occur in up to 65% of patients with glioma during the end of life phase [10]. Patients can have seizures from the point of diagnosis onwards, but it is also possible that seizures occur for the first time in the later phases of the disease trajectory. Seizures can have great impact on the patient and their relatives. Anti-epileptic drugs (AEDs) are mostly prescribed to minimise the risk of further seizures developing. Seizure management at the end of life is often hampered by swallowing difficulties, as was the case with Mrs. Murdock. In such instances, alternative routes to administer the drugs are necessary, such as intranasal midazolam or buccal clonazepam [4].

Part of a nurse's responsibility is to monitor the type and frequency of seizures and discuss observations with the treating physicians, and to keep the patients and their relatives informed about seizures and their intended management.

## 19.1.2  Advance Care Planning

There is an increasing body of evidence that early involvement of palliative care services improves both quality of life and mood of cancer patients [11, 12]. Discussions are held around what is important for the patient (life-prolongation, quality of life or a combination) and what his/her (medical) wishes are. These wishes can be documented in an advance directive (AD), at a time when the patient still has formal mental capacity to make informed decisions about future care, without being neurologically compromised by the glioma. However, an AD alone is not enough to make wishes known—they also have to be communicated to physicians, relatives and other important persons. One way to achieve this is by a process known as advance care planning (ACP).

ACP is a process which involves patients and their relatives at an early stage when discussing future (palliative) care, which also includes care in the last months of life [13].

ACP in elderly patients has been shown to improve the quality in end of life care; improve satisfaction with care for both the patient and family; and decrease stress, anxiety and depression among relatives of deceased patients [14]. Furthermore, by using ACP, the level of agreement between patients' preferences for care and actual received care increased in patients with chronic diseases (such as end-stage congestive heart failure and renal disease) [15].

Several studies investigated the effects of ACP in glioma patients specifically, with one study suggesting ACP could improve symptom control and quality of life in patients with a glioma [16]. Other studies found if patients with a glioma indicated their wishes regarding end of life care, including their preferred place of death, these were met in 90% [17, 18]. Furthermore, dying in the preferred place of death was associated with dignity, and it may help avoid hospitalisation at the end of life [19].

Glioma patients have an incurable disease and can deteriorate very rapidly from a cognitive perspective. This cognitive decline begins at the point of diagnosis and only increases as the disease progresses. Part of the glioblastoma patients (38%) have difficulty in making treatment decisions prior to surgery because of mental incapacity [20]. During the course of the disease trajectory, more patients are unable to make appropriate decisions, as was the case with Mrs. Murdock: she needed help with daily activities, she could only speak a few words like 'yes' and 'no', but most of the time she was unable to find the right words. Most patients will at some point be unable to participate in ACP discussions. The majority of patients with a high-grade glioma have a reduced decision-making capacity due to delirium, cognitive decline and/or decreasing consciousness in the last weeks—this increases in the last days before death [21]. Therefore an early implementation of ACP discussion with patients with a glioma is warranted, starting at the time of diagnosis in the hospital environment. The possible role of ACP and the importance of its timing for patients with a glioblastoma is discussed in a recent study aimed at treating disease-specific symptoms (such as somnolence and dysphagia, epileptic seizures, headache, and personality changes, agitation and delirium) towards the end of life phase in this patient population [22].

The optimal timing to introduce ACP discussions is unknown. Tools to start a conversation about ACP—for example, PAUSE [6, 23]—could be used to determine if the patient is open to start ACP conversations, to ascertain their goals (what they consider as important), to appoint a legal representative and to provide emotional support. The nurse in the case description asked both Mr. and Mrs. Murdock if they would listen to what could be expected during the last months of life, and to find out if they were open to discuss this last phase of life.

Through shared decision-making, the patient and their loved ones can discuss with the doctor or another team member what wishes and thoughts they have and how to meet them. ACP is a continuous process during the disease course. Oncology nurses work closely together with patients and it is very important to keep in touch on a regularly basis with the patient and their proxies about ACP and its implementation. This is also demonstrated in the case description, where the nurse frequently discusses future plans with both the patient and her husband. For instance, after every MRI, the results were discussed, along with how this impacted future treatment options.

During the end of life phase, when there is less contact with the hospital, patient preference and control of symptoms can be guided by the general practitioner and/or by the oncology nurse via telephone, as highlighted by the case description.

Nowadays, many tools for ACP are available, for instance, in the USA Respecting Choices® [24] or in Australia Respecting Patient Choices® [25]: these are general programmes, and not specific for glioma patients, but they can give guidance for nurses and treating physicians to commence ACP in patients with a glioma.

## 19.1.3 Psychosocial and Spiritual Care

A patient undergoing anticipatory grief can include a very comprehensive sense of loss: loss of functions; loss of working satisfaction; loss of support by the partner or spouse; loss of communication with colleagues; loss of social interaction; and loss of income, combined with an increasing social isolation, a feeling of uselessness, with the inability to perform daily tasks.

Mrs. Murdock also talks about loss of future perspective, where she says: 'My life is of good quality, but when I am thinking of the fact it will not last long enough to see my children grow older, to see them go to university and graduate, start a relationship, marry, to see them become parents, to become a grandmother...then I become very upset, very sad, very angry and I regret the fact this disease is my fate....and the fact I am empty handed.....'

During the disease process, psychological adjustment to the new situation is a continuously dynamic process, in which nurses can play an important role. Patients faced with life-altering (and life-shortening) news experience distress and need honest, personalised information to help promote and adjust their future hopes and adaptive coping strategies. A nurse can listen to a patient and his/her relatives, support them in their grief and help them make informed decisions.

An incongruent or incompatible coping style between a glioma patient and his/her relatives could be an extra source of tension and distress, which would require a lot of psychological support and counselling from other healthcare professionals. This need for ongoing support might best be served by having one dedicated point of contact with a healthcare professional (most likely a specialist nurse).

There are several tools to measure distress and support needs in patients, for instance, the distress thermometer and problem list for patients [26]. It measures distress in all care domains (physical, psychosocial and spiritual) and can help gain insight into the problem(s) and determine which problems to focus on.

Studies have shown that information on end of life issues is of importance, and when healthcare professionals are open and sensitive on these issues, they will be able to guide patients and relatives and fine-tune communication [27]. The overall aim of psychosocial care and guidance is to enable the patient to take control of their last months of life, supported by his or her relatives.

## 19.1.4 Care for Relatives

As previously described, most patients with a glioma encounter physical, psychosocial and spiritual problems, but the disease also has great impact on relatives, such as a partner, children and other loved ones. Patients are often relatively young; many have young children which can make the overall impact even more complicated. Palliative care and care in the last months of life includes caring for the relatives and nurses have an important role in supporting them.

Anxiety, exhaustion and reduced quality of life are frequently reported concerns by relatives of patients. Partners are often the main carer, and they can face heavy burden. These concerns have been reported as being related to the changing sense of identity—going from a partner or spouse (for instance) to assuming a carer's role, loss of a relationship with the patient (due to the cognitive changes as previously described), a sense of social isolation and (survivors) guilt and fears regarding the eventual death of the patient. Specialist nurses can support relatives by including them in the caregiving process, for instance, at appointments, requesting their feedback and acknowledging their essential role in caring for the patient [28].

In the case description of Mrs. Murdock, the nurse saw the patient alongside her husband. She included Mr. Murdock in the conversations about his wife and asks how they are coping at home and talks about their joint future uncertainties. When the disease progresses, most glioma patients will need an increasing amount of support, as Mrs. Murdock did.

There are several tools to measure support needs of relatives. One of these tools is the Caregiver Strain Index, measuring level of strain in relatives [29]. Another more recently developed tool is the Carer Support Needs Assessment Tool (CSNAT) [30]. The CSNAT is an evidence-based tool that facilitates support for relatives (for instance, partners, children and friends/carers) of adults with life-limiting conditions. It is comprised of 14 broad domains in which carers commonly say they require support. Carers may use this tool to indicate further support they need in relation to enabling them to care for someone at home (needs as 'co-worker'), as well as support for their own health and well-being within their caregiving role (needs as 'co-client') [30]. One study in which nurses used this tool in home care showed that they were very positive about it. They described the CSNAT as providing guidance, focus and structure to facilitate discussion with relatives and as identifying needs and service responses that would not otherwise have been undertaken in a timely manner [31].

The tool is foremost meant to screen for needs, it does not give solutions. Further conversations with the relatives are needed to see how to best support their individual needs. For instance, respite care can be an option to give a partner some rest or time for himself/herself, but introducing professional caregivers is not the solution for each individual. In a study about palliative home care, for instance, it was found that introducing professional caregivers caused burden, because the carer doubted the professionals would give good care or because their privacy at home was at stake [32]. Therefore, it is important to look at individual support needs and create a shared action plan.

## 19.1.5  Multidisciplinary Teams and Transfer from Hospital to Home Care

Since patients with a glioma and their relatives have care and support needs in all care domains, a multidisciplinary team approach is important throughout the disease trajectory. Oncologist, neurologist, neurosurgeons and (specialist) nurses are the main professionals in the hospital team that care for the patient in the phase of diagnosis and life-prolonging treatments. But, as mentioned in this chapter, physiotherapists or psychologists, but also social workers or occupational therapist, might be necessary to give the patient the best care possible. Often, the specialist nurse has a key role in the team and is often in the best position to monitor the patient's and relatives' needs and discuss these with the wider team.

In the last 10 years or so, integration of oncology care and palliative care is developing. Involvement of specialised and experienced palliative care teams in the care of patients with cancer is found to improve symptom management, quality of life in patients and satisfaction in relatives [11].

When hospital treatment options have been exhausted, most patients with a glioma are handed over to the general practitioner and community home care teams. Specialised (hospital) nurses often keep in touch with the patient and/or their relative, by having regular telephone meetings, as was the case with Mr. and Mrs. Murdock. In this way needs can be monitored at home. It is important that specialists in neuro-oncology and professionals in home care keep in touch, since a glioma is a relatively rare disease and general practitioners and home care teams do not often encounter this specific patient group. The hospital nurse plays a pivotal role in bringing the expertise of neuro-oncology to the home care. It is advised to already have contact with the general practitioner during treatment and care in the hospital.

Many patients with a glioma want to remain at home during the final stages of their disease and the majority of patients also prefer to die at home [17]. Absence of hospital transitions in the last month of life is predictive for a dignified death [19]. Therefore, hospital admissions in this last phase of life are best avoided as much as possible. When patients get optimal care at home, admission to the hospital can often be prevented, even at the end of life.

In the case description, the hospital nurse stays in regular contact with Mrs. and Mr. Murdock. She continued to monitor their needs and was able to help when Mrs. Murdock developed seizures at home. By intervening they were able to prevent any further seizures and subsequent admissions, and Mrs. Murdock was able to remain at home until her death.

# References

1. WHO. http://www.who.int/cancer/palliative/definition/en/.
2. Zwinkels H. Grief, bereavement and mourning. Eur Assoc Neuroncol. 2013;3:70–1.
3. Stupp R, Mason WP, van den Bent MJ, Weller M, Fisher B, Taphoorn MJ, Belanger K, Brandes AA, Marosi C, Bogdahn U, Curschmann J, Janzer RC, Ludwin SK, Gorlia T, Allgeier A, Lacombe D, Cairncross JG, Eisenhauer E, Mirimanoff RO, European Organisation for Research and Treatment of Cancer Brain Tumor and Radiotherapy Groups; National Cancer Institute of Canada Clinical Trials Group. Radiotherapy plus concomitant and adjuvant temozolomide for glioblastoma. N Engl J Med. 2005;352(10):987–96.
4. Pace A, Dirven L, Koekkoek JAF, et al. European Association of Neuro-Oncology palliative care task force. European Association for Neuro-Oncology (EANO) guidelines for palliative care in adults with glioma. Lancet Oncol. 2017;18(6):e330–40.
5. Grant R, Brown PD. Fatigue randomized controlled trials – how tired is "too tired" in patients undergoing glioma treatment? Neuro-Oncology. 2016;18:759–60.
6. Walbert T, Chasteen K. Palliative and supportive care for glioma patients. In: Raizer J, Parsa A, editors. Current understanding and treatment of gliomas. Cancer Research and treatment volume 163. Dordrecht: Springer; 2015.
7. Armstrong TS, Gilbe MR. Practical strategies for management of fatigue and sleep disorders in people with brain tumors. Neuro-Oncology. 2012;14(Suppl 4):iv65–72.
8. Sizoo EM, Braam AM, Postma TJ, et al. Symptoms in the end-of-life phase of high grade glioma patients. Neuro Oncol. 2010;12:1162–6.
9. Rooney AG, McNamare S, Mackinnon M, et al. Frequency, clinical associations, and longitudinal course of major depressive disorders in adults with cerebral glioma. J Clin Oncol. 2011;29:4307–12.
10. Sizoo EM, Koekkoek JA, Postma TJ, Heimans JJ, Pasman HR, Deliens L, Taphoorn MJ, Reijneveld JC. Seizures in patients with high-grade glioma: a serious challenge in the end-of-life phase. BMJ Support Palliat Care. 2014;4:77–80.
11. Lorenz KA. Progress in quality-of-care research and hope for supportive cancer care. J Clin Oncol. 2008;26(23):3821–3.
12. Temel JS, Greer JA, Muzikansky A, Gallagher ER, Admane S, Jackson VA, Dahlin CM, Blinderman CD, Jacobsen J, Pirl WF, Billings JA, Lynch TJ. Early palliative care for patients with metastatic non-small-cell lung cancer. N Engl J Med. 2010;363(8):733–42.
13. Andreassen P, Neergaard MA, Brogaard T, Skorstengaard MH, Jensen AB. The diverse impact of advance care planning: a long-term follow-up study on patients' and relatives' experiences. BMJ Support Palliat Care. 2015;7:335–40.
14. Detering KM, Hancock AD, Reade MC, Silvester W. The impact of advance care planning on end of life care in elderly patients: randomised controlled trial. BMJ. 2010;340:c1345.
15. Kirchhoff KT, Hammes BJ, Kehl KA, Briggs LA, Brown RL. Effect of a disease-specific advance care planning intervention on end-of-life care. J Am Geriatr Soc. 2012;60(5):946–50.
16. Walbert T. Integration of palliative care into the neuro-oncology practice: patterns in the United States. Neurooncol Pract. 2014;1:3–7.
17. Koekkoek JA, Dirven L, Reijneveld JC, Sizoo EM, Pasman HR, Postma TJ, Deliens L, Grant R, McNamara S, Grisold W, Medicus E, Stockhammer G, Oberndorfer S, Flechl B, Marosi C, Taphoorn MJ, Heimans JJ. End of life care in high-grade glioma patients in three European countries: a comparative study. J Neuro-Oncol. 2014;120(2):303–10.
18. Flechl B, Ackerl M, Sax C, Oberndorfer S, Calabek B, Sizoo E, Reijneveld J, Crevenna R, Keilani M, Gaiger A, Dieckmann K, Preusser M, Taphoorn MJ, Marosi C. The caregivers' perspective on the end-of-life phase of glioblastoma patients. J Neuro-Oncol. 2013;112(3):403–11.
19. Sizoo EM, Taphoorn MJ, Uitdehaag B, Heimans JJ, Deliens L, Reijneveld JC, Pasman HR. The end-of-life phase of high-grade glioma patients: dying with dignity? Oncologist. 2013;18(2):198–203.
20. Kerrigan S, Erridg S, Liaquat I, Graham C, Grant R. Mental incapacity in patients undergoing neuro-oncologic treatment: a cross-sectional study. Neurology. 2014;83:537–41.

21. Sizoo EM, Pasman HR, Buttolo J, Heimans JJ, Klein M, Deliens L, Reijneveld JC, Taphoorn MJ. Decision-making in the end-of-life phase of high-grade glioma patients. Eur J Cancer. 2012;48:226–32.
22. Fritz L, Dirven L, Reijneveld JC, Koekkoek JA, Stiggelbout AM, Pasman HR, Taphoorn MJ. Advance care planning in glioblastoma patients. Cancers (Basel). 2016;8(11):pii:E102.
23. www.vitaltalk.org.
24. https://www.gundersenhealth.org/respecting-choices/.
25. https://www.advancecareplanning.org.au/ACP-projects.
26. Van Hoose L, Black LL, Doty K, Sabata D, Twumasi-Ankrah P, Taylor S, Johnson R. An analysis of the distress thermometer problem list and distress in patients with cancer. Support Care Cancer. 2015;23:1225–32.
27. Cavers D, Hacking B, Erridge SE, Kendall M, Morris PG, Murray SA. Social, psychological and existential well-being in patients with glioma and their caregivers: a qualitative study. CMAJ. 2012;184(7):E373–82.
28. Applebaum AJ, Kryza-Lacombe M, Buthorn J, DeRosa S, Corner G, Diamond EA. Existential distress among caregivers of patients with brain tumours: a review of the literature. Neurooncol Pract. 2016;3:232–44.
29. Robinson BC. Validation of a caregiver strain index. J Gerontol. 1983;3:344–8.
30. CS NAT. http://csnat.org/.
31. Aoun S, Toye C, Deas K, Howting D, Ewing G, Grande G, Stajduhar K. Enabling a family caregiver-led assessment of support needs in home-based palliative care: Potential translation into practice. Palliat Med. 2015;29:929–38.
32. De Korte-Verhoef MC, Pasman HR, Schweitzer BP, Francke AL, Onwuteaka-Philipsen BD, Deliens L. Burden for family carers at the end of life; a mixed-method study of the perspectives of family carers and GPs. BMC Palliat Care. 2014;13(1):16.

# Glossary

**1p/19q co-deletion** Loss of part of the short arm of chromosome 1 and the long arm of chromosome 19. This abnormality is seen in oligodendrogliomas.

**Adjuvant therapy** Additional cancer treatment given after the primary treatment to lower the risk that the cancer will come back.

**Afferent fibers** Fibers that carry impulses from sensory structures or organs toward the central nervous system (typically sensory fibers).

**Agnosia** Inability to process sensory information.

**Alopecia** Hair loss.

**Angiogenesis** The physiological process through which new blood vessels form from pre-existing vessels.

**Astrocyte** The most common cell type in the central nervous system and regarded as an important supporting cell with many different functions.

**ATRX** A protein encoded by a gene on the X chromosome. Mutations in ATRX are identified in diffuse astrocytomas.

**Central nervous system (CNS)** The brain and spinal cord.

**Chromosome** The large molecules in the cell nucleus that contain DNA.

**Communicating hydrocephalus** Increased cerebrospinal fluid volume due to decreased absorption.

**Concomitant therapy** Two or more cancer treatments given at the same time, for example, chemotherapy and radiotherapy (chemo-RT).

**Cytoplasm** The material within the cell excluding the nucleus.

**Cytotoxic chemotherapy** Use of anticancer drugs to kill cells.

**Deoxyribonucleic acid (DNA)** The molecule that carries the code for the growth, development and function of living cells and organisms.

**Desquamation** Shedding of the outer membrane of the skin can be termed as dry when there is no evidence of skin breakdown or moist where the skin in not intact and evidence of weeping.

**Efferent fibers** Fibers that carry impulses away from the central nervous system to peripheral structures such as muscles and glands (typically motor fibers).

**Erythema** Redness of the skin caused by the radiotherapy can be graded from mild to brisk depending on severity.

**Expressive aphasia** Language compromise characterized by loss of ability to produce speech or written word in the presence of adequate comprehension.

© Springer Nature Switzerland AG 2019                                                    313
I. Oberg (ed.), *Management of Adult Glioma in Nursing Practice*,
https://doi.org/10.1007/978-3-319-76747-5

**Extra-axial** Descriptive term to denote lesions that are external to the brain parenchyma.

**Haematogenous spread** Distributed or spread by way of the bloodstream, as in metastases of tumours or in infections.

**Haematoxylin and eosin (H&E)** The principal tissue stain used in histopathology.

**Heterogeneous** Consists of visibly different substances.

**Homogeneous** The same uniform appearance and composition throughout.

**Hyperintense** An area of high signal on MR imaging, typically represented by the colour white or light grey.

**Hypointense** An area of low signal on MR imaging, typically represented by the colour black or dark grey.

**Intra-axial** Descriptive term to denote lesions within the brain parenchyma.

**Immunohistochemistry** A specialist technique that uses antibodies to visualise specific proteins.

**Isocitrate dehydrogenase (IDH)** An enzyme involved in cell metabolism. Mutations are seen in low-grade gliomas and secondary glioblastomas.

**Isoform** A member of a group of similar proteins that perform the same function in a cell.

**Krebs cycle** Part of a cell's metabolism that makes energy for the cell.

**Microvascular proliferation** The abnormal growth of blood vessels often encountered in high-grade gliomas.

**Mitotic figure** A microscopic feature of a cell seen when the cell is in the process of dividing and has copied its chromosomes and is separating them into two daughter cells. Seeing lots of mitotic figures generally means that a tissue (or tumour) is growing rapidly.

**Necrosis** Cell death.

**Nucleus** The part of the cell that contains the DNA.

**O6-methylguanine-DNA methyltransferase (MGMT)** A protein involved in DNA repair.

**Obstructive hydrocephalus** Increased cerebrospinal fluid volume due to blockage of flow out of the ventricular system.

**Oligodendrocyte** A type of glial cell that provides support and insulation of nerve fibres in the central nervous system.

**p53** A protein with important anticancer functions. p53 mutations are typically seen in astrocytomas and glioblastomas.

**Palisading necrosis** Cell death (necrosis), surrounded by a layer of tumour cells. This pattern of necrosis is often seen in glioblastoma.

**Proliferation** Growth of tissue through cell division (reproduction).

**Promoter** Part of a gene that controls whether that gene is switch on or off.

**Receptive aphasia** Language compromise characterized by impaired comprehension of spoken or written word; speech is usually fluent.

**Telomerase reverse transcriptase (TERT)** A DNA repair protein. Mutations are identified in oligodendrogliomas and glioblastomas.